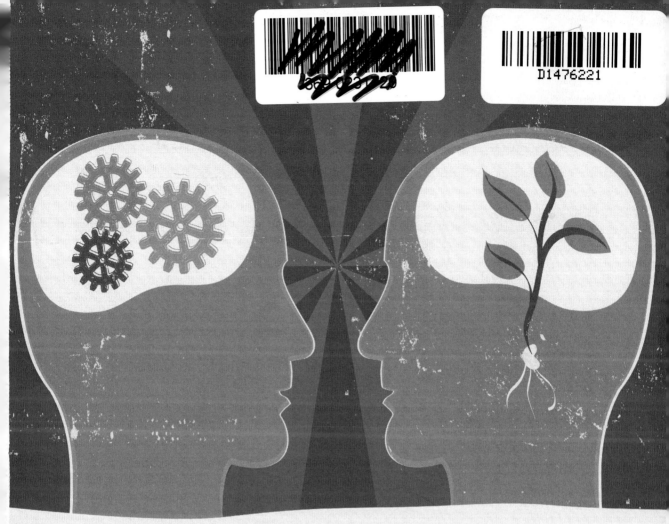

Understanding and Caring for People with Brain Disorders

A handbook for frontline staff, carers and students

Declan Mc Nicholl and Robert Poppleton

Pavilion

Understanding and Caring for People with Brain Disorders

A handbook for frontline staff, carers and students

© Declan Mc Nicholl and Robert Poppleton 2011

The authors have asserted their rights in accordance with the *Copyright, Designs and Patents Act 1988* to be identified as the authors of this work.

Published by:
Pavilion Publishing and Media Ltd
Rayford House
School Road
Hove
BN3 5HX
UK

Tel: 01273 434943
Fax: 01273 227308
Email: info@pavpub.com
Web: www.pavpub.com

First published 2011, 2013

A catalogue reference for this book is available from the British Library.

ISBN: 978-1-84196-279-5

Pavilion is the leading training and development provider and publisher in the health, social care and allied fields, providing a range of innovative training solutions underpinned by sound research and professional values. We aim to put our customers first, through excellent customer service and good value.

Editor: Sanaz Nazemi
Cover design: Emma Garbutt
Page layout and typesetting: Emma Garbutt
Printed on paper from a sustainable resource by: Printondemand-worldwide

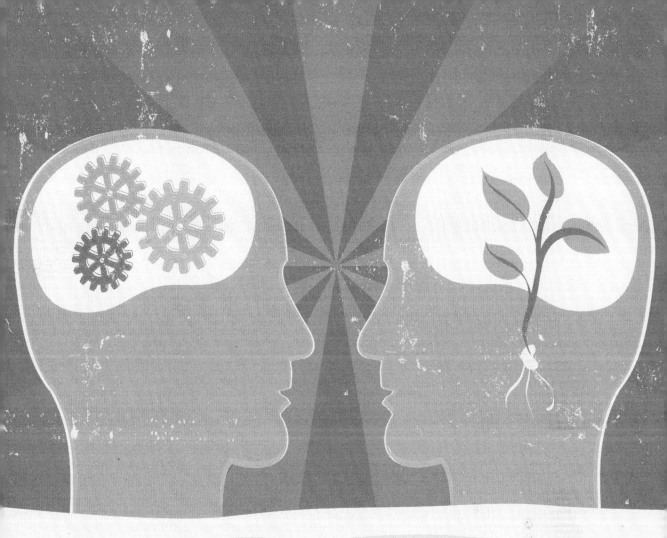

Understanding and Caring for People with Brain Disorders

A handbook for frontline staff, carers and students

Declan Mc Nicholl and Robert Poppleton

Contents

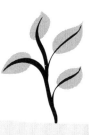

Part 3: Two further applications

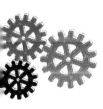

Acknowledgements

This book, like all my individual endeavours, is the culmination of a collective process with the people who have encouraged and supported me. Some of those people have been part of my life since an early age, my parents Patricia and John, and my teachers. Others are more recent in my personal and professional life. In particular I would like to thank the authors of each of the chapters; my colleagues at Leicestershire Partnership NHS Trust and Leicester General Hospital and Joanne Applewhite for her perseverance and administrative skills. I would also like to thank Sanaz Nazemi at Pavilion Publishing for her support, guidance and editorial skills. Finally, my thanks and gratitude to my wife, Catherine, and children Liam, Connor and Owen.

Declan Mc Nicholl

I am fortunate to be have been brought up, taught and worked with many people who provided me with great inspiration and encouragement in my life. From early on in life, my parents John and Margaret and my brothers and sisters have given me love and support. I would also like to thank the authors of the chapters for their hard work and my colleagues at Royal Leamington Spa Rehabilitation Hospital for their advice and support in particular Aimee Green, Vicki, Edward Gulliver, Gagan Chohan, Richard Lawson and Karen Melrose. I would also like to thank Sanaz Nazemi for all her support, advice and editorial skills in the development of this book. Lastly I would like to express my greatest gratitude and my love to my wife, Gill, and our wonderful children Aaron, Beth and Alice for their valuable help and support.

Robert Poppleton

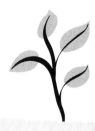

Contributors

Claire Pavlou is a clinical psychologist at the Royal Leamington Spa Rehabilitation Hospital in Warwickshire and has worked in the field of clinical psychology and neuropsychology for 11 years. She obtained an MA in health psychology at Coventry University followed by a clinical doctorate at Coventry University and Warwick University. Claire's interest in working with people with multiple sclerosis (MS) began 15 years ago when volunteering and working at a specialist care centre for people with MS. She now delivers clinical neuropsychology interventions as part of a specialist community neurorehabilitation team for people with MS. Claire also works for younger adult inpatient and outpatient services providing neurorehabilitation for people with a range of brain injuries and neurological conditions, including people in minimally conscious states. She also lectures on the clinical psychology doctorate course at Coventry University and the University of Warwick, Warwickshire. Between 2002 and 2006, Claire was a trustee for Headway Coventry where she was involved at every level with the organisation and taking a lead role in raising awareness of the needs of people with 'hidden disabilities' caused by brain injuries.

Declan Mc Nicholl studied Psychology at Queen's University, Belfast and obtained an MSc in clinical psychology at Leicester University. Initially he worked in adult mental health and then specialised in clinical neuropsychology. He later completed his doctorate of clinical psychology at Salomon's, Canterbury Christ Church University. He is also a trained psychotherapist in the Personal Construct Psychology approach. He currently works as a consultant clinical neuropsychologist and is the Head of Department of Clinical Neuropsychology at Leicestershire Partnership NHS Trust. He is an honorary lecturer in the Department of Clinical Psychology, University of Leicester. He works with people who have a wide range of neurological disorders and neuropsychological challenges. Declan has many links with voluntary sector organisations and is a trustee of his local Headway House.

Gerald Burgess is a clinical psychologist at the Department of Clinical Neuropsychology within the Leicestershire Partnership Trust. He works predominantly with adult acquired brain injury patients in both acute inpatient and outpatient clinic settings. As a part of this work, Gerald has conducted trainings for frontline staff in health and social services and for family and carers of brain-injured patients on issues of personality, behaviour,

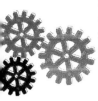

and emotional changes following brain injury. He was a mental health clinician in the United States before returning to university to earn his doctorate in clinical psychology in 2004, and is now completing a post-doctorate MSc in clinical neuropsychology from the University of Nottingham.

Karen Treece is a chartered clinical psychologist and a full member of the Division of Clinical Psychology of the British Psychological Society, and a registered practitioner of the Health Professions Council. She obtained a neuropsychology MPhil at the University of Nottingham and works in the field of adult clinical neuropsychology within the Department of Clinical Psychology and Neuropsychology of Nottingham University Hospital NHS Trust. She qualified with a doctorate of clinical psychology at the University of Birmingham and has recently completed a post graduate diploma in clinical neuropsychology at the University of Nottingham. Prior to entering clinical psychology training she held a research post at the Clinical Research Group of the University of Nottingham for five years. She contributed to neuropsychological research studies with patients with stroke, multiple sclerosis and pituitary tumours. As a clinical psychologist Karen has worked within the specialism of clinical neuropsychology, both in acute hospital-based settings and within community multidisciplinary rehabilitation teams.

Liam Gilligan has an MSc in Research Methods in Psychology and his dissertation looks at autism and gender dysphoria. Alongside this he has worked as an assistant psychologist at the Royal Leamington Spa Rehabilitation Hospital, working with young adults with traumatic and acquired brain injury and with older persons with dementia and other organic diseases. His wants to continue working in clinical psychology, with future plans to do further training in neuropsychology to work with people with acquired brain injuries.

Louise Braham is a consultant clinical and forensic psychologist. She currently works part time at Nottingham University on the Trent doctorate in Clinical Psychology and is acting lead psychologist for the Mental Health Service at Rampton Hospital. Louise developed an interest in neuropsychology and cognitive functioning during her clinical practice and to further this, went on to complete her MSc in Clinical Neuropsychology at Nottingham University. She has a special interest in the neuropsychology of those with mental health problems (particularly schizophrenia) and its application and use within a mental health setting. This interest is evident within her clinical work within a mental health, forensic setting, applying neuropsychological ideas to forensic

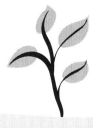

patients and providing neuropsychological assessment and rehabilitation. Violent behaviour and emotional difficulties are both common within these populations and neuropsychological ideas can be helpful aiding understanding. Louise has over 15 years experience working within the NHS with people with severe and enduring mental health problems, and many years of experience in utilising cognitive models and neuropsychological functioning within the psychological arena.

Melanie Stevens is a chartered clinical psychologist at Glenside Hospital in Salisbury, which is a specialist neurological rehabilitation centre where she works on the neurobehavioural pathway. Melanie also works at Newbridge House in Sutton Coldfield, which provides specialist treatment for anorexia nervosa. Melanie has several years of experience working in neurorehabilitation including NHS inpatient and outpatient service and a vocational rehabilitation service. She has worked with people at all stages of their injury or illness. She obtained an MSc in Health Psychology at Coventry University followed by a doctorate in Clinical Psychology at the universities of Coventry and Warwick. In addition she has undergone specialist training in EMDR in the treatment of trauma and compassion focused therapy and is a chartered scientist. Melanie has used cognitive remediation therapy for five years in the treatment of anorexia nervosa whilst working in the field of eating disorders thus linking both of her specialist areas of interest. She also lectures on the clinical psychology doctorate at Birmingham University and is now completing a post-doctorate MSc in Clinical Neuropsychology at Glasgow University.

Nigel Schofield is an NHS consultant clinical neuropsychologist. He is a chartered clinical psychologist and an associate fellow of the British Psychological Society, being a full member of the Division of Clinical Psychology and a practitioner member of the Division of Neuropsychology. In 1990, he established the Department of Clinical Neuropsychology in Derby and is now head of speciality based at the Royal Derby Hospital. Through his work he has gained considerable experience in the general field of neurorehabilitation, working primarily with patients suffering from neurological conditions or brain damage. He teaches on neuropsychology and physical disability to clinical psychology doctoral students at Leicester University; and the topics of sleep problems and medico-legal work to MA students at the University of Nottingham. He is a member of a number of local multidisciplinary and multi-agency neurorehabilitation strategic planning and operational groups, and has also been a member of a number of similar groups at a regional level.

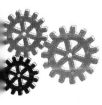

Patrick Vesey is consultant clinical neuropsychologist at the neurosciences unit of Nottingham University Hospitals NHS Trust where he is jointly responsible for adult neuropsychology services. As a full member of the Divisions of Clinical Psychology and Neuropsychology of the British Psychological Society, his routine clinical practice involves the provision of diagnostic and interventional neuropsychology services for people with neurological illness or neurological injury including acquired brain injury, multiple sclerosis, epilepsy, neurodegenerative conditions and neurodevelopmental conditions. He teaches at the Universities of Nottingham and Leicester and his research interests include the outcomes of acquired brain injury, carer strain in families of people with acquired brain injury, cognition and emotion in motor neuron disease, psychosocial outcome after hypoxic-ischaemic brain injury, adjustment in multiple sclerosis, and psychological aspects of functional neurological conditions.

Rachel Mills is an assistant psychologist in the South Sheffield Community Learning Disability Team where she works with adults with varying levels of learning disabilities. She has worked in this field for nearly four years, previously working as a support worker for Mencap after completing her undergraduate degree at the University of Manchester. Rachel spends a lot of time working with people who may have dementia and with their families/carers. She is also part of the Dementia Practice Development Group in Sheffield, contributing to the care pathway that is currently being developed for the assessment of dementia referrals to the community learning disability team.

Robert Poppleton is a qualified neuro-psychologist at the Royal Leamington Spa Rehabilitation Hospital, a regional NHS centre for people with acquired brain injuries. Having trained in the Oxford In-Service Clinical Psychology Training Course, he is a registered neuro-psychologist with the British Psychological Society. He is particularly interested in working with people who have suffered from acquired brain injuries and the related implications in living with these conditions and their effects upon families. He also provides neuro-psychology training to doctorate clinical psychology students from Coventry University and also works with research students from Birmingham University Doctorate Clinical Psychology course.

Roshan das Nair is a consultant psychologist working with the Department of Clinical Psychology and Neuropsychology at Nottingham University Hospitals NHS Trust, where he runs a specialist HIV and

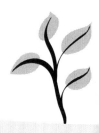

sexual health service. He is also a research tutor on the Trent doctorate in clinical psychology at the University of Nottingham, where he teaches research methods and supervises trainee clinical psychology research projects. His PhD studies included a randomised controlled trial of memory rehabilitation for neurological disabilities, funded by The Stroke Association and Remedi. Roshan is also a special lecturer with the Institute of Work, Health and Organisations, where he teaches on the MSc in clinical neuropsychology programme. His current research interests include sexuality and disability, and neuropsychological deficits and rehabilitation for people living with HIV/AIDS.

Shirley Thomas is a health psychologist and lecturer in rehabilitation psychology at the University of Nottingham. She has previously worked as a research tutor on the Trent Doctorate in Clinical Psychology where she taught research methods and supervised research projects for clinical psychology trainees. Her PhD studies were focused on emotional distress after stroke and she has published journal papers and book chapters on this topic. Shirley's recent research interests have included assessment tools and the treatment of mood problems after stroke. She is particularly interested in improving mood assessments and psychological treatments for people with aphasia. She is currently managing a multi-centre research study, funded by The Stroke Association, which is evaluating behaviour therapy for low mood in people with aphasia following a stroke. Alongside her research she teaches and supervises students across MSc courses in applied psychology.

Suzie Beart is a clinical psychologist working in the South Community Learning Disability Team in Sheffield where she works with a wide range of people with learning disabilities. She has also worked for four years within the brain injury rehabilitation services in Sheffield and teaches on the clinical psychology course at Sheffield University. She is particularly interested in researching issues of identity and transition while working alongside people with learning disabilities. She is also interested in the different ways to use neuropsychological models and assessments in partnership with people with learning disabilities and those who care for and about them. She is involved in developing a care pathway in Sheffield for assessing people with learning disabilities for dementia.

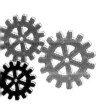

Introduction

Declan Mc Nicholl

About this handbook

Our ability to detect, diagnose and survive brain disorders has greatly improved in recent years. Those who suffer traumatic brain injuries (TBI) from road traffic accidents (RTA) or serious falls are surviving more frequently and, because of our aging population, more people are developing disorders in older age, for example, the dementias (see chapter 5). Brain disorders such as stroke – cerebrovascular disease (CVA) – epilepsy, multiple sclerosis and Alzheimer's disease are now common in the adult population. Furthermore, the increased use of recreational drugs, such as cannabis and cocaine, and significant alcohol use increases the likelihood of developing brain-related difficulties.

There are a wide variety of brain disorders ranging from those with a sudden onset, such as resulting from a traumatic blow to the head, to those with a slow onset, such as Alzheimer's disease. Some can stay fairly static for long periods of time while others progress (see chapter 5).

Brain disorders can give rise to a wide variety of very disabling and ongoing physical, psychological and social difficulties. There can often be a wide range of health and social care professionals involved with people with brain disorders. Along with general practitioners, these can include a range of medical personnel including neurologists, stroke and other physicians; generic and specialist nurses; occupational therapists; physiotherapists; speech and language therapists; various psychologists, including clinical and neuropsychologists; case managers and social workers. These professionals endeavour to work with the individual and their wider social network, often using a multiple-disciplinary team approach. However, of critical importance are those people who work directly with or live alongside the person on a day-to-day basis, namely, direct carers, family members and friends.

People with significant brain disorders often need substantial amounts of care and the need for this care within the general population as a whole is

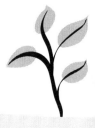

growing year on year. Care services, whether they are helping people stay in their own homes or live in residential establishments, are springing up in order to meet this increasing need. With the advent of community-based care and recent initiatives such as 'personalisation', an increasing burden of care will fall on families and frontline professional carers. With this comes an increased need for appropriate knowledge and understanding of what happens to people whose brains are injured and the effects brain changes have on behaviour, emotions and cognitions and how to help and support such people.

This book endeavours to provide important aspects of this knowledge and to help demystify some of the issues around brain injury and disorder. In particular the book sets out to make available to a wider audience some of the knowledge and insights into brain disorders gained through the practice of clinical neuropsychology.

It is hoped that by reading this book a fuller understanding of the person with a brain injury and their disorder will be obtained along with ideas and practical suggestions about how to help them.

Who this book is for and how it is structured

This book is aimed at a number of different but related groups of people, including the family members, friends and direct carers of people with acquired neurological disorders and students and trainees from the various health and social care professions. Qualified professionals who do not specialise in working with people with brain disorders will also find parts of it useful.

Existing books and educational materials on the subject tend to be aimed at only one of these groups. This is often for good reason as the level of existing knowledge is often very different for each group. However, there is a need for families, friends and direct carers to be able to understand and share the language, conceptual frameworks and ways of intervening used by professionals in the field and to have ways of developing more sophisticated understandings, if they so wish. This book aims to address this need and help bridge some of the gaps between families, 'hands on' carers and other professionals. It is a resource that any of those parties could bring to an appointment, consultation or case review as a way of facilitating discussion, increasing understandings of or helping a person with a neurological disorder. It could also be used in a range of educational settings.

The book is set out in three sections. The first section entitled 'Covering the basics' looks at some very complex material in a way that someone with a good secondary level education, but limited previous exposure to or understanding of the material should be able to grasp. This section contains chapters on the main parts of the brain and their functions; the major neurological disorders; the impact of these disorders on a person's emotions and cognitive functions, that is, the mental processes associated with attention, perception, language, learning and memory and the ability to plan, carry out and reflect upon day-to-day tasks and experiences (Loring, 1999).

The second section 'Getting into more details' mainly considers how cognitive functions can be assessed and some of the interventions useful in addressing deficits; but it also looks at the important issues of fatigue and a person's wider social network.

The final section 'Two further applications' considers how the information and approaches set out in the previous chapters can be used to understand some matters related to mental health and learning disabilities.

The language used in the book has been made as accessible and understandable for a lay reader, especially in the earlier chapters. However, as the book progresses a number of chapters are included, especially in sections two and three, which are more challenging in terms of the concepts and terminology used. This has been done for a number of reasons including the nature of the issues these chapters address; to challenge the reader who has read the previous chapters to move to a further level of understanding and appreciation of the issues, and to give readers with some existing knowledge the opportunity to understand better how clinical neuropsychologists and other professionals who work in the field think and why they do what they do.

The reader will probably find it easiest to start at the beginning and work through the book systematically. However, each chapter is designed so that it can be read, depending on existing knowledge, in a reasonably 'stand alone' manner.

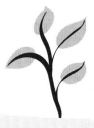

Each chapter follows a general overall format as follows.

▶ The aims of the chapter are made explicit.

▶ An introduction to the chapter is provided.

▶ The main information of the chapter is then given. Some chapters use highlighted boxes that contain case studies, examples of good practice or other additional information.

▶ A quiz or series of questions to get the reader thinking about the subject matter of the chapter.

▶ Reference section/suggestions for further reading and resources.

A few words about terminology

The reader may not have come across some of the terms used in this book before, or if they have, they may not understand them fully. Furthermore, some terms used about brain disorders are defined and used differently by different people in different contexts, and different terms are sometimes used for the same thing. Do not allow this to put you off trying to understand. The authors have endeavoured to use terminology consistently and a glossary of terms is given at the back of the book.

A few words about 'cognition'

This book focuses on and gives particular emphasis to cognition. 'Cognition' can be defined in a number of different ways but for the purposes of this handbook the following definition is applicable: '*Intellectual functions including perceiving, remembering, imagining, conceiving, understanding, judging and reasoning*' (Ayd, 2000).

References

Ayd F (2000) *Lexicon of Psychiatry, Neurology and the Neurosciences.* Philadelphia: Lippincott, Williams and Wilkins.

Loring D (Ed) (1999) *International Neuropsychological Society Dictionary of Neuropsychology.* New York: Oxford University Press.

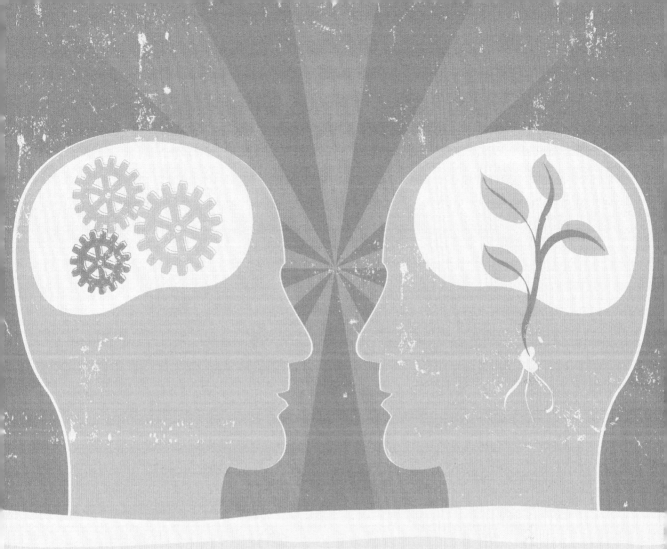

Part 1:
Covering the basics

Chapter 1:

A way of understanding human functioning: the biopsychosocial-functioning model

Declan Mc Nicholl

Aims of the chapter

This chapter aims to:

▶ give a framework for understanding human functioning

▶ explain the biopsychosocial model, its different parts and how these parts interact with each other

▶ explain the World Health Organization's International Classification of Functioning, Disability and Health

▶ present a new framework to understand and help those with an acquired neurological disorder that combines the biopsychosocial model with the International Classification of Functioning, Disability and Health. This is referred to as the biopsychosocial-functioning model

▶ encourage the reader to reflect on the argument that empowerment needs to be the goal when offering support and rehabilitation.

Introduction

This chapter discusses the biopsychosocial-functioning (BPS-F) model of human functioning, which provides useful background information for anyone delivering care to a person with a brain injury. This model highlights the different aspects that affect a person's experience of disease

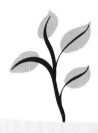

or injury, and also considers areas of strength and need. This model is a combination of two existing models, which is the biopsychosocial model (BPS), and the World Health Organization's Classification of Functioning, Disability and Health (ICF). The chapter begins by explaining the biopsychosocial model; the ICF is then explained and, finally, the combined BPS-F model is discussed. The fictitious case example of 'Alfonso' is used to help the reader understand how the model can be applied to someone with a brain injury or disease so that better care can be delivered. Finally, the chapter finishes by briefly discussing empowerment.

Separating things up: splitting mind and body

A great deal of Western scientific thinking involves taking ideas, dividing them up and breaking them down into smaller pieces in order to analyse the details. The reader might conclude after reading the later chapters of this book that Western scientific thinkers overuse the left side of their brains. One such person who stressed the divisions was the 17th century French philosopher and mathematician, René Descartes who suggested that there is a difference between 'mind' and 'body', between what someone thinks and the brain that thinks it. This has been referred to as the 'mind-body split' or 'mind-body dualism'. 'Mind-body dualism' suggests that human psychological life is somehow separate from the body and, therefore, the brain.

In this chapter and during the course of this book, discussions on the brain, psychology and social relationships are sometimes dealt with separately. However, this separation is used only in order to try and help explain a particular topic. The reader needs to keep in mind that these different topics are part of a wider understanding; part of a more holistic and 'joined up' way of thinking where the bits need to be put back together again.

Putting them back together: the biopsychosocial model

One of these joined up ways of thinking is known as the biopsychosocial model. As suggested in its name, the 'bio-psycho-social' model attempts to understand the person and especially their health, well-being and illness by combining knowledge from the physical sciences such as *biology*; understandings and insights from *psychology* along with approaches developed within sociology, the *social* aspect (Loring, 1999).

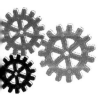

What is meant by the word 'model'?

The word 'model' refers to a way of representing and explaining the real, external world in a theoretical way. This understanding of the outside world can then guide behaviours and actions such as how to prevent, treat or intervene with particular problems or diseases, in this case how to deal with injuries to the brain. There are many other models mentioned throughout this handbook.

History of the biopsychosocial model

Although the basis of the biopsychosocial model has been around in Asia and Europe for centuries, if not millennia, its modern origins generally have been attributed to George Engel (Engel, 1997). Engel, who was a medical doctor with an interest in both physical medicine and psychiatry, pointed out that physical disease such as heart disease is often the end product of a large number of cultural, social, genetic and personal factors (Gilbert, 2002). Let's look now at the three different aspects of the model.

The biological aspect

The biological aspect of the model uses biological or 'organic' explanations for health and illness. It recommends carrying out physical or medical investigations in order to identify whereabouts in the body or brain there is damage, that is, where things have gone wrong biologically. The focus is on the physical causes of disease, for example, personal and family history of disease and the history of symptoms, pain and discomfort.

Biological malfunction is taken to be the underlying reason for any difficulties a person might have. For example, the reader will see in later chapters comments on what is referred to as 'disinhibited behaviour' which can be sometimes seen in people who have damage to particular areas of their brains, especially parts of their frontal lobes. The biological aspect of the biopsychosocial model emphasises this brain damage and dysfunction as a way of explaining disinhibited behaviour (see chapter 4).

Furthermore, biology also has been used to explain feelings or disturbing internal experiences such as hallucinations. Some go so far as to describe other psychological phenomenon such as anxiety or depression as disturbances of physical processes, for example, in the disruption of chemical processes in the brain (Fleminger *et al*, 2003). Therefore, when using only the biological aspect of the model to explain things, everything is 'boiled down' to biological mechanisms.

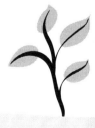

The psychological aspect

The psychological component of the biopsychosocial model encourages us to look at psychological causes or explanations for health problems. Psychological aspects are to do with how the person thinks and feels about a situation. Theories, ideas and approaches developed within psychology about emotions and cognitions are used to understand the individual and their difficulties. For example, in trying to understand someone who is depressed after acquiring a brain disorder a psychological explanation does not look for changes in brain structure and chemistry, but to changes in how the person understands, views and thinks about themselves and the disorder they have acquired. The theories of Freud and those from other psychoanalytic traditions, self-psychology, cognitive and behavioural psychology – often combined into what is referred to as cognitive behavioural therapy – can be considered in order to understand the person.

In addition, personality prior to the development of a brain disorder is considered important in how a person copes after brain injury. Whether or not a person had a positive outlook on life can determine their reaction to injury. For example, there is a great deal of evidence that suggests that the outcome of mild traumatic brain injury, where a person loses consciousness just for several minutes or less, may be significantly influenced by pre-injury personality (McCrea, 2008).

The social aspect

The third and final component of the biopsychosocial model is the social part. This considers how factors such as social and economic status, employment, poverty, culture, technology, relationships, family and religion can influence health and well-being. This social aspect considers the individual in their wider grouping and social context. Here sociological ideas and theories about society and group psychology are considered important in understanding illness and its treatment. One of the most widely read texts in neuropsychology written by Muriel Lezak and colleagues (2004) states, '*Brain injury is a family affair*' suggesting that the person's family and other relationships are both affected by and have an effect on brain disorder and its recovery.

Putting the three aspects together

Therefore, the three aspects – the psychological, social and biological – combine to give the biopsychosocial model. However, it is important to see them not as three separate components but that they interact with

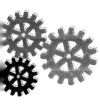

and are interdependent on each other (see **figure 1**). Unlike 'mind-body dualism' mentioned earlier, this model suggests that the body can affect the mind and vice versa; a person's physical state affects how they are as a person and how they get along in social situations and vice versa. This model states that the biological, personal and social aspects of disease must be understood effectively and addressed in order that health can be maintained and illness avoided.

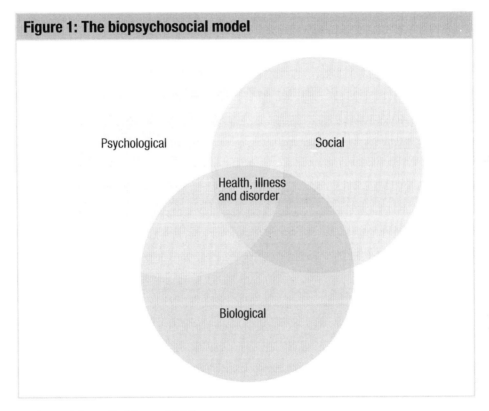

Figure 1: The biopsychosocial model

Psychological

Social

Health, illness and disorder

Biological

(Adapted from Lakhan, 2006)

Examples of using the different aspects of the biopsychosocial model

Biological aspect

It is known that if there is a family history of certain disorders, such as Alzheimer's or Huntington's disease, then this will increase the likelihood

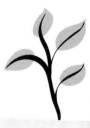

of someone in the next generation inheriting the disease in other words, some diseases have a genetic component. Furthermore, the area of brain that is damaged by disease is important because, as shown in Chapter 2, different parts of the brain are associated with different parts of the body and different mental functions. For example, if someone has an injury to the area in the right side of their brain that controls movement of the left arm then they are likely to have difficulties with mobility in their left arm.

With Alzheimer's disease, parts of the brain associated with memory function are often damaged. With Huntington's disease, parts of the basal ganglia lying underneath the frontal lobes (see Chapter 3) in that help control bodily movements are damaged, and this accounts for the jerky movements seen in this disease. With traumatic brain injury, which is an injury that happens after a traumatic event such as a car accident or fall, the part of the brain damaged will often determine important aspects of the disabilities that a person experiences (see Chapters 3 and 5). So if a person has damaged the back of their brain or the nerves from their eye that carries information to the back of the brain, they are likely to have problems with vision; if they have damaged the left side of their brain at the front, they may experience difficulties with language such as expressing themselves. Therefore, the biological aspects of a neurological disease are important in understanding and explaining both the disease and its outward symptoms.

Psychological aspect

Every adult with an acquired neurological disorder has had a personal history ie. a life, before they acquired or developed their disorder. Over the years they will have developed outlooks, attitudes and ways of doing things. These pre-injury aspects of personality and behaviour will influence how they see their disorder. For example, someone who liked to be in control of others may become depressed after acquiring a disease because they cannot have the same influence over people, whereas someone who just liked being around others and freely shared their feelings with others may continue to do so after acquiring their disorder, which could shield them from low mood or depression. If someone believes the only meaning to life is being one with an able body acquires a physical disability, then they are likely to cope very differently from someone with a similar disability but who emphasises what they can do and tries to work to his or her strengths. Therefore, two people who have the same or similar disorders can view that disorder very differently because of their psychological makeup. This, in turn, will influence how they cope with and adjust to the disorder.

Social aspect

A person who lives alone and has few friends when they acquire a disorder may become very isolated afterwards. For example, consider someone who has had a stroke but beforehand was living with his or her partner and had a lot of support from adult children and after their stroke their family continued to be supportive and helpful. Compare that person with one who lived alone before their stroke and had no family support afterwards. These two people are likely to cope very differently.

Furthermore, compare someone who is reasonably wealthy and can afford to pay someone to help them cook, clean and shop; who can afford to make adaptations to their home, with someone who lived and continues to live on state benefits or in relative poverty – these two people with a similar disorder are likely to have very different lives. Therefore, a person's level of social support and financial resources will influence the impact of any neurological disorder.

In summary, the part of the brain that is damaged, the person's psychological makeup and their social circumstances are all important in how each individual deals with neurological disorder. Furthermore, these three factors combine and interact with each other to determine outcomes and quality of life (Gilbert, 2002).

The World Health Organization's International Classification of Functioning, Disability and Health (ICF)

The World Health Organization

The World Health Organization (WHO) is the body within the United Nations responsible for directing and co-ordinating health. It provides leadership on global health matters, looks at the evidence for effective treatments and makes recommendations for health policies to promote healthy lives globally (WHO, 2010).

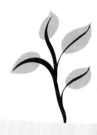

The International Classification of Functioning, Disability and Health

The WHO has produced a document called the *International Classification of Functioning, Disability and Health* known more commonly as the ICF. This provides a framework and standard language for the description of health-related conditions from the point of view of functioning of the whole person. The ICF not only considers and classifies illness or disease from a medical point of view but considers the consequences of such disease and disorder in terms of the impact on the person and on their social circumstances (WHO, 2002).

Physical health, personal activity and social participation

The ICF states that human functioning, health and disability arise from an interaction between (a) health conditions such as diseases, disorders and injuries; (b) personal activities and abilities and (c) the person's participation in social and community life. The interaction between these factors gives rise to three levels of functioning, namely; the level of the *physical body*, the level of *activity* carried out by the person and the level of *participation* of a person in wider social networks and society (see **figure 2**). ICF refers to this as, '*Functioning at the level of body or body part, the whole person and the whole person in a social context. Disability involves dysfunction at one or more of these same levels; impairments of body or brain, activity limitations and participation restrictions*' (WHO, 2002). Within services for people with neurological disorders, with some notable exceptions (Wade, 2003) there has not been a great deal of work in using and applying the ICF model.

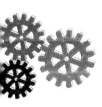

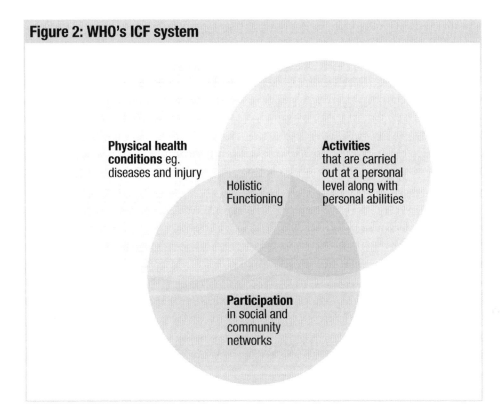

Figure 2: WHO's ICF system

Physical health conditions eg. diseases and injury

Holistic Functioning

Activities that are carried out at a personal level along with personal abilities

Participation in social and community networks

Two other important matters: capacity and performance

The ICF also introduced two very important matters for further consideration. The first of these is the *capacity* of an individual to carry out a particular activity or task. Capacity is the highest possible level of functioning that an individual can achieve on any particular task. The second important matter ICF introduced was that of *performance* which describes what an individual does in the particular environment in which they find themselves. Therefore, 'capacity' is about what an individual is able to do and 'performance' is about what they actually do. The ICF refers to capacity and performance as 'qualifiers' because they qualify or influence physical health, personal activity and social participation.

Comparing capacity and performance

Comparing capacity with performance and deciding whether or not there is a gap between them gives some very important information. If an individual's capacity is less than performance this means that the environment has, most likely, helped or enabled that individual to

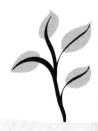

perform at a level above their capacity; in other words the environment has helped them. However, if a person's performance is less than capacity this means that a person is performing at a level less than they are capable or less than their optimum; therefore their environment is probably holding them back or limiting their performance. Following on from this it can then be determined whether or not a person needs changes to their environment, aids, or personal assistance so that their performance matches or outperforms their capacity.

Putting together the biopsychosocial and ICF approaches to give the Biopsychosocial-Functioning (BPS-F) model

The combined model

The three aspects of the biopsychosocial model and the three levels of the ICF can be combined to give six separate but interconnected and overlapping *dimensions* namely the *biological, physical, psychological, activity, social* and *participation* dimensions.

These dimensions can be applied to people with neurological disorders and defined as follows (see **figure 3**): the *biological* dimension refers to the internal organic, physical structure and functioning of the body, especially the brain and the nervous system; the *physical* dimension refers to the person's external bodily functioning (eg. mobility levels) and any physical strengths or limitations a person might have; the *psychological* dimension refers to a person's emotional and cognitive abilities and functioning; the *activity* dimension refers to the things a person does in their personal lives in order to care for themselves, including activities of daily living; the *social* dimension refers to an individual's close and immediate relationships and social network, such as family and friends; *participation* refers to the person's involvement in wider society and includes their social, leisure, financial, housing and employment situation. **Figure 3** and **table 1** show the interlocking nature of the six dimensions and their descriptions respectively.

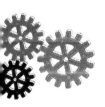

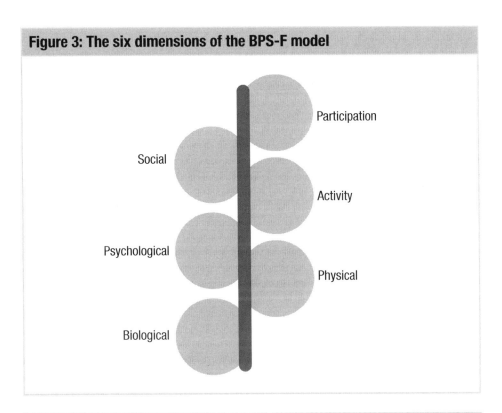

Figure 3: The six dimensions of the BPS-F model

Table 1: Descriptions of the six dimensions of the BPS-F model

Dimension	Description
Biological	Biology or internal organic make-up especially structure and functioning of the brain
Physical	Bodily strengths, weaknesses and limitations
Psychological	Emotional and cognitive abilities and difficulties
Activity	What a person does day-to-day in their personal lives, including activities of daily living
Social	Close relationships such as contact with family and friends
Participation	The individual and wider society, including leisure activities, financial, housing and employment matters

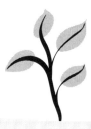

Therefore, a person's biological disease or disorder; their physical and psychological strengths and limitations; their social circumstances, housing, finances and those they have around them to support them are all important matters.

Different dimensions are important at different times

It is also the case that each dimension may be more or less important at different stages in a person's recovery. Just after injury or the appearance of symptoms it may be most important for the person to have the appropriate medical treatment in hospital or have access to investigations that will help give the correct diagnosis. At such times the biological and physical dimensions may be more important. However, two years later it may be the psychological, social and participation dimensions that are prominent. One way to think about this is to view the person as being on a 'journey' or 'pathway' following acquiring their brain disorder and different things are needed at different points along the way (see also chapter 11).

Case example

Alfonso, a plumber by trade, is a 33-year-old man who one weekend had been working on the roof of a friend's house fixing some slates when he slipped, fell and banged his head on the ground and as a result he was unconscious for several minutes. He eventually became conscious and started to talk with those who had gathered around him. An ambulance had been called and when the paramedics arrived they checked Alfonso's basic medical signs all of which appeared normal. The paramedics were with him for approximately 25 minutes during which he got up on his feet and was walking around but complaining of a headache. Given what had happened to him it was decided to take him to the local accident and emergency department to investigate him further and rule out any other injuries.

When Alfonso was waiting in the accident and emergency unit his headache got significantly worse and he began to experience some difficulties with his speech. He was seen by medical doctors and nurses on several occasions at 15 minute intervals; he appeared to be deteriorating. He reported getting 'funny' sensations in his right arm and leg and also was having difficulty moving them; he also had difficulty concentrating and his speech became slurred. When his headache got so severe and he lost part of his sight he was taken for a brain scan, the results of which showed the presence of a large haematoma (or bleed) on the left side of his brain.

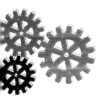

When Alfonso fell off the roof he burst a blood vessel on the left side of his brain, which slowly bled into surrounding areas, putting pressure on his brain. As a result, he gradually deteriorated both physically and psychologically.

Alfonso had emergency surgery to release the pressure on his brain by draining the blood, and on waking from surgery he had lost the ability to talk fluently, although he seemed to understand what others said to him, and he had difficulty with moving his right arm and leg.

Over the coming weeks and months some of Alfonso's difficulties improved. He was able to use more words and he moved from using a wheelchair to walking with crutches. However, three months later Alfonso was still having difficulties with walking and he had restricted movement in his right arm. Furthermore, he continued to have difficulties expressing what he wanted to say and at times he could be aggressive towards members of his family and those caring for him.

Using the BPS model, Alfonso's situation can be understood as follows.

Biological

From a biological perspective, Alfonso's difficulties can be viewed as being a direct result of the haematoma or bleed into his brain, which damaged some of his brain cells. This caused damage to the parts of the brain that control the right side of his body and speech, resulting in mobility problems in his right arm and leg, and problems with talking. His aggressive behaviour may be, totally or in part, a direct result of damage to the front part of his brain.

Physical

The physical or bodily impairments related to the haematoma included restricted movement on the right side of his body, which reduced his mobility and resulted in problems with speech production.

Psychological

Alfonso is frustrated by his physical difficulties and reduced ability to talk. He finds it difficult to express this frustration which results in him being hostile towards others.

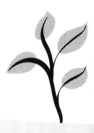

Activities

These physical impairments meant that he was unable to continue with daily activities, for example, walking his dog, eating, dressing and undressing, and holding a drink with his right arm.

Social

Alfonso was unable to hold conversations with other people. Joining in with family and group activities was difficult. His aggression made others wary of him.

Participation

Alfonso could not work and was unable to be involved in the range of social activities that he had participated in before. His language problems excluded him from many social situations and he was seen increasingly by others as aggressive and hostile, which led to social isolation and withdrawal and a further lack of participation in social activities. His withdrawal included lack of engagement with physical and occupational therapies which meant that he gained less from the help that was offered to him.

Here, at three months post injury, we see a downward spiral of decreased body function, decreased activity and reduced social participation.

Twelve months post-injury

Twelve months on and Alfonso is now very aware of the injuries he has sustained and he is embarrassed by his disabilities. Although he is not now using a wheelchair he uses a crutch or walking stick to get around and has difficulty doing anything which he feels is worthwhile with his right arm. He has been unable to return to work; he is very irritable and depressed and spends a lot of time in his bedroom staring out the window or watching television. His partner is unsure of what to do and any attempts to help result in him becoming aggressive. Although he realises he needs help he does not want it because it reminds him of his difficulties, disabilities and dependence on others. Alfonso compares the life he has now to the life he had before his injury, which leaves him feeling worthless and unable to offer anything to other people, or in his relationships, neither to his partner nor to wider society.

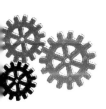

Biological and physical

Alfonso's brain recovery has slowed down and he may have recovered most of what he is going to recover by this stage. His physical abilities have improved but his strength and ability to use the right side of his body remain reduced and the extent to which this is improving has levelled off. His lack of engagement with physical and occupational therapy has not helped.

Psychological

Alfonso's awareness of his injuries, how he views them and the changes they have meant for his life, mean that there is an important psychological aspect to his irritation, aggressive behaviour and low mood. It may be the case that Alfonso's organic brain injury cannot be directly changed or cured, but his reaction to it, how he views himself and his life may be open to some change to help him improve the quality of his life.

Activities

Although Alfonso could do more for himself he is not motivated to do so and spends a lot of time alone doing nothing much in particular. He is understimulated and does the minimum of things for himself.

Social

Alfonso remains, and is increasingly isolated from others. He sees only his immediate family and professional carers and keeps them at an emotional distance. His relationship with his partner is very strained.

Participation

Alfonso has now been made redundant. He has no job, no source of income other than state benefits and this adds to his low mood, depressed state and social isolation.

Two years post injury

At two years post-injury, Alfonso's long-term partner is now on the verge of leaving him because of the stress of living with him and because of financial burdens. The daily grind of caring for Alfonso and trying to coax him into doing more for himself has led to frequent arguments and his partner feeling increasingly 'worn down'. His partner is

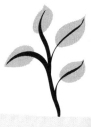

now the main earner in the household, which means working long hours at times. For his partner, work has become a refuge from the stresses and conflict at home. Alfonso is embarrassed to go out as he feels that others look at him differently, seeing him as somewhat 'damaged goods' and unable to adequately contribute to relationships and society. He feels that he is seen as an economic liability and burden rather than someone who is contributing positively to the economy. Society judges him as inferior, which in turn, makes him more isolated and depressed. Alfonso's friends do not know how to help him so they avoid him as he makes them feel uneasy.

Here we can see Alfonso spiral downwards into a state of depression. His exclusion from society started with his brain injury but is now exacerbated and made more complex both by his emotional reactions, social withdrawal, lack of activity and how he is viewed and treated by others.

In conclusion, it would seem that some of the major issues for Alfonso two years post-injury are psychological ones that centre on his struggle to come to terms with the changes in his body and his life. Such difficulties are sometimes referred to as 'issues of transition', that is making the transition between pre- and post-injury lives. It would seem that unless Alfonso can help himself or be helped by others to deal with his emotional response to his injuries he is unlikely to engage with his partner or in activities that will help him physically, socially or in his participation in wider society. He may need medication, eg. antidepressants or the help of a psychological therapist. Furthermore, his partner may also require help to deal with changes in Alfonso and their relationship.

The BPS-F model and capacity and performance levels

Building on the ICF approach each of the six dimensions in the BPS-F model also have related 'capacity' and 'performance' levels. These can be used to assess and understand a person's abilities and restrictions and to make decisions about the appropriate rehabilitation activities to be offered so that an individual can use all of their capacity and maximise their performance.

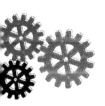

The biopsychosocial-functioning model in table format

The biopsychosocial-functioning model's six dimensions, their capacity and performance aspects and the gaps between capacity and performance are represented in **table 2**. This table also includes some relevant issues and questions to be considered for each dimension. This table can be completed and used as a method to understand a person with an acquired neurological disorder; their abilities, limitations and the issues that may need to be addressed.

and performance for each dimension can highlight gaps and needs, and identifies ways of addressing these gaps, that is, the things that need to be done. **Table 3** shows an example using Alfonso at two years post injury.

How the biopsychosocial-functioning model can help carers and family members

This combined BPS-F model gives carers and family members a framework to understand the person with a brain injury or disorder and helps identify what needs to be done in order to help them. The model can also help identify gaps in the service when a person is performing at a level less than their capacity and when further support, professional or informal, is needed. It also offers the reassurance that there are often many things to be done to help each person with an acquired neurological disorder and there is a role for everyone. Therefore, although not everyone is qualified or licensed to treat the medical and physical aspects of a brain disorder or hold professional roles that enable them to carry out extensive psychological or social assessments or interventions, each can have an important part to play in helping with the physical, psychological and social components of brain disorder and rehabilitation.

For example, as in Alfonso's case, the treatment of depression following a brain injury sometimes needs a biological treatment or the application of a particular psychological therapy, such as cognitive behavioural or personal construct therapy. Both of these treatments require trained professionals, but the support that a person gets from their family and wider social group along with the amount of finance they have at their disposal is also very important, perhaps more important. Such support and help can be and often is offered by frontline carers and family members.

The model and this handbook

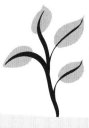

Table 2: The six dimensions of the biopsychosocial-functioning model along with their qualifiers and gaps

Dimension	Qualifier		Any gaps?	What can be done about the gaps?
	Capacity	Performance		
Biological	What is the brain disease/injury? What remains intact? Is the disease/disorder likely to get better, worse or stay the same?	What (medical) treatments are available?	Is there a difference between capacity and performance?	Are the biological aspects of the person's condition fully investigated and understood? Do they need a new/different medical treatment/medication? eg. to see a neurologist or other medical specialists.
Physical	What physical abilities/ limitations do they have? eg. to mobility, sight, language?	Do they use their physical abilities to their optimum level?	Is there a difference between capacity and performance?	Do they get physical and occupational therapy? What aids do they use? What adaptations have been made?
Psychological	What are their cognitive and emotional strengths and limitations? What were their cognitive abilities and personality characteristics before injury?	Are they using all their cognitive abilities as much as they can? Do they need support or advice in order to deal with any emotional or cognitive problems?	Is there a difference between capacity and performance?	Have they seen a neuropsychologist, psychiatrist or therapist? Are they using strategies to compensate for problems?

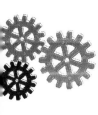

Table 2: The six dimensions of the biopsychosocial functioning model along with their qualifiers and gaps (continued)

Dimension	Qualifier		Any gaps?	What can be done about the gaps?
	Capacity	Performance		
Activities	What can a person do for themselves? eg. activities of daily living (ADL) skills such as dressing, cleaning, cooking.	Has the person had the opportunity to do ADL for themselves? Are they supported if need be? Does their environment help or hinder?	Is there a difference between capacity and performance?	Do they have a care package that allows them to be as independent as possible? Have they seen an occupational therapist?
Social	What is their family, and domestic situation?	Does their family and social network help or hinder their development?	Is there a difference between capacity and performance?	Do family and friends know how to cope? Have they been given advice, information and training? Does the family need support?
Participation	What groups do they belong to? What is their housing and financial situation?	What groups could they belong to or would like to belong to? What do they do outside their home?	Is there a difference between capacity and performance?	Has the person access to the right supports? eg. transport, technology. Do they have adequate housing (with adaptations if needed)? How much money do they have? Can they afford carers, holidays etc.? Do their finances need to be reviewed?

As can be seen from **table 2**, each dimension of the model has a capacity and performance component. Comparing capacity

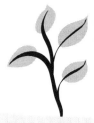

Table 3: The six dimensions of the biopsychosocial-functioning model with qualifiers and gaps applied to Alfonso's situation at two years post injury

Dimension	Qualifier		Any gaps?	What can be done about the gaps?
	Capacity	Performance		
Biological	Left frontal haematoma. Most biological aspects have been dealt with and medical interventions stopped apart from six month reviews.	The right and back of Alfonso's brain remain intact meaning that he has a good understanding of his situation, his perceptual and language comprehension remains intact.	Is Alfonso using the parts of his brain that remain intact in any structured therapeutic way and to the best of his ability?	Is Alfonso getting the appropriate medical treatment? eg. medication. To what extent is his aggression due to biological changes? Can any medication help with this? Given the nature and extent of his brain injury, are expectations of him both challenging and realistic?
Physical	Reduced mobility on his right side and problems with producing speech. However, able to use left side, walk with aids, understand others and write down what he wants to say.	Refuses to use crutches. Does not try to walk. Does not use a notebook or other aids to communicate.	Is not doing what he could do in terms of ability to move around and communicate. Large gap between capacity and performance.	Any additional aids needed, for example, to help with communication? If a psychological therapy and/or medication is offered, Alfonso's mood may improve and he may engage with physical and occupational therapies. Refer to speech and language therapy?
Activities	Can complete most of his ADL skills on his own; can cook and is mobile enough to leave home on his own.	Stays at home most of the time; watching television a lot.	Significant differences between capability and performance.	Perhaps Alfonso could visit local Headway Group or go with the physiotherapist to the hospital therapy pool or local swimming pool – either general public or 'closed' sessions. Look at ways of increasing independence.

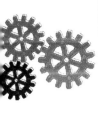

Understanding and Caring for People with Brain Disorders: A handbook © Pavilion Publishing (Brighton) Ltd 2011

Table 3: The six dimensions of the biopsychosocial-functioning model with qualifiers and gaps applied to Alfonso's situation (continued)

Dimension	Qualifier		Any gaps?	What can be done about the gaps?
	Capacity	Performance		
Psychological	Aware of emotional and cognitive difficulties. Problems with attention, memory, expressive language.	Low in mood, aggressive. Does not try to communicate a great deal.	He is aware of deficits but not using strengths to the best of his abilities.	Psychological therapy to look at issues of transition, mood and decreased tolerance for frustration. Help to use cognitive strengths and compensate for cognitive difficulties. Refer to neuropsychology?
Social	Could be involved in social situations by listening and writing. Enjoyed others' company before injuries.	Withdrawn emotionally and socially. Could have increased social roles but does not. Partner really struggling: now relationship one of carer and cared for.	Significant gaps.	A major issue is the potential breakdown of Alfonso's relationship with partner. Can they as a couple or his partner be offered further support or counselling? Is his partner getting adequate support? Could they go to carers group? Have his friends been given information? Do they want information? Are there any social groups he could attend? Could friends be engaged more?
Participation	Could think about voluntary work; could go swimming or join lobby group on disability.	Does not do any leisure or other activity he finds meaningful.	Not fulfilling potential	Alfonso's reduced income is a major issue. Is he getting all the benefits he is entitled to? Are there charitable organisations that can help with other matters? eg. transport. Can some of society's attitudes and prejudices about people with disabilities be challenged?

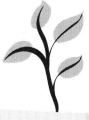

This biopsychosocial-functioning model underpins many aspects of the remaining chapters that follow in this handbook. All six dimensions emerge throughout the title with each chapter highlighting one or more of the six dimensions. The biological and physical dimensions are particularly emphasised in chapters 2, 4 and 5; the psychological dimension is emphasised in chapters 3, 4 and 11; the activity dimension in chapters 5, 6, 7, 8, 9 and 10; the social and participation dimensions feature in chapter 11. Chapters 12 and 13 use the information from the other chapters that has been traditionally used to understand people with acquired neurological disorders, and applies it to aspects of mental health and learning disability. After reading the other chapters in this book, the reader could come back and look at **table 2** again and use the information and knowledge from the other chapters to help them complete this table for someone they know.

A few words about empowerment

Arguably, the final outcome of rehabilitation should be the empowerment of the individual because the more a person is empowered the more they will want to do for themselves and the more they will be able to contribute to society. Yates (2003) states that empowerment has got three important elements; first, the perceived and actual power of an individual having choice and control; second, the process of reinvolvement and integration of a person with a disability back into their community and third, access to valued social roles such as in education, employment and financial security. Neath and Schriner (1998) describe these three types of power as being 'person power', that is, the power of the individual to influence their circumstances; second, power over others and circumstances or 'social power' and the third form of power is where people get together with others as equals as expressed in friendships and social and political groups. Likewise McColl *et al* (1998) define successful community integration as '*having something to do; somewhere to live; and someone to love*'.

The biopsychosocial-functioning model is a framework that can give rise to actions that endeavour to empower a person with disabilities at these three different levels. It is designed to help the person overcome or adapt to their illness; make psychological adjustments; compensate for difficulties; find new ways of expressing themselves along with confronting and helping others confront the disabling aspects of the society in which they live.

Take away message

People with neurological disorders and brain injuries can be helped in a wide variety of ways by many different people, including professional and informal carers and especially by families and friends. The biopsychosocial-functioning model is one way to understand a person and their context and to think of ways in which they might be helped and supported.

Quiz

1. What is the World Health Organization?

2. Describe the three aspects of the biopsychosocial model.

3. What are the three main components of the *International Classification of Functioning, Disability and Health?*

4. What are the two 'qualifiers' in the *International Classification of Functioning, Disability and Health?*

5. If someone has greater capacity than performance, what does this mean?

6. What are the six dimensions of the biopsychosocial-functioning (BPS-F) model?

7. What needs to be the goal of rehabilitation?

8. Think about someone you know who has a disability and fill out the empty BPS-F table about them in the appendix at the end of this chapter.

References

Engel G (1997) The need for a new medical model. *Science* **196** 129–136.

Fleminger S, Oliver D, Williams H & Evans J (2003) The neuropsychiatry of depression after brain injury. *Neuropsychological Rehabilitation* **13** (1/2) 65–78.

Gilbert P (2002) Understanding the biopsychosocial approach: conceptualisation. *Clinical Psychology Forum* **14** 13–17.

Lakhan S (2006) The biopsychosocial model of health and illness. *BioPsychoSocial Health* [online]. Available at: www.brainblogger.com (accessed December 2010).

Lezak M, Howieson D & Loring D (2004) *Neuropsychological assessment.* Oxford: Oxford University Press.

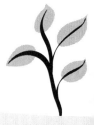

Loring D [Ed] (1999) *International Neuropsychological Society Dictionary of Neuropsychology*. Oxford: Oxford University Press.

McColl M, Carlson P, Johnston J, Minnes P, Shue K, Davies D & Karlovitz T (1998) The definition of community integration: perspectives of people with brain injuries. *Brain Injury* **12** (1) 15–30.

McCrea M (2008) *Mild Traumatic Brain Injury and Post Traumatic Syndrome*. Oxford: Oxford University Press.

Neath J & Schriner K (1998) Power to people with disabilities: empowerment issues in employment programming. *Disability and Society* **13** (2) 217–228.

Wade D (2003) *Neuropsychological Deficits within the World Health Organization's Model of Illness*. In: P Halligan, U Kischka & J Marshall (Eds) (2003) *Handbook of Clinical Neuropsychology*. Oxford. Oxford University Press.

World Health Organization (2002) *International Classification of Functioning, Disability and Health*. Copenhagan: World Health Organisation.

World Health Organization [online]. Available at: www.who.int/en/ (accessed December 2010).

Yates P (2003) Psychological adjustment, social enablement and community integration following acquired brain injury. *Neuropsychological Rehabilitation* **13** (1/2) 291–306.

Further reading

Johnstone B & Stonnington H (2009) *Rehabilitation of Neuropsychological Disorders*. London: Psychology Press.

Williams H & Evans J (2003) *Biopsychosocial Approaches in Neuro-rehabilitation: Assessment and management of neuropsychiatric, mood and behavioural disorders. Neuropsychological rehabilitation*. Hove: Psychology Press.

Acknowledgment

I would like to acknowledge and thank Ashley Verheyden and Jacqui Brown for discussions on aspects of this chapter.

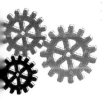

Appendix

An empty biopsychosocial-functioning (BPS-F) table, which can be photocopied and used by the reader to complete with a relative or client.

Table 4: Biopsychosocial-functioning (BPS-F) table				
Dimension	**Qualifier**		**Any gaps?**	**What can be done about the gaps?**
	Capacity	Performance		
Biological				
Physical				
Psychological				
Activities				
Social				
Participation				

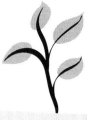

Chapter 2

Understanding the brain

Declan Mc Nicholl

Aims of the chapter

The chapter aims to:

▶ give an outline of the nervous system

▶ consider the evolutionary nature of the brain

▶ explain the main parts of the brain and their associated functions

▶ explain that although each area of the brain has evolved specialist functions, the parts are interconnected.

Introduction

Systems in the human body

The human body has a number of systems involved in maintaining life. The digestive system breaks down food to give nutrition to feed the body and give it energy. The respiratory system allows for the intake of oxygen and breathing out of carbon dioxide. The circulatory system involves the heart pumping blood around the body in artaries and veins to supply all cells with nutrients and oxygen and take away waste products and carbon dioxide. The excretory system removes waste and poisonous substances from the blood, which are filtered out in organs such as the liver and kidneys and excreted in the form of urine and faeces. The reproductive system gives the capacity to reproduce. The human skeletal system offers support to other organs and soft tissue and in some places provides a tough barrier to protect other delicate organs, for example, a skull to protect the brain. A system of muscles attached to bones gives the body the ability to move as they contract and relax.

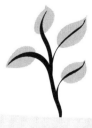

Message systems

There also are two message systems in the body; the endocrine and nervous systems. The endocrine system produces chemicals called 'hormones' that are put into the blood stream from a number of glands around the body such as the thyroid gland and pancreas and, in the brain, the pituitary gland. Hormones control things like growth, sexual characteristics and the menstrual cycle in women. Each hormone has particular cells around the body with which they interact and have an effect, known as 'target cells'. An example of one hormone is adrenaline, which is secreted into the blood in response to a threatening external stimulus or situation. This increases breathing and the heartrate and blood supply to the muscles allowing the person to move faster and run away or prepare to fight. These chemical messengers of the endocrine system provide a slow acting message system which is sustained over a long period of time.

The final system, the nervous system, produces very fast messages over a relatively short period of time, using mainly electrical impulses. The nervous system includes the sensory organs, including the eyes, ears, nose, tongue and skin that pass information from the surrounding environment to the spinal cord and the brain. The brain then co-ordinates a response and sends electrical messages back via the motor system of the brain and spinal cord to create a response.

The nervous system

The body is made up from many different types of cells, one of which is nerve cells, also called 'neurons'. Surrounding nerve cells are glial cells ('glia' in Greek means glue) which offer support and make neurons more effective. Neurons can be of different shapes and sizes but they generally have a number of similar parts including a cell body containing the nucleus, dendrites which receive information from other nerve cells that carry information to the cell body, and axons that carry information onto the next nerve cell (see **figure 1**). Axons are often covered in a white fatty substance known as 'myelin', which acts as an electrical insulator and increases the speed with which electrical impulses pass along the axon. In some conditions it is depleted, such as in multiple sclerosis, which causes information to be passed along the neuron much slower. There is a little gap between cells known as a 'synapse' across which information is carried using chemicals called 'neurotransmitters'.

Figure 1: A nerve cell or neuron

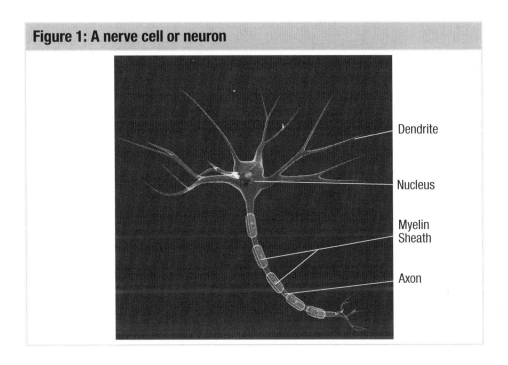

Dendrite

Nucleus

Myelin Sheath

Axon

Neurons form many complex connections with each other as **figure 2** shows.

Figure 2: Interconnecting neurons

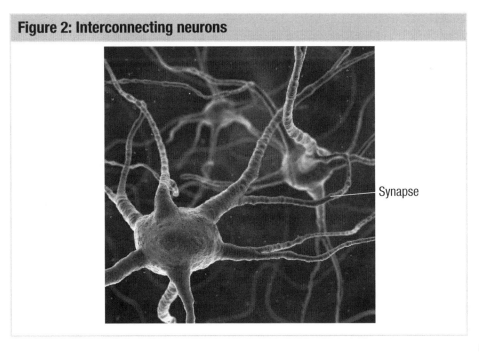

Synapse

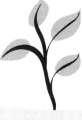

Peripheral and central nervous systems

The nervous system is made up of two main sections namely the central nervous system and the peripheral nervous system. The central nervous system consists of the brain, which is encased in the skull, and the spinal cord which runs down the centre of the back. The peripheral nervous system is made up of the nerves that come off the central nervous system, for example, nerves that go from the brain and spinal cord into the head, face, arms and legs.

Messages are carried along nerves to and from the brain to all parts of the body. Those that carry messages to the brain are known as 'sensory' neurons and those which carry messages back to the body are called 'motor' neurons. An example of the work of a motor neuron would be carrying a message from our brain to move the muscles around the eyes to move them across the page of a book so it can be read.

The brain

The brain is a very complex organ that is slowly being better understood due to recent scientific developments. The human brain weighs over one kilogram (about three pounds) which is around two per cent of the total body weight of the average adult. The brain consists of billions of nerve cells which communicate with each part of the body and with each other enabling us to process information and initiate activities. It is split into two hemispheres linked by the corpus callosum.

Areas of the brain that contain cell bodies are grey in colour and hence they are called 'grey matter', while those containing mainly axons and glial cells are called 'white matter' because axons are covered in a white fatty coating known as the 'myeline sheath' (see **figure 1**) which make them white in colour.

The evolution of the brain

Most people today understand that human beings have evolved from more primitive species and the structure of the human brain reflects this process of evolution. The brain can be seen to have evolved three main levels. The first and most 'primitive' level is the part of the brain which is shared with reptiles and evolved for self-preservation, including the processes of

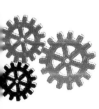

 Understanding and Caring for People with Brain Disorders: A handbook © Pavilion Publishing (Brighton) Ltd 2011

aggression and reproduction. On top of this primitive brain sits what is often referred to as the 'intermediate' brain which contains the limbic system. The limbic system, which is explained more fully later in this chapter and in chapter 5, is thought to be closely associated with emotions. Finally, on top of the limbic system is a third level, which is the last part of our brain to evolve and is sometimes referred to as the neocortex or new cortex. This new cortex contains the highest order of human functioning, for example, intellectual abilities. It is here that much of the intermediate and primitive brain is controlled and regulated which allows humans to operate in a much more sophisticated way compared to other animals. It includes the capacities that allow humans to socialise, communicate and use language.

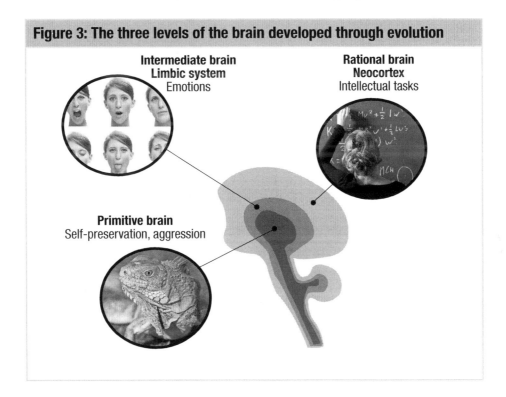

Figure 3: The three levels of the brain developed through evolution

The different halves of the brain

Front and back

There is a division line that runs across the top of the human brain, roughly from ear to ear, which divides the brain into front and back halves. Behind this line is the part that is mainly to do with information coming in to the

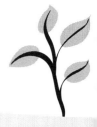

brain, that is the sensory part of our brain. This part of the brain then puts this sensory information together so that each individual can understand what is happening around them and in their body. In front of this central line is the part that deals with output or telling the body what to do, or motor commands. Here information is co-ordinated to allow us to move around, talk and respond to things going on in our environment.

Figure 4: Diagram of the brain showing the back (sensory) and front (motor) parts

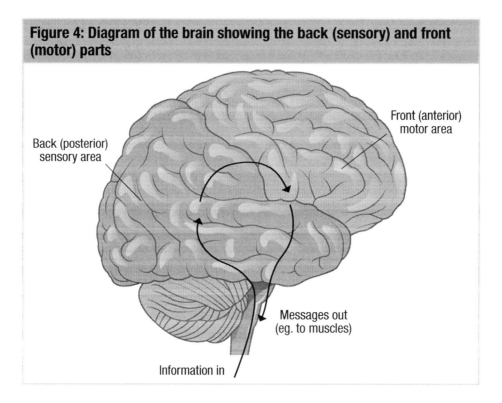

Front (anterior) motor area

Back (posterior) sensory area

Messages out (eg. to muscles)

Information in

Left and right

There is also a line running from the front to back of the brain, which divides it into the left and right sides. For most people the left-hand side contains verbal and language skills, such as the ability to hear and understand what other people say; the ability to speak; write and read. The right-hand side deals mostly with non language-based tasks. These include aspects of perception and understanding space, for example, the ability to have an internal 'map' of and move around in the environment; understand and appreciate music, humour and the subtleties of social relationships, for example, sarcasm and irony.

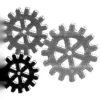

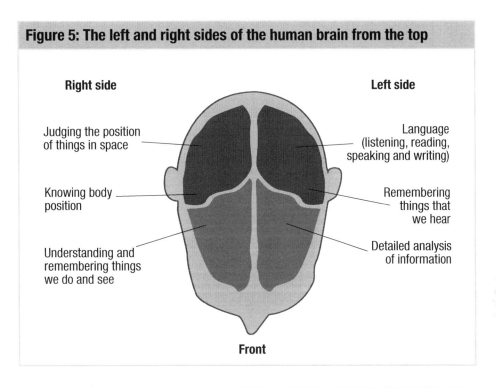

Figure 5: The left and right sides of the human brain from the top

Right side

Left side

Judging the position
of things in space

Language
(listening, reading,
speaking and writing)

Knowing body
position

Remembering
things that
we hear

Understanding and
remembering things
we do and see

Detailed analysis
of information

Front

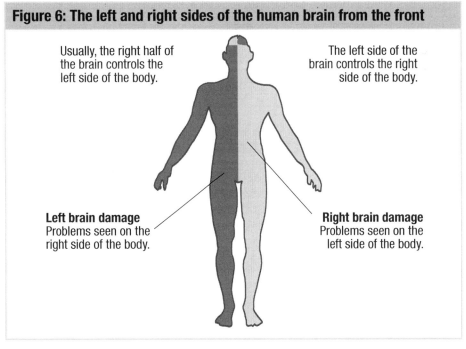

Figure 6: The left and right sides of the human brain from the front

Usually, the right half of
the brain controls the
left side of the body.

The left side of the
brain controls the right
side of the body.

Left brain damage
Problems seen on the
right side of the body.

Right brain damage
Problems seen on the
left side of the body.

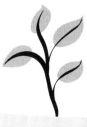

The three main divisions and other important parts of the brain

One of the most common ways of understanding the brain is to break it down into three main divisions namely the forebrain, midbrain and hindbrain.

The hindbrain

Just above the spinal cord at the base of the skull sits the hindbrain which is made up of the pons, medulla oblongata and cerebellum (see **figures 7, 8 and 9**). The hindbrain is that part of the brain that maintains functions vital for life, including control of breathing, heartbeat and blood pressure. Significant injury to this part of our brain usually results in death.

The cerebellum performs a number of functions including the control of fine movement, for example, the ability to walk smoothly. Damage to the cerebellum often results in unsteady walking or an inability to control or make fine movements. However, because of its connections to other parts of the brain, damage to the cerebellum can also affect non-motor abilities and can disrupt aspects of attention, speech, reasoning and emotional regulation. The hindbrain also contains what is referred to as the reticular activating system (RAS) which is part of the network which controls wakefulness and sleeping patterns, alertness and the ability to be focused at times of threat. This is one of the areas important in being conscious. Damage to this area can result in anything from sleep disorders right through to states of semi-consciousness or coma.

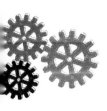

Figure 7: The main parts of the brain as viewed from the side

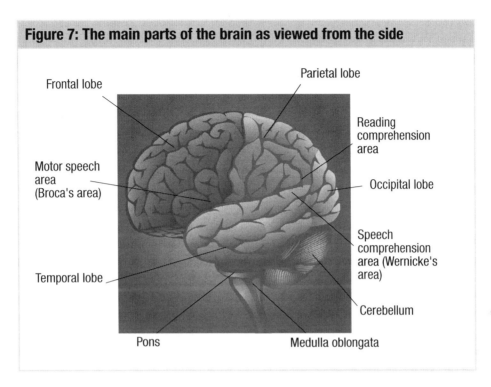

Frontal lobe

Parietal lobe

Reading comprehension area

Motor speech area (Broca's area)

Occipital lobe

Speech comprehension area (Wernicke's area)

Temporal lobe

Cerebellum

Pons

Medulla oblongata

Figure 8: Components of the brain stem as seen from underneath

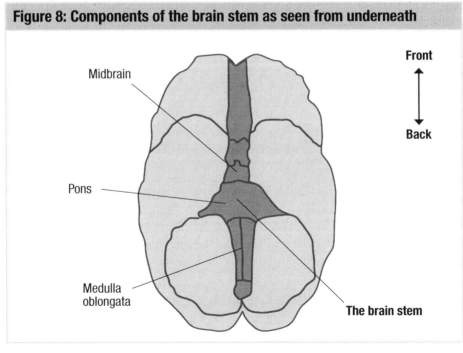

Front

Back

Midbrain

Pons

Medulla oblongata

The brain stem

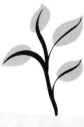

The midbrain

On top of the hindbrain is the midbrain, which is short and narrow and connects the hindbrain to the forebrain. This area also contains a major part of the reticular activating system and is also important in regulating consciousness.

Taken together the pons, medulla and midbrain are often referred to as the 'brain stem'. The brain stem is the part of the brain which is evolutionary the oldest and, as mentioned above, performing functions that are associated with reptiles.

The forebrain

The forebrain is the largest part of the nervous system in humans. It consists of the two cerebral hemispheres with four lobes on each side that contain the cerebral cortex, the grey matter, and below this the white matter (see **figure 9**). Also buried deep within the white matter of the brain and not visible from the outside are a number of smaller but very important grey matter structures called the basal ganglia, thalamus and hypothalamus (see **figures 9** and **10**). Like most other structures in the brain we have one of these on each side.

The thalamus

The thalamus has a lot of information passing through it. The thalamus interconnects with many different parts of the brain, and information from all the main senses apart from smell passes through the thalamus. Therefore, damage to the thalamus can cause major disruption to the processing of sensory information. The thalamus is also the end point of the reticular activating system and therefore is also involved in the process of consciousness. It also has connections with areas that are important for memory, especially with the remembering of new information. For example, people who develp Korsakoff's disease lose the ability to learn new information or to remember recent events. This disease results from a Vitamin B1 (thiamin) deficiency and is most often found in people who abuse alcohol. It is also found in people with other difficulties such as eating disorders.

The thalamus is also involved with higher order cognitive functions such as reasoning, flexible thinking or what is referred to as 'executive functioning' (see chapter 4). Damage to the thalamus can also disrupt emotions; in particular a person can develop apathy or lack of motivation which can lead to changes in personality.

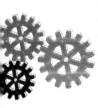

Some people suffer a stroke in the thalamus (see chapter 5). Even small strokes in the thalamus can have a devastating effect on a person's abilities because the thalamus is highly interconnected with different areas of the brain.

The hypothalamus

Just underneath the thalamus is the hypothalamus, which is also an important regulatory centre. The hypothalamus acts as a control for the endocrine system that deals with the regulation of hormones as mentioned earlier in this chapter. Although this is a very small structure it regulates very important functions such as appetite, sexual arousal and thirst. Patterns of behaviour associated with fear, anger and rage are also regulated by the hypothalamus. Bodily reactions associated with fright are regulated in the hypothalamus, which helps us to prepare for emergency or threatening situations.

Disruption to the functioning of the hypothalamus can result in disturbances in temperature regulation, sexuality, food and water intake such as obesity or change in sex drives. Mood may also be affected by changes in the hypothalamus. The brain stem and hypothalamus together allow an organism to eat, drink, reproduce and sleep.

Figure 9: The major parts of the brain as seen from the inside

Parietal lobe

Cerebrum

Occipital lobe

Temporal lobe

Corpus callosum

Thalamus

Hypothalamus

Cerebellum

Pituitary gland

Frontal lobe

Pons

Medulla oblongata

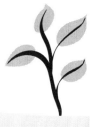

The basal ganglia

Situated in the white matter of the cerebral hemisphere there are a number of structures known as the basal ganglia (see **figure 10**), which include the caudate, putamen, and globus pallidus. The caudate and putamen are thought to be part of the system that turns our thoughts into actions (Lezak *et al*, 2004). The basal ganglia is very important in motor control and is also important in the learning of skills that eventually become automatic, for example, riding a bike or performing a skilled craft. Damage to this area will result in motor dysfunction and particularly the occurrence of involuntary movements such as tremors when a person is at rest. Two disorders in particular, Parkinson's disease and Huntington's disease, both of which are associated with changes in a person's ability to control their bodily movements, are associated with damages to these areas. As the basal ganglia connects with other parts of the brain, changes here can also have an impact on emotions and the ability to problem solve. As a result of some other very distressing disorders such as obsessive compulsive behaviours, Tourette's syndrome and attention deficit disorders are also associated with changes in the basal ganglia (Lezak *et al*, 2004).

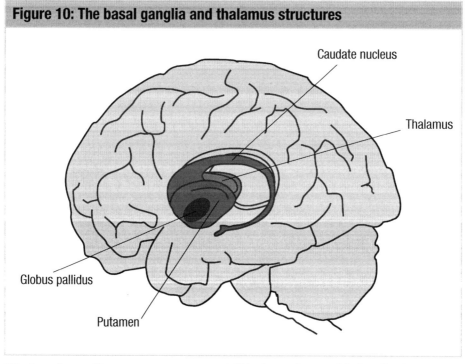

Figure 10: The basal ganglia and thalamus structures

Caudate nucleus

Thalamus

Globus pallidus

Putamen

The basal ganglia structures are not visible from the outside but lie deep within the brain. The thalamus is included in this diagram to help locate the basal ganglia in the brain.

The cerebral cortex

The cerebral cortex is divided into two hemispheres, left and right and these two hemispheres are connected to each other by the corpus callosum. Each hemisphere is divided into four major lobes – the frontal, parietal, temporal and occipital (see **figures 8** and **9**). The frontal lobe is concerned with motor control and movement. The parietal lobe is concerned with receiving and co-ordinating information from our senses especially taste, touch and hearing; the occipital lobe is concerned with the processing of vision; the temporal lobe has a number of functions, including the processing of what is heard or auditory information.

In the cerebral cortex, information to and from the left side of the body is dealt with by the right side of the brain and vice versa. Therefore, each side of the cerebral cortex controls and receives information from the opposite side of the body. This is called 'contralateral control', 'lateral' meaning 'side' and 'contra' meaning 'opposite' (see **figure 5** and **6**). Exceptions to this contralateral rule include some aspects of vision and hearing functions.

Each lobe has what is referred to as 'primary areas', which are involved in the crude analysis of information coming in from the body (sensory) or the beginnings of a motor response (motor). These primary areas connect with what are called 'association areas'. Here the information is put together either from a single sense or from different senses.

There are a number of these association areas that carry out higher order information processing, and language is a particularly good example of a higher order function. Information from the primary auditory (listening) or visual (reading) language areas feed into an association area in the temporal lobe known as Wernicke's area, which is the area that deals with understanding language. This area connects with an area in the frontal lobe known as Broca's area, which controls the production of language (see **figure 9**). Damage to Wernicke's area would mean that a person would have difficulty in comprehending what has been said and damage to the Broca's area would mean difficulty with language production. A difficulty with language, especially the production of language, is often associated with particular types of strokes and can be a cause of a great deal of distress for people who have suffered left-sided strokes (see chapter 5).

Lesions or damage in parts of the parietal lobe in the left hemisphere can produce a number of difficulties with reading and writing language, making calculations, and causing an inability to recognise objects by name.

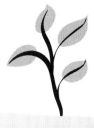

Difficulties in the non-dominant, usually right hemisphere of the parietal lobe can cause neglect of the opposite side of the body. Patients with this difficulty often ignore objects on the left-hand side, for example they may draw a house with the left part of the house missing or may be completely unaware of the left side of their body. In extreme cases people can think that their left arm belongs to someone else or they may not even be aware that they have got paralysis or weakness in the left side of their body.

So many areas are associated with the planning of complex motor behaviours that change to a wide number of different areas can give rise to the disruption in the planning and carrying out of complex motor tasks, a condition known as 'dyspraxia'.

The frontal lobes contain the biggest areas of association cortex, and difficulties in these areas can mean disruption of complex motor functions but also changes in personality. For example, depending on where the lesion is, a person may find it difficult to initiate behaviours, they may have difficulty monitoring their behaviour or they may have difficulties finishing tasks (see chapter 5). They may also have difficulty switching their attention or may tend to focus on one particular thing and find it difficult to think of other things. Some people become increasingly disinhibited and they have difficulty stopping themselves from doing things, for example, when they think of doing something or saying something they go ahead and say or do it without considering the consequences.

What is 'executive functioning'?

The term 'executive' means the ability to plan, carry out and complete a task, like the chief executive in a company overseeing production from start to finish. Executive functioning is what makes up goal directed activity, for example, to do shopping or laundry, or arranging to see friends. This ability is thought to be primarily located in the frontal lobes. In the frontal lobes we organise what to do, how to do it, when to do it and why to do it, which includes planning, organising and problem-solving. For example, making a cup of tea involves a number of steps: fill the kettle with water, switch on the kettle, get out a cup, put in the teabag, pour the water into the cup, get a teaspoon, squeeze the teabag with the teaspoon, take the teabag out, pour in some milk and, for some, put in some sugar and stir. The frontal lobe acts as the overseer of all these steps so that they happen in the right order; it would be unhelpful to put the water into the cup before boiling the kettle. The disruption of executive functioning could upset the sequencing of tasks so that the person is unable to plan the steps and unable to carry out these steps in the proper sequence. The frontal lobes are a common site of injury from accidents resulting in what is called 'dysexecutive syndrome' or, in other words, the disruption of executive abilities.

The limbic system

Deep within the brain, with connections to the thalamus, hypothalamus and frontal lobes are a number of grey matter bodies known as the 'limbic system' (see **figure 11**). These structures include the amygdala, fornix, hippocampus and mammillary body. The limbic system, 'limbus' meaning 'near' in Latin, is near the cerebral cortex, also includes some certain areas of the cerebral cortex including the inner and lower temporal and frontal lobes. Some parts of the limbic system, such as the mammillary body and the hippocampus, have been shown to have very important roles in the learning of new information and retaining it in long-term memory.

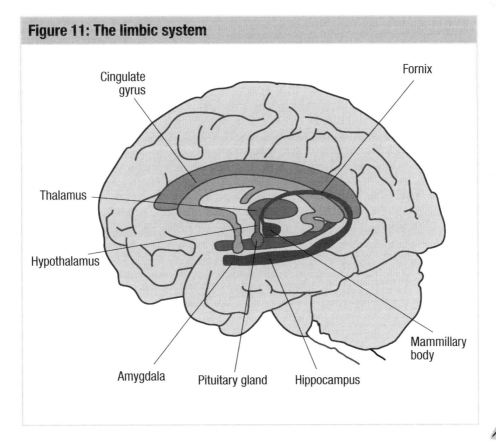

Figure 11: The limbic system

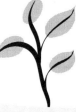

Limbic structures are also very important in the regulation of emotions (see chapter 4). Some limbic system structures, such as the hypothalamus, regulate drives like thirst, appetite and sexuality. Through connections with the frontal lobes, the limbic system is also involved in reasoning, problem-solving and initiation of behaviours. Damage to the limbic system often causes changes in personality and patterns of behaviour. Two conditions that particularly affect the limbic system are temporal lobe epilepsy and encephalitis. These conditions can cause upset in the regulation and expression of emotions and severe memory deficits (Bigler & Clement, 1987). Epileptic seizures often arise within these limbic structures in the temporal lobe and can begin with sensations or 'auras' such as the emotion of fear, déjà vu experiences or experiencing a particular smell.

There is a very important connection between emotion and memory and people often remember emotionally laden material better than that which has no emotion attached to it, hence the ability to remember how one felt about what someone else said more than what was actually said. The amygdala, in particular, plays an important part in emotional processing and learning (Lezak *et al*, 2004). It is thought to be important in reacting to fear or seeing fear in another person's face; it is also thought, because of its association with emotions that dysfunction in the amygdala may be involved in specific disorders. For example, Kluver-Bucy Syndrome occurs with the destruction of the amygdala and people with this disorder, which can occur through disease or brain injury, find it difficult to learn and eat excessively and indiscriminately.

The vascular system

The brain needs a rich supply of oxygen and nutrients, which is carried to it by its blood supply. The control systems for this supply are extremely sophisticated but can be rendered completely ineffective if an artery ruptures or is closed off in some way; this is referred to as a cerebrovascular accident or stroke (see chapter 4).

There are three main arteries that carry blood to the front, middle and back of the brain and these are called the anterior, middle and posterior cerebral arteries respectively (see **figures 11** and **12**). All these arteries connect up underneath the base of the brain and form a circle, like a roundabout with roads leading into it and off it. This circle is known as the 'Circle of Willis' (see **figure 13**).

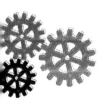

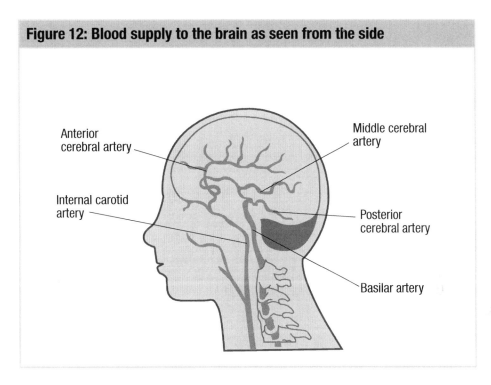

Figure 12: Blood supply to the brain as seen from the side

Anterior cerebral artery

Middle cerebral artery

Internal carotid artery

Posterior cerebral artery

Basilar artery

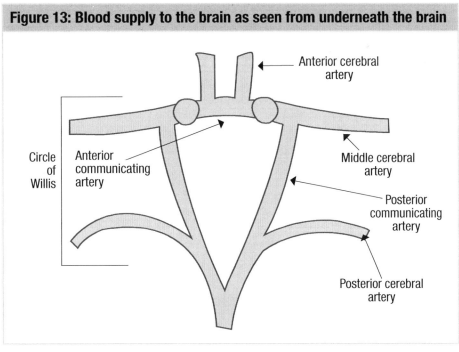

Figure 13: Blood supply to the brain as seen from underneath the brain

Anterior cerebral artery

Circle of Willis

Anterior communicating artery

Middle cerebral artery

Posterior communicating artery

Posterior cerebral artery

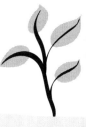

A stroke or cerebrovascular accident is a disruption of the blood supply to the brain and can happen quickly with symptoms having a quick onset and persisting for 24 hours or more. It can be caused by a haemorrhage or bleeding from an artery, or by the closing up of an artery through progressive narrowing, for example, with the build up of fatty material on the walls of the arteries, which is known as 'ischemia'. In addition a piece of this fatty material can break off to form an 'embolus', which can then become jammed in an artery causing a blockage.

Strokes are caused in areas where brain cells are damaged, or an 'infarct', and depending where the damage is in the brain this will disrupt different functions. For example, an infarct in the area that is responsible for speech production at the front of the brain will disrupt speech. A 'posterior' or stroke at the back of the brain usually results in nausea or vomiting, difficulties with balance and vision, unsteadiness and difficulty walking. A stroke in the brain stem can result in a coma or death.

Cerebral spinal fluid and the ventricles

Surrounding the brain and contained within cavities inside the brain is the ventricles and there is a fluid known as cerebral spinal fluid (CSF). This fluid also surrounds the spinal cord. This is a clear liquid and it serves as a cushion to protect the brain from impacts to the skull when the head is subject to external forces, for example, during a fall or car accident. Some diseases and some strokes can result in some waste material or blood getting into the CSF. Therefore tapping into cerebral spinal fluid through the spine is one of the tests that can be done to detect some disorders, such as multiple sclerosis or stroke. This is called a 'lumbar puncture' and where the term 'spinal tap' comes from.

If too much CSF is produced or one of the pathways in which it flows becomes blocked then this produces enlarged ventricles, a process known as hydrocephalus. Some babies are born with enlarged ventricles, which can result in learning disabilities.

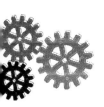

The interconnectedness of the brain

It is important to understand that although specific areas of the brain are more or less involved in specific functions most human behaviour and higher order functioning involves many different areas within the brain. This interconnectedness has been emphasised at various times throughout this chapter. Therefore, it is important to be very careful when trying to map any particular behaviour or human activity onto one particular brain area, as complex behaviour often involves many different parts.

Take away message

The human brain has evolved into an extremely complex organ that allows us to carry out highly specialist behaviours. It is made up of many parts which often have particular functions but these parts form an interconnected whole. Understanding the different parts, what they do and what can go wrong when they do not function properly, can help us understand a person with a neurological disorder.

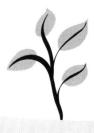

Quiz

1. What are the three main parts of the brain that have come about through evolution?

2. What are the four lobes of the brain called and what are their main functions?

3. What is the limbic system and what does it do?

4. Where and what is the thalamus?

5. The hypothalamus and brain stem allow human beings to carry out what activities?

6. What is an infarct?

7. Describe the purpose of a 'spinal tap'?

References

Bigler E & Clement P (1987) *Diagnostic Clinical Neuropsychology*. Austin: University of Texas.

Lezak M, Howieson D & Loring D (2004) *Neuropsychological Assessment*. Oxford: Oxford University Press.

Further reading

Carter R (2003) *Mapping the Mind*. London: Phoenix.

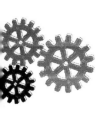

Chapter 3

Cognitive functions

Robert Poppleton and Liam Gilligan

Aims of the chapter

The chapter aims to:

▶ obtain a better understanding of some of the main cognitive functions

▶ provide an understanding of problems related to brain injuries and how they may affect cognitive functioning

▶ think about the ways in which people may overcome these problems.

Introduction

Before discussing the main cognitive functions, it is important to have a quick overview of the brain (see also chapter 2). The brain consists of 100 billion living nerve cells, also known as neurons, and each neuron is connected to 100s of other neurons, which use electrical impulses to pass information across the brain. No other part of our body has such a complexity and density of nerve fibres; it is like a very sophisticated telephone exchange centre with billions of cables.

The brain (cerebrum)

The brain is the most complex organ in the human body and enables us to use complicated tools, build complex houses and have highly developed languages. However, the brain is the least understood of all our organs, for example, we do not know exactly how memories are made and stored. The brain is presently the focus of much research and as we try to understand it in greater depth, it is hoped that in the future we will be able to treat and

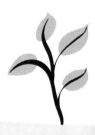

repair brain damage and restore functioning more successfully. There are some relatively new experimental treatments such as brain cell implants and the use of stem cells, which are being tested in order to see if they can repair damaged areas of the brain. The results to date have not been very successful, but there is hope for the future.

Damage to the brain can have dramatic effects on a person's everyday functioning, for example weakness in one side of the body or even not being able to move an arm or leg at all; not being able to talk fluently or not being able to remember important information.

These impairments can occur following incidents such as a stroke or brain injury following a road traffic accident (see also chapter 5). The brain is the centre of cognitive processes: it is the central location of learning, knowing and our personalities. It controls the skills and tasks we undertake in everyday life such as studying, working, interacting with our friends and families and undertaking sports and leisure activities.

Different parts of the brain are involved in different specialised skills (see also chapter 2). For example, in the front of the brain (ie. the frontal lobes) there are areas that play a large role in speaking, reasoning and fine motor skills, where as the back of the brain is more associated with vision and visual processing (see **figure 1** below).

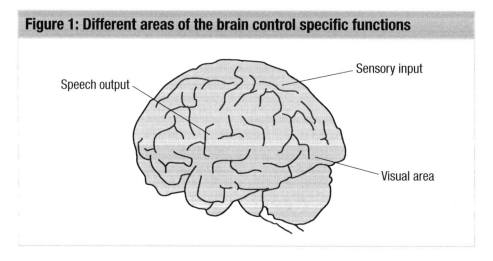

Figure 1: Different areas of the brain control specific functions

Speech output

Sensory input

Visual area

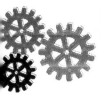

It is very common for cognitive abilities and functions to be adversely affected as a result of a brain injury. The affects this has on an individual's everyday life depends on the severity of the injury and the areas of the brain that have been damaged. Furthermore, an individual's age, health and cognitive ability before the injury are also important and therefore the cognitive problems caused by a brain injury are unique to each individual person (see also chapter 1).

Why is it important to know about the consequences of brain injuries?

If we can understand the consequences of brain damage and its implications on a person's life we can:

▶ provide help and support to facilitate and aid recovery

▶ provide better quality of care, taking into account each individual's specific needs

▶ try to minimise the risks a person may face, for example, change their living environment to reduce the risk of them falling.

Some quick facts and figures about brain injuries

One in six people in the UK will suffer a traumatic brain injury which requires treatment at some point in their life, with the highest risk group being older people due to falling over, young men due to road traffic accidents and children. This number is much larger if you take into account acquired brain injuries such as strokes (Daisley *et al*, 2008). It has been estimated that there are around half a million adults in the UK who live with disabilities as a result of a head injury at anyone time (Daisley *et al*, 2008).

The most common cases of traumatic brain injury are:

▶ falls

▶ road traffic accidents

▶ assaults

▶ sports injuries

▶ home or occupational accidents.

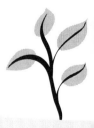

The most commonly reported cognitive changes include:

▶ compromised concentration abilities: 'I cannot concentrate as well as I used to'

▶ reduced memory function, for example, 'I cannot remember what others have said to me'

▶ personality changes: 'He is not the person I married'

▶ reduced speed of processing: 'I cannot think as quickly as I used too'.

The only way to fully understand how someone is affected by injury is through observations and assessments of their everyday lives.

Cognitive functions

Figure 2 below highlights some of the main cognitive functions. For a definition of the term 'cognitive' see chapter 1.

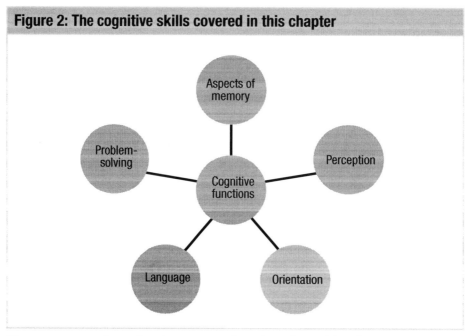

Figure 2: The cognitive skills covered in this chapter

There are a number of main areas or domains of cognitive functioning. These include orientation, attention, memory, language and executive functions. These will now be considered individually.

Orientation

Orientation is the awareness of a person in relation to their surroundings. Being orientated and not confused is fundamental in our everyday lives as it is important to know where we are, what we are supposed to be doing and where we need to be. It is very common for someone who has suffered a brain injury to be confused for a while afterwards. The length of time the person is confused is usually a good indicator of the severity of their brain injury.

Becoming orientated after a brain injury is important to aid recovery. It can be assessed by enquiring about the person's ability to learn new information, for example, where they are and what they have been doing recently, knowledge of their relationships and current events. Levels of orientation can be used to monitor a person's progress and guide rehabilitation.

Different aspects of orientation

There are different aspects of orientation as shown below in **figure 3**.

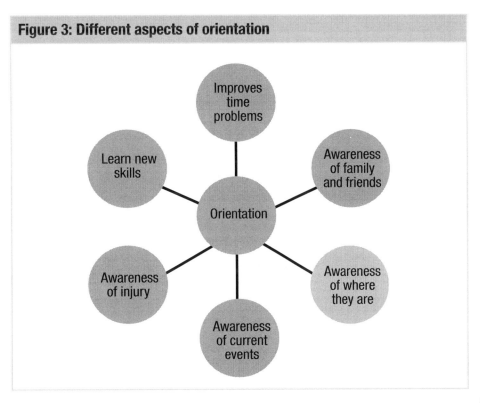

Figure 3: Different aspects of orientation

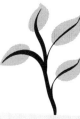

Time

Many people with brain injuries are often 'lost' in time. They are unaware of the current time (eg. whether it is morning/afternoon/evening) and date. When asked, they may guess a date from the past and not being orientated to time can affect the activities that they undertake – if they are confused they may get out of bed at 2am for a job that starts at 9am or turn up for an appointment several hours after it.

Current events

Another matter related to the issue of time is being aware of current events. For example, people may not realise who the current Prime Minister is or that well known public figures are no longer alive.

Past life

Some people with significant retrograde amnesia may not recognise or remember members of their family, friends or aspects of their past life.

Injuries

Some people are not aware of the extent to which they have been injured or damaged and some do not realise that they are injured at all. This can lead to much confusion and may lead to an individual not seeing a need for rehabilitation services such as physiotherapy, occupational therapy and neuropsychology. This lack of awareness can make them very vulnerable as they do not compensate for the difficulties they have. For example, if they have difficulties with mobility they are more likely to fall over if they try to walk without support, and this could result in further avoidable injuries such as a broken hip.

Location

Some people with brain injuries are unaware of their current location and where they live. This can be a problem as some do not realise they are in hospital or may not realise the type of treatment that they should receive to help them reduce the consequences of their injuries. For example, one person who had moved to a rehabilitation facility thought she was in the hospital that she was at previously and this resulted in her getting lost when she wandered around the ward, as rooms were in different locations on the new ward.

Orientation in a clinical context

If someone is struggling with orientation then it is very difficult for them to get the most out of their rehabilitation programme as they may not see the need for it. Therefore, initially trying to improve orientation may be essential in helping them to understand why they need and will benefit from the rehabilitation process. For an example of an orientation programme see **figure 4** below.

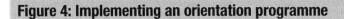

Figure 4: Implementing an orientation programme

To help orientate the person, focus on important personal details eg. your son Harry is coming to see you today.

↓

Also use important and often mentioned news events, especially ones the person may have been previously interested in eg. football scores.

↓

Use an errorless learning approach, which is presenting information in a way that the person is not likely to make a mistake (see page 73 for more information).

↓

After an allocated time, assess if the person has learnt the relevant information and whether the approach should be discontinued, or whether it should focus on helping the person learn other important information eg. an approaching appointment.

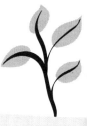

Case study 1

A middle-aged woman who had contracted meningitis suffered from problems with orientation. Her main problem was confusion and adjusting to the fact that it was now 2010 and not the 1980s. She believed that she was younger than she was and struggled to repeat the date even though she had just been reminded of it. She could, however, remember clearly that she had one daughter and she could remember her birth date accurately. The majority of the time she could remember why she was in hospital and where she was. When her daughter visited her she did not recognise her as she was not the right age.

Case study 2

A 55-year-old man who had suffered from a heart attack resulting in an anoxic brain injury (lack of oxygen to the brain) had severe problems with his orientation. The damage was so severe that he struggled to remember any time-related information such as the date and his age. He also struggled with remembering how many children he had and what their names were and was unable to recognise them when they came to visit. Even though he was severely impaired he had little understanding of his impairments, especially the fact that he could not walk unaided. Consequently he required constant supervision (ie. one-to-one care) to maintain his safety.

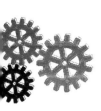

There are many methods that can be used to help orientate people and one way is the use of an orientation programme like in **figure 5** below.

Figure 5: Example of orientation programme

Orientation programme 25/11/2009

Aims: To help re-orientate Liam and to measure his new learning skills.

Method: Please read the enclosed passage twice daily with Liam and score as necessary.

Liam, you are presently in hospital after you suffered a heart attack. You can be confused at times. You are in Sussex hospital. Today is (day of week) Monday (day of month) 10th of November 2010. You were born on 18/03/1959, which makes you 50 years of age. You have two children, Carrie, who is 13 and Sian who is 11. The current prime minister is David Cameron. My name is Dr Jones, do not hesitate to contact me if you need anything.

Date	Answers	1/12/09	Date	Date
What is your full name?	Liam Smith	Liam Smith		
How old are you?	50	38		
What is the day today?	Monday	Don't know		
What is the date?	29th	Don't know		
What is the month?	November	August (hesitated)		

Attention and concentration

Introduction

When someone gives full attention they tend to 'block out' everything else going on around them – they are 'focused'. There are many things in our environment to which we pay little attention, for example, the feel of our clothes on our skin or the number of stairs on a staircase, but we can turn our attention to them if we choose to do so.

Attention can be thought of as the cognitive process of selectively concentrating on one aspect of the environment whilst ignoring others.

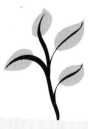

This requires a conscious effort to attend to a piece of information while ignoring many other stimuli. Sometimes a person with a brain disorder can have their attention abilities disrupted or damaged and they may find it difficult to concentrate or remain focused, or to cut out distractions especially in busy environments or situations.

It is important to understand that many everyday tasks can be difficult when attention and concentration abilities are compromised, especially as attention abilities are linked closely with other cognitive processes such as the ability to learn new information.

Types of attention

The 'hierarchy of attention'

The psychologists Sohlberg and Mater (1989) suggested a 'hierarchy of attention' model, which outlines five types of attention of increasing complexity that are used in everyday functioning. Each level is associated with different tasks (as shown below in **figure 6**).

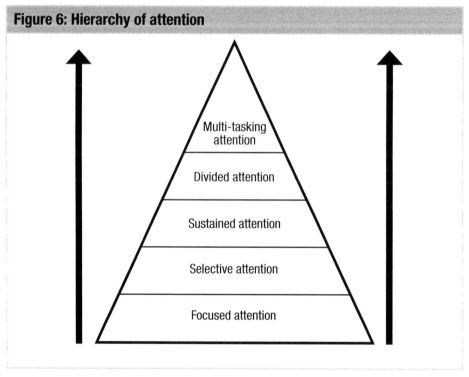

Figure 6: Hierarchy of attention

Multi-tasking attention

Divided attention

Sustained attention

Selective attention

Focused attention

Focused attention

Focused attention is the ability for someone to focus their awareness on a particular task when there are no other distractions, for example, looking at a personal photograph of a holiday in a quiet room for a few seconds. This is the first level on the hierarchy and is also the least complex.

Selective attention

Selective attention is the process of filtering stimuli in your internal and external environment and focusing on a specific one. This allows someone to focus on one stimulus whilst blocking out other distractions, for example, talking to a friend in a pub. This occurs regularly in our everyday lives as there are constantly multiple stimuli causing many distractions, for example, reading the newspaper without being distracted by someone else's conversation.

Sustained attention

Sustained attention is more complex when compared to selective attention as it involves being continually focused on one task for an extended period of time, for example, reading a short story without being distracted by other stimuli.

Divided attention

Divided attention involves being able to focus on two things simultaneously, for example, opening the door whilst on the telephone.

Multi-tasking

Multi-tasking is the most complex level of the 'hierarchy of attention' as it involves being able to respond to multiple tasks or demands simultaneously, for example, cooking a roast dinner whilst doing the washing up and talking to family members.

What can affect levels of attention?

Now that the different types of attention have been broken down it is important to look at some of the things that can affect attention and at some suggestions for how attention skills can be improved.

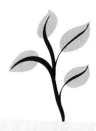

Variation in ability

The ability to attend to a task varies throughout the day. Most people state that their attention is at its best during the morning, with increasing tiredness during the day and consequently some people feel less able to concentrate in the afternoon. In order to help someone with attention difficulties it is important to try to assess when they are at their most attentive and plan activities accordingly. If they are a 'morning person' then more complex jobs should be completed in the morning with easier, less complex jobs left for the afternoon. Some are able to complete many tasks in a big chunk whereas others may need to break down tasks into smaller chunks to be able to complete them. This ability varies from person to person.

Time

A lot of research has looked at how long people are able to concentrate on a task, finding that most people concentrate well for about 15–25 minutes (see **figure 7**). After 30 minutes, research on students in lectures found that they either ceased to take in any new information or they forgot what they had memorised earlier. This is why structuring the day to get the most out of someone's abilities and skills, and pacing activities, ensuring frequent breaks, is important.

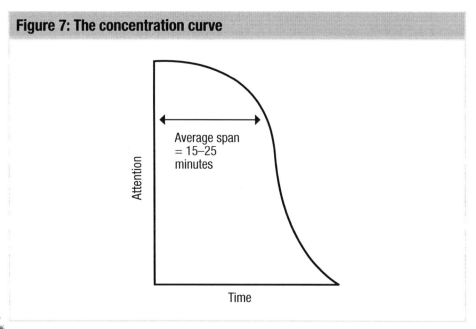

Figure 7: The concentration curve

Average span = 15–25 minutes

Attention

Time

(Taken from Blight, 1998)

Learning style

Research has also looked at the best ways in which people absorb and hold on to information. One way suggested is to vary the format of how information is presented and learned. Researchers who compared television news to radio news found that people recalled more from television, which was attributed to the addition of the visual stimulus that television allows. What this means is that, especially in boring tasks, varying the information format improves learning. Therefore, reading pages of text may be less effective than reading and using visual aids. Others find that hearing information helps them attend better so reading aloud may be a good way to hold on to information.

Environment

The environment can potentially have positive or detrimental effects on people's ability to attend to a particular task. Research has shown that noisy environments can cause a significant decrease in attention abilities, and most prominently in tasks that require people to split their attention across several tasks. Another factor that has been linked to task performance is the temperature of the environment. Whilst research in this area is not extensive it has been shown that for some, more complex tasks and an environment that is either too hot or too cold can adversely impact on ability to attend to a task – so it's important to ensure that environment is as comfortable as possible.

Sleep

A good night's sleep is vital in maintaining attention. Research shows that not only does it have health benefits and reduces stress, but not getting enough sleep has quite a negative effect on a person's ability to attend and react quickly on a task (also see chapter 6). Reduced sleep can lead to a higher number of lapses in attention, which occur for longer periods of time. It is important, therefore, to ensure plenty of sleep, especially the night before a day filled with lots of jobs that need to be achieved.

Motivation

Motivation can be described as the incentive to work towards achieving a desired goal. Motivation can be further sub-divided into two types, intrinsic and extrinsic. Intrinsic motivation comes from internal factors such as the rewards of doing well at a task and achieving a certain

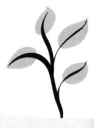

level of performance. This is the feeling of achievement after solving a tricky puzzle, or completing a particularly hard piece of work. To be well motivated, it is important that it is understood that the results are directly related to the amount of effort put in rather than being determined by luck. Therefore, rehabilitation tasks and goals need to be meaningful to each individual person if motivation is to be monitored. One motivation can be the reward of becoming more cognitively able and overcoming limitations. Extrinsic motivation is that which comes from outside the person and this involves receiving rewards for performance achieved on a specific task, for example, being paid depending on how many items you have made.

Helping with concentration: five golden rules, or 'FOCUS'

Fiercely pace yourself – Structure/plan your time; take frequent breaks, alternate between physical and mental tasks.

Only do tasks for up to a period of 20 minutes (or whatever is best for each person) then take a short break.

Caution arousal or raised alertness helps to focus attention whereas general anxiety reduces the ability to concentrate and retain information.

Unusual events that have a distinct meaning can help a person keep motivated and sustain concentration. When completing boring and repetitive activities it can be more difficult to keep focus.

Survey when you feel more alert during the day and use this knowledge to plan when to complete tasks that require more sustained concentration.

Putting FOCUS into practice
F – Make a list of what needs to be completed in the time available and devise a timetable. Use your day more efficiently by getting enough sleep and waking up early.
O – Work in 20 minute blocks with breaks in between to allow the person to re-energise their attention skills.
C – Make sure the person does not become too stressed. Encourage them to use relaxation techniques when needed, however, people need to be slightly aroused to keep focus on the tasks required.

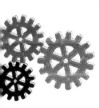

U – Ensure work is varied and interesting, for example, when studying change topic and revision method frequently.

S – Complete the most difficult and demanding tasks at the time of day when their concentration skills are at its best such as in the morning.

Problems with attention and how to improve it

Many problems can occur following a brain injury and attention difficulties are one of the more commonly reported problems. Different problems can affect each of the five different levels of attention.

Focused attention

Individuals who have problems with their focused attention skills are usually in a severely cognitively impaired state. They usually have large periods where they are inactive and unresponsive to their environments, which may be referred to as being in a 'vegetative' state. They are inactive because they fail to have the ability to respond to basic stimuli (touch, smell, taste) ie. flinch in response to pain, blink in response to an object coming towards them or respond to an unpleasant smell.

Selective attention

Individuals who have problems affecting selective attention tend to get easily distracted by stimuli around them. They find it difficult to attend to a stimulus whilst ignoring distractions, for example, trying to hold a conversation whilst the television is on in the background as the television noise may interfere with their attention abilities. They tend to have poor concentration and may frequently divert their attention onto something apart from the task in hand. When working with people with poor selective attention it is important to make sure they are free from as many distractions as possible and that work sessions are kept short.

Sustained attention

Individuals who have problems with sustained attention have the ability to select what they want to focus their attention on, but do not have the ability to keep their attention on that task for long periods of time. They tend to drift away because they cannot maintain their train of thought, for example, reading a newspaper article or focusing on one topic of

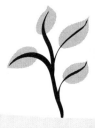

conversation. Forgetfulness is often associated with problems of sustained attention because individuals find it difficult to retain information long enough for it to be encoded and stored. These individuals need clear, precise and simple instructions that are easy to follow. Short sessions and varying tasks are required to help maintain their interest.

Divided attention

Individuals who have problems with divided attention find it hard to switch their attention between two tasks so can only concentrate on one thing at a time. If they are attending to one task (eg. cooking) and another stimulus (eg. the telephone ringing) attracts their focus then they may forget the original stimuli, which can be very dangerous and frustrating for them.

People with such difficulties need to be supported in focusing on one task at a time and doing one thing well before moving onto another task. They may need guidance in sequencing tasks and often need others to be around to do the things they cannot do.

Multi-tasking

Individuals who have problems with multi-tasking find it difficult to switch their focus between many different stimuli whilst completing them at the same time. As it is the most complex level of attention it is usually one of the main problems that those who have suffered a brain injury experience. They may find it difficult to cook, watch the children and prepare a shopping list all at the same time. It can also apply to an activity such as driving a car which requires attention on the road and surroundings simultaneously.

Memory

Introduction

Memory is not a single entity; rather it is a process that allows for the encoding, manipulation, storage and retrieval of information. It is the mental process involved in acquiring, organising and using knowledge and information of any type. Atkinson and Shiffrin (1968) devised a model to explain this and they suggested memory has three main stages as shown in **figure 8**.

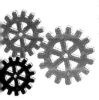

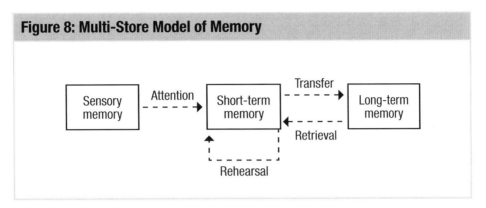

Figure 8: Multi-Store Model of Memory

(Taken from Atkinson & Shiffrin, 1968)

Sensory memory

Sensory memory is the information we get from our environment through our sensory organs, which are our ears (hearing), eyes (vision), tongue (taste), finger tips (touch) and nose (smell) (see chapter 2) and each sense has its own separate store. It has a large capacity but is of a short duration and the information is not really processed here but is held until the brain decides whether to attend to it and transfer it into our short-term memory (STM) or lose it.

Short-term memory

There is some debate about how to define STM, but it has a shorter duration than most people think, at most about 20–30 seconds and has a capacity to hold about seven items or chunks of information, for example, a telephone number. The encoding of STM is mainly visual (things we see) and acoustic (things we hear).

Long-term memory

Long-term memory is different from STM as it has a potential to be infinite in capacity and duration. Its encoding is semantic in that things are stored using meaning and understanding and how they are linked with other existing memories.

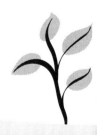

Types of memory

Although there are many ways information can be transferred to a person's long-term memory, it can be broken down into two major sub-divisions; implicit and explicit. These can be further broken down into specific types of memories such as episodic, semantic and procedural as shown in **figure 9** and **figure 10**.

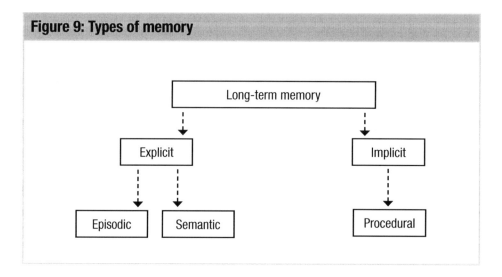

Figure 9: Types of memory

Long-term explicit

Explicit memory means that a conscious effort is required to recollect factual experiences and information. We use explicit memory throughout the day when remembering a doctor's appointment or naming animals that live in the desert. It is explicit memory that people think of when they say they have a 'good' or 'bad' memory because it involves the process of consciously thinking of something. Explicit memory allows us to link memories together, for example, thinking of a holiday can bring back a host of associated memories that are linked together.

Long-term implicit

Implicit memory is different to explicit memory as it does not require conscious effort; rather tasks or skills can be carried out with the aid of previous experiences without having to think about it and these memories are somewhat automatic. Implicit memory allows us to brush our hair or ride a bike without consciously thinking about these activities.

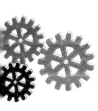

Figure 10: Types of learning

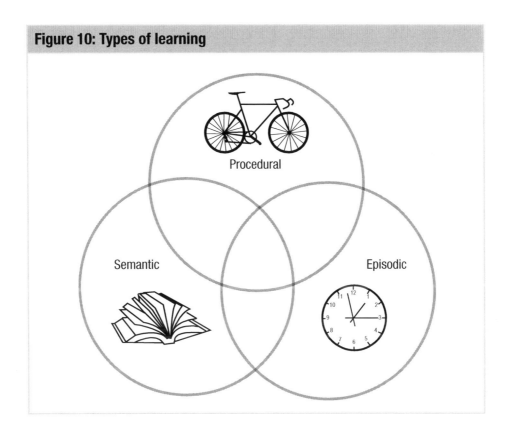

Episodic memory

Episodic memory represents our memory of personal events in time or 'episodes' in our lives. It allows us to reconstruct the personal experiences that occur in people's lives. It is episodic memory that allows us to remember a trip abroad, what we ate for dinner last night or winning an important sports game. Any past event in which we played a part and remember as a scene can be stored as an episodic memory.

Semantic memory

Semantic memory is sometimes referred to as our 'textbook' or general knowledge about the world. It is a structured record of facts and concepts that we have acquired through meaning. It is what enables us to say, without knowing exactly when and where we learned it, what a bike is, that a fish has scales or that London is the capital of England.

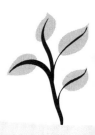

Procedural memory

Procedural memory can be referred to as our 'how to' memory that is the knowledge that enables us to carry out commonly learned tasks without thinking about them. It allows us to put our memories into action, for example, how to ride a bike or how to write a letter. Even 'natural' tasks such as walking require procedural memory. As procedural memory uses a different part of the brain to episodic memory, after a brain injury it is possible to lose the ability to remember past events but still remember how to park a car, ride a bike or use a fork. We take these skills for granted but following a brain injury these automatic skills can be affected so previous tasks can become very difficult and effortful.

Types of memory problems

Memory difficulties can occur in any of the areas described above. Another important distinction to make is whether someone who has had a brain injury has difficulties with remembering 'new' information – that is information received after their injury – or 'old' information, which is information received before their injury. The former is referred to as 'anterograde' amnesia, for example, difficulties in remembering what the person had for breakfast or who told them what yesterday, while the latter is referred to as 'retrograde' amnesia. Anterograde episodic memory is most important in allowing each of us to function on a day-to-day basis and difficulties in this area can mean that someone will need a great deal of support and can make them very dependent on others.

Some people can have extensive retrograde memory problems and have lost important memories from several years of their lives before their injury. For example, they may not remember the death of a loved one, starting a relationship or getting married. Therefore, some people with brain injuries can sometimes forget that they have partners or children; depending on how badly their retrograde memory has been affected. Sometimes they can remember close relations but they may not be able to recognise them as they feel they have aged or changed in appearance.

For example, one woman who had a 16-year-old son could remember his name, but when she saw him she did not recognise him as she only remembered him as a five year old.

Another patient was asked what the current year was; he believed it was 1989 when it was actually 2010 and he thought his daughter was nine when she was actually 29.

Errorless learning

We know that people who have memory difficulties after a brain injury may find it more difficult to learn new information. Evidence shows that people with memory difficulties may not benefit from trial and error learning because they may not remember their mistakes. However, helping them learn new information and skills without making mistakes, in so far as possible, can be important in helping them learn more accurately (Wilson *et al*, 1994). Indeed getting something wrong spontaneously, even if corrected immediately, such as is the case in 'trial and error' learning, may mean a person with compromised memory abilities will be more likely to retain the wrong information.

Take, for example, trying to teach someone who has difficulty learning that their physiotherapist is called Catherine. A trial and error approach might involve the physiotherapist saying to the person, '*The last time we met I told you my name. Can you tell me what it is?*' If the person is not able to remember they may be encouraged to guess.

An errorless learning approach on the other hand might involve the physiotherapist saying something like, '*The last time we met I told you my name. I would like you to try and remember it but if you are in any way unsure about what my name is, please do not say anything because I will tell you again*'. If the person cannot remember the therapist might say, '*My name is Catherine. Could you repeat it please?*' They might do this a few times until the person indicates that they are able to repeat it correctly. On the next occasion they meet the therapist might say, '*I would like you to tell me my name but if you cannot remember it I do not want you to guess. I will give you a clue*'. If the person cannot remember them the therapist might say. '*It begins with "Cather", can you remember?*' If the person cannot remember the therapist tells them her name immediately before they guess. If the person gets it right then on future meetings the therapist continues with ever decreasing clues, for example using 'Cath' and then, 'It begins with a C', until the person is able to say the therapist's name correctly without cues.

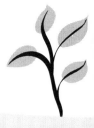

Language

What is language?

Language is a process by which symbolic information is used to communicate between two or more people. Even animals have systems of communication between each other but humans have by far the most complex communication system. Language can take many forms including written, spoken and gestural, such as sign language.

There are many stages involved in understanding and using language and disruption to any one part of this process can cause significant communication difficulties. There are a variety of common causes of language difficulties, such as traumatic or acquired brain injury, autism, cerebral palsy, cleft palate, dyslexia, head and neck cancer, learning disability, mental health problems, progressive neurological disorders (eg. multiple sclerosis, Parkinson's disease), stammering and voice disorders. There are two main areas where difficulties can occur as follows.

Motor difficulties

Difficulties with language may be related to problems in the making of sounds to produce verbal language due to poor motor co-ordination and control (that is, the 'mechanical' aspects of language); this can be caused by damage to the brain stem. Patients often recover these abilities, although some individuals may be left with long-term difficulties.

These disorders involve the following.

▶ **Apraxia** – not being able to make the appropriate mouth movements.

▶ **Dysarthria/dyspraxia** – difficulties with muscles that control speech including slowness, weakness and lack of co-ordination that prevent the individual from forming words. People can also have difficulty controlling the pace and volume of speech production and their speech may be slurred and monotonous; it can also affect writing and gesturing.

▶ **Dysphagia** – problem with swallowing and for example may choke when eating.

▶ **Dysphonia** – the muscles of the voice box are affected making it hard to make speech sounds.

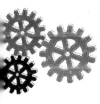

Cognitive difficulties

'Aphasia' (total loss) and 'dysphasia' (partial loss) refer to problems with the use of language. There are several broad types of problems including the following.

▶ **Receptive dysphasia** – the inability to understand language when individuals may not be able to make sense of what is said to them even when hearing and thought processes are normal.

▶ **Expressive dysphasia** – the inability to produce speech when individuals struggle to find the right words, have shortened sentences or a complete loss of speech.

▶ **Global dysphasia** – is the reduced understanding of speech (receptive aphasia) and cannot produce speech or read or write (expressive aphasia).

▶ **Nominal dysphasia** – is the difficulty in naming objects appropriately even though they are recognised.

Specific areas of the brain control specific skills and with most people, language is controlled by the left hemisphere of the brain. For example, Broca's area (between the frontal and temporal lobes) is involved in producing speech, and damage to this area can result in expressive dysphasia. Wernicke's area (further back between temporal and parietal lobes as shown in **figure 1**) is involved in understanding the speech of others and damage to this area results in receptive dysphasia (see also chapter 2).

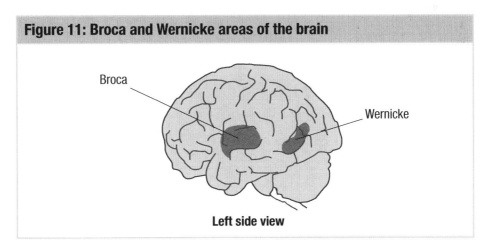

Figure 11: Broca and Wernicke areas of the brain

Broca

Wernicke

Left side view

Expressive language problems can occur with spoken and written language and receptive language problems can occur with verbal understanding and reading.

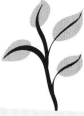

Prevalence of language problems in acquired brain injury

Language is disturbed in 75% of cases after brain injury (McKinlay *et al*, 1981) but estimates of actual dysphasia range from 2–32%. This is because language difficulties after brain injury are often due to general memory and other cognitive deficits rather than true dysphasia, although the problems often have a similar presentation. This should be taken into account during treatment as often treatment for people with dysphasia assumes the presence of memory, cognitive and communication problems.

Individuals of any age can experience communication problems but it is more difficult to identify the causes in children. This is because children's language skills are still developing, whereas in adults we can compare an individual's current ability to their ability before injury. In children it may be noticed that their language skills are not developing as expected and there's a delayed development. It is thought that six in 100 children have some form of language difficulty, and that one in 500 children will experience this in the long term.

Case study 3

Peter was a 44-year-old man who suffered a closed brain injury after falling down the stairs at his workplace. After rehabilitation he recovered quite well, however he was left with fairly severe language difficulties, particularly in finding the right words to express himself and pronouncing words.

Once Peter returned home he realised the extent of his difficulties as he found it almost impossible to complete daily tasks such as shopping, making a phone call, reading, following a film and joining in conversations. He found this extremely frustrating as before the accident he had been a very sociable and independent person. He became distant from many of his close friends and relationships with his wife and children became strained as he could never seem to find the right words to speak to them. He describes the experience as being 'locked inside my own head'.

He was unable to return to his previous job due to the language difficulties and consequently worried about the family's financial security. This caused Peter to become stressed, which in turn made his language difficulties worse. After seeing a speech and language therapist he was diagnosed with global aphasia and received information about support groups and coping strategies to help improve the communication within his family and integrate him back into the community.

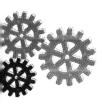

Perception

What is perception?

Perception is the process of obtaining information about our environment through our senses, which can include sight, hearing, smell, taste and touch. Our perception is determined by how our brain tries to make sense and organise the information we receive, rather than what our sense organs, which are the eyes, ears, skin, tongue and nose actually experience. Therefore, perceptual problems usually occur due to brain injuries to the sensory cortex, which is predominantly located within the parietal and occipital lobes (see **figure 12** below). These areas process and interpret information from our senses.

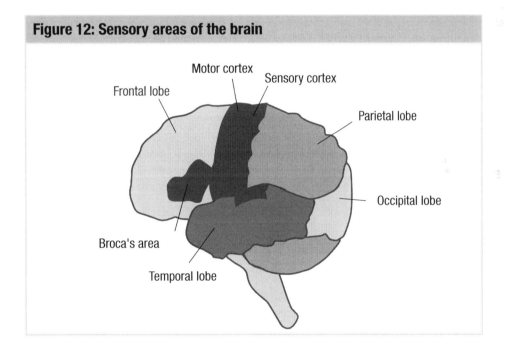

Figure 12: Sensory areas of the brain

There are five main parts of the sensory cortex:

▶ visual cortex (sight)

▶ auditory cortex (hearing)

▶ somatosensory cortex (touch)

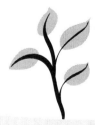

▶ olfactory cortex (smell)

▶ gustatory cortex (taste)

The perceptual problems a person experiences will depend on which area or areas of the sensory cortex are damaged. The recovery of the sensory cortex will depend on the extent and severity of damage. If the sensory cortex has been bruised then there will often be a gradual improvement over time. However, if the cells in this area are killed, this area is unlikely to return to being fully functional.

Vision

Sense organ: eyes

Area of brain: occipital lobes

The occipital lobes contains both a left and right side (in each hemisphere), so if only one of these hemispheres is damaged then only part of vision/ visual field may be affected. An example of this is when the left hemisphere is damaged patients may experience difficulties with their right visual field.

Hearing difficulties

Sense organ: ears

Area of brain: temporal lobes

The temporal lobes are responsible for the basic processing of sound and hearing.

Sensation

Sense organ: skin, skeletal muscles, joints, internal organs and cardiovascular system

Area of brain: somatosensory system in the parietal lobes

The somatosensory system processes a variety of mechanisms including touch, temperature sensation, body position and pain.

Smell

Sense organ: the nose

Area of brain: entorhinal and pyriform cortexes

Loss of smell usually occurs in cases of facial injury or any injury that leads to damage of the olfactory nerves and tracts located in the upper parts of the nose that run underneath the frontal lobes. It may also occur due

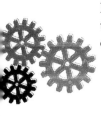

to damage to the parts of the brain that process olfactory information, in which case recovery of smell is unlikely.

Loss of taste

Sense organ: upper surface of tongue and other areas within the mouth and upper throat
Area of brain: temporal lobes
The tongue is used to detect tastes such as sweetness and bitterness. The sensation of smell and taste are intimately connected and taste largely depends on smell. The latter is much more sensitive and has the ability to detect subtle flavours and therefore, loss of smell and taste often occur together. After severe head injury 20% of people permanently lose their sense of smell (Daisley *et al*, 2008).

Type of symptoms arising to sensory damage

Table 1: Types of symptoms that can occur with damage to different sensory systems	
Sense	**Symptoms**
Visual difficulties	Problems judging distances and having blurred or double vision. Severe damage can cause blindness. If one side of the visual field is damaged then this results in the patient neglecting that side and for example bumping into door frames or only eating half their dinner
Hearing difficulties	Not comprehending what people say or misunderstanding what people say
Loss of touch sensation	Finding it difficult to pick up sensation and finding it difficult to grasp an object picking up sensation, and very hard to grasp an object (may grasp too hard/soft). This can include having issues in the perception of temperature (feeling too hot/too cold).
Loss of taste and smell	Appreciation of subtle tastes is often impaired, which can lead to a reduction in appetite and appreciation of food. Physical problems involving saliva production may also appear, leading to difficulty in eating food. Depression may also result as enjoyment of food is removed.

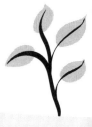

Case study 4

Harry was a 25-year-old male who was involved in a road traffic accident and suffered a moderate brain injury including problems with his vision. He was admitted to hospital and later transferred to a rehabilitation hospital where he stayed for four weeks.

Although he had recovered most of his physical and mental abilities he was left with some residual symptoms. The hospital staff noticed that Harry would often only eat the food on one side of his plate or would shave only one side of his face. He lost pleasure in reading, had problems in judging distances and often missed objects when he reached out to pick them up. He was found to have a hemiopia: a large hole in his visual field, and therefore he could not see things in the right side of his visual field.

Executive functions

Introduction

Executive functions are the most complex part of the brain's activities and are primarily but not exclusively associated with the frontal lobes. The cortex and underlying white matter of the frontal lobes is the site of the richest inter-connections and feedback loops between the major sensory and motor systems, linking and integrating all components of behaviour at the highest level. Thus they are very important in making sense and interpreting external and internal information at a conscious and unconscious level. They are the centre of our personality (see also chapters 2 and 4).

Damage to the frontal lobes is common after acceleration followed by deceleration events such as in road traffic accidents. Damage is more likely in this area as the skull is not smooth under the frontal lobes and the abrupt cessation of motion causes the brain to impact against the inside of the skull. This is very likely to send shockwaves through the front part of the brain (see also chapter 5).

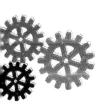

Figure 13: Location of the frontal lobes

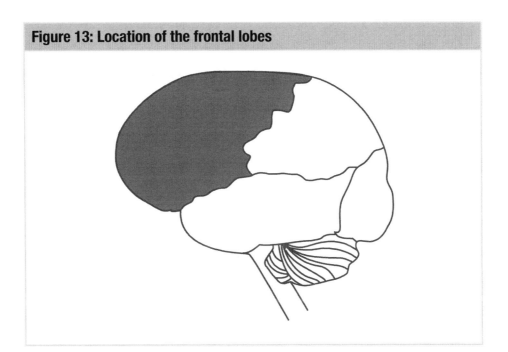

One of the most famous examples of frontal lobe damage is the Phineas Gage case study in 1848. Gage was a railway construction worker who had an accident involving an iron bar which was forced through his head piercing his frontal lobes. Physically his health was fine as the frontal lobes are not essential in maintaining life, however, his behaviour and personality radically changed. He became angry and started swearing and getting into fights regularly, especially when he was stopped from doing the things he wanted to do. This change in his behaviour has been documented with a famous quote: '*In this regard, his mind was radically changed, so decidedly that his friends said he was no longer Gage.*' (Cited in Damasio *et al*, 1994)

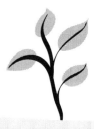

There are a number of important executive skills and some of these include the following.

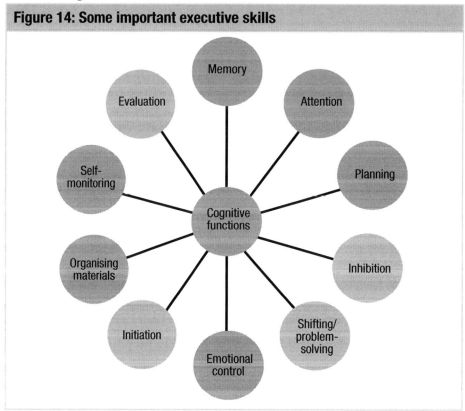

Figure 14: Some important executive skills

▶ **Initiation** – being able to start an activity without being prompted by anyone else.

▶ **Planning** – being able to break down a final goal into smaller steps, which can be achieved more easily, and then being able to follow those steps until the task is completed. This also involves being able to 'see' what is important and what is not and being able to put all this together as part of a plan.

▶ **Prospective memory** – this involves memory for future events and planning them in a time-related order.

▶ **Attention** – multi-tasking, attending to and being able to manage multiple things at any one time and taking account of ongoing changes in the situations and changing focus as needed.

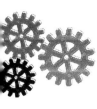

- ▶ **Organisation skills** – the ability to structure tasks and arrange items in order to achieve a goal.

- ▶ **Emotional control** – the ability to regulate emotions appropriately to the context or situation, for example, a person with frontal lobe damage may laugh inappropriately at a sad event, for example at a funeral.

- ▶ **Insight** – being able to realise and understand one's own strengths and limitations; also, to be able to adapt plans taking personal abilities or difficulties into account.

- ▶ **Self-monitoring** – being able to change performance in real time; self-correct mistakes and ask for help when needed.

- ▶ **Shifting and problem-solving** – being able to adapt to errors and setbacks to plans; then working out alternative solutions and being able to shift resources in implementing a new plan or a change of strategy.

- ▶ **Inhibition** – having the ability to block expressing thoughts and behaviours that may cause disruption or offence to others.

- ▶ **Evaluation** – once an activity has been completed, being able to look at the outcome, weigh up the positives and negatives and adapt future plans taking into account these outcomes and possibly achieving the same task more effectively.

- ▶ **Control of impulsiveness** – to inhibit acting on the spur of the moment without thinking through the consequences.

- ▶ **Abstract reasoning** – the ability to think creatively or beyond the current, concrete situation.

- ▶ **Moral reasoning** – this lets us weigh up the pros and cons of situations to make an ethical decision.

Supervisory attentional system

The supervisory attentional system (SAS) is a model proposed by Norman and Shallice (1986) to explain the cognitive processes used in controlling the actions people undertake. For example, in order to wash clothes in a washing machine, the steps need to be completed in a specific order, ie. collect the washing, sort it into colours, load the machine, add powder and conditioner, turn to the required setting and then turn on. If these are completed in the wrong order, multiple colours and fabrics could be washed

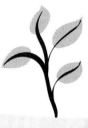

together with no powder or on the wrong setting, which could be disastrous. This model is shown in **figure 15** below.

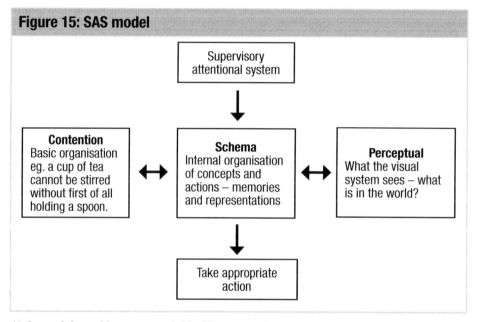

Figure 15: SAS model

(Adapted from Norman and Shallice, 1986)

The model suggests that when someone sees an object such as a washing machine they immediately begin to activate what are known as 'schemas'. These are our individual representations of the world and the objects in it. If we are asked to think of a 'typical dog' for example, there are certain characteristics which we always associate with dogs, such as four legs, fur and wagging tails; this is the schema 'dog'.

When we think of a particular object then related objects are also activated or associated alongside it. The schema 'doctor' may also activate 'nurse', 'hospital' and other medical items – it is like a web in which the objects connect together. In the example of washing clothes, when the person sees the washing machine, schemas relating to all aspects of using a washing machine become activated and compete for the person's attention. All unsuitable schemas have to be stopped to make sure the focus is on one schema at a time.

The model claims that this is not the only process which influences behaviour. There is also 'contention scheduling' where certain actions automatically stop others as part of the process. For example, a person can't put clothes in the washing machine without already picking them up. In addition to this, Norman and Shallice (1986) also postulated that the 'perceptual system', which is what is seen in the environment, can influence the schema(s) which are activated. Taken together, these three processes allow for actions to be stopped and started at specific times and in a specific sequence in order to correctly complete tasks.

In the model, the supervisory attentional system is a higher level system which is able to control and override aspects of these three subsystems. In the case of the competing schema, it tells the person to load the dirty washing into the machine before closing the door, loading the drawer or adjusting the dials to set the programmes. It is also able to inhibit the automatic process of contention scheduling. Rather than loading all the washing at once, if someone is doing a dark wash it allows them to stop and separate the clothes into different sorts.

Damage to the frontal lobes disrupts the SAS which is why, according to this model, those with frontal lobe damage often have a hard time structuring events and putting plans into a coherent order.

Factors affecting executive functioning

Environment
The environment in which a person works can have serious implications for their ability to plan and organise tasks. Noisy environments can decrease attentional abilities, which may mean that they may find it harder to concentrate. This in turn may result in them failing to identify problems and shortfalls which could affect how successful their plan turns out to be. Visual noise, in the form of a crowded environment, can also drain attention resources.

Timing and planning
It is important to spend an appropriate amount of time planning a task otherwise important information may be missed and there could be failure in properly accounting for factors which may limit the success of a plan. When thinking about this, it is a good idea to imagine what it's like trying to find car keys when late for work, compared to when there is time to

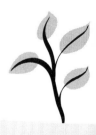

spare. When trying to find something quickly important details are often missed and therefore the keys are not found. It is important to take time when planning activities and remember the five Ps: Planning and prevention prevents poor performance.

Ways of improving and managing executive skills

▶ **Time:** Do not rush into tasks; first take a few moments to think and plan.

▶ **Tasks:** Set clear goals and the order in which they need to be completed to achieve best results. Identify the main areas and remain focused on these, not on tasks which are not needed to reach the final outcome.

▶ **Attention:** Remove distractions. Make sure the environment is clear. Make sure the most difficult tasks are being completed at the time of day when most attentive. Remember to take breaks and rest.

▶ **Evaluation:** Make sure to review and evaluate the progress and make changes as needed to complete the task. At the end look back over the task and think about what should be changed next time the same task comes up.

There are many tasks that people undertake daily without applying much thought, such as making a cup of tea, but following an acquired brain injury it is possible for a person's skills and abilities to change for a variety of reasons. The person may be unable to sequence tasks and for example may be unable to put parts of a task in the right order, or they may become more impulsive, for example, the person starts doing the task before they have the ingredients ready. **Figure 16** shows how a person can take the steps to problem solve using the example of making a cup of tea.

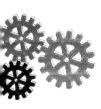

Figure 16: Steps involved in problem-solving

Identifying what the problem is ensures only the problem in hand is the focus of a person's attention.

I would like a cup of tea

Go through the different components and solutions, and work out the stages required to complete the task.

Identify the tasks involved in making a cup of tea, eg. putting water in the kettle, getting a tea bag, etc.

Choose the best plan and identify the steps to reach the final solution. There may be many different approaches to tackling the problem so to stay focused the best plan is needed, the stages identified need to be organised into a systematic order.

Put the stages into the correct order, so first put water in the kettle, then boil the water, then get a mug, then put a tea bag in the mug etc.

Carry out the plan.

Start to make the cup of tea.

Assess your progress and if required adjust the plan. While completing the plan keep evaluating how it is going as situations can change and the original plan may require adjusting to reach the desired outcome.

After the water is poured into the cup, it is noticed there is not enough water so you have to boil more water to make the required amount of tea.

Evaluate: was the plan a success? Look at both the positives and negatives so the plan can be adjusted for when it is next required.

Next time put more water into the kettle for the right amount of tea.

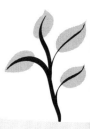

Take away message

The brain is the most sophisticated and complex part of the human body and damage to the brain can cause a wide range of difficulties and problems which may have a significant impact in a person's day-to-day life and the lives of close relatives. Areas of cognitive function such as attention, memory, language, perception and executive function are vulnerable to brain injuries. Cognitive difficulties can cause some of the most disruptive and long-term consequences of brain injuries. Understanding cognitive functions, what can go wrong with them and how people with cognitive difficulties can be supported is very important.

Quiz

1. What is orientation?
2. Name and describe two areas of impairment that can benefit from conducting an orientation programme?
3. What is the difference between selective and sustained attention?
4. What is divided attention?
5. What does the hierarchy of complexity show?
6. What are the three main stages of memory?
7. What are the three main types of memory?
8. What are the two main types of language difficulties?
9. What is perception?
10. What are the five main parts of the sensory cortex?
11. Where are the executive skills located in the brain?
12. What is the supervisory attentional system (SAS)?

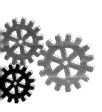

References

Atkinson R & Shiffrin R (1968) Human memory: a proposed system and its control processes. In: JT Spence & KW Spence (Eds) (1990) *The Psychology of Learning and Motivation* (Volume 2). London: Academic Press.

Blight D (1998) *What's the Use of Lectures?* San Francisco: The Jossey-Bass Higher Adult Education Series.

Daisley A, Tams R & Kischka U (2008) *Head injury: The facts*. Oxford: Oxford University Press.

Damasio H, Grabourski T, Randall F, Galaburda AM & Damasio AR (1994) The return of Phineas Gage: clues about the brain from the skull of a famous patient. *Science* **264** 1102–1105.

McKinlay W, Brooks DN, Bond MR, Martinage DP & Marshall MM (1981) The short term outcomes of severe blunt head injury as reported by relatives of the injured persons. *Journal of Neurology, Neurosurgery, and Psychiatry* **44** 527–533.

Norman DA & Shallice T (1986) Attention to action: willed and automatic control of behaviour. In: RJ Davidson, GE Schwartz & D Shapiro (Eds) (1986) *Conscious Control and Self Regulation (Volume 4)*. New York: Plenum Press.

Sohlberg MM & Mateer CA (1989) *Introduction to Cognitive Rehabilitation*. New York: Guilford Press.

Wilson B, Baddely A, Evans J & Shiel A (1994) Errorless learning in the rehabilitation of memory impaired people. *Neuropsychological Rehabilitation* **4** (3) 307–326.

Further reading

Powell T (2004) *Head Injury: A practical guide*. Milton Keynes: Speechmark.

Sterling J (2001) *Introducing Neuropsychology*. Hove: Psychology Press.

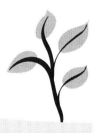

Chapter 4

Emotions: a brain-based perspective

Gerald Burgess

Aims of the chapter

This chapter should allow you to:

▶ identify the main brain structures that play a role in emotion

▶ recognise several social and emotional disability syndromes associated with brain damage or disease

▶ appreciate and understand the importance of emotions and emotional processing to successful everyday functioning.

Introduction

Emotions and the brain

Like motor movements or memories, emotions come from and are controlled within the brain. Additionally, like motor movements or memories, people's emotional functioning may become impaired when disease or damage encroaches upon certain areas of their brains, areas sometimes referred to as the 'emotional centres' (ie. primarily but not exclusively located in the limbic system and frontal lobes, with a supporting role from the brain stem).

Carrying this thought a bit further, disease or damage to areas of the brain that control motor movements may lead to disabilities such as being unable to walk or having tremors. Disease or damage to areas of the brain involved in memory and learning may cause people to forget what was said to them five minutes ago, to forget appointments, to misplace items, or errors of a similar nature.

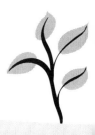

Disease or damage to areas of the brain that control emotion can also cause disabilities of a social and emotional nature. The causes of these disabilities can be much more elusive, harder to understand and explain, and this is because they are often entangled with a host of 'external' changes (eg. loss of job, relationship strain, isolation) that are extremely challenging. However, independent of this, social and emotional disability can be caused by a specific problem of the brain, and this occurs in many neurological conditions. What is usually clear in cases of emotional impairment is that family or friends who knew someone well before and after the onset of a neurological condition will say that person is changed, for example, their personality, their social behaviour or even their apparent level of maturity. Throughout this chapter case studies will be presented to illustrate some of the ways brain damage or disease may be directly responsible for social and emotional disabilities. These case studies are included so that you may begin to recognise some of the signs when you see them. Here's the first case study to provide an overview of acquired emotional (and social) impairment.

Case study 1

A 54-year-old man who was a successful manager of a distribution company and a husband and father of three had a cardiac arrest and suffered a hypoxic brain injury. Oxygen was deprived to his brain for 15 minutes causing extensive damage to areas responsible for both memory and emotion. As he came out of his coma, it became clear that he was no longer the same person – he alternated between being passive and raging, and displayed paranoia. He could no longer effectively manage being in crowds, and got too easily irritated and misinterpreted the actions of others (often as hostile, though this wasn't actually intended by those he came into contact with). His previous ability to look after his children, including one with a disability, was no longer possible. In fact, he acted like a child himself, asking his wife's permission to eat, drink, or go to the bathroom with interspersed moments of rage because he felt controlled and dictated to. He was not able to understand the feelings of others and lacked empathy, which was a devastating change from his previous self. He would treat his wife of 26 years with disdain and showed no evidence of appreciation for the care she provided or for her losses and sacrifices. When asked how he felt, his emotional range was limited to feeling paranoid-related fear (that someone meant to harm him) anger, or apathy. His motivation to do anything, other than eat, drink or use the toilet was limited but he often stared blankly at daytime television. If carers or his wife suggested that he go into the garden like he used to instead of watching television, he would go into a rage, screaming to leave him alone.

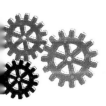

Two aspects of emotion

In order to begin to appreciate and understand the importance of emotions for successful everyday functioning, we will now look at two aspects of emotions that could (and often do to some degree) become impaired when disease or damage encroaches upon the 'emotional centres' of the brain. These include the internal, subjective experience of 1. emotions/feeling states, and the externalised emotional actions, otherwise known as 2. emotional behaviours. Let's look at each of these in turn:

1. Emotions/feeling states

There are six universal emotions or feeling states that human beings worldwide are 'hard-wired' (in the mind) to experience and to recognise in others. These include a) happiness, b) anger, c) surprise, d) fear, e) sadness and f) disgust. When we experience these feelings, there are corresponding chemical releases into the blood stream and neural (brain) circuits, fine and gross muscle movements resulting in facial expressions and other nonverbal cues, and often characteristic thoughts or actions that accompany the particular emotion. **Figure 1** shows a few facial expressions and descriptions for each of the six primary feeling states.

Figure 1: Nine facial expressions

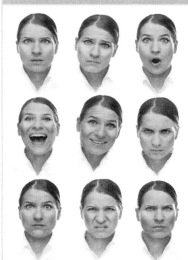

Happiness = joy, ecstatic, amused or content

Anger = rage, indignant, irritated or frustrated

Surprise = pleasantly or unpleasantly surprised

Fear = terrified, scared, worried or anxious

Sadness = sorrow, regret, grief or depressed

Disgust = dislike, distasteful, sick or put off

Can you find the faces that express the six primary emotions?

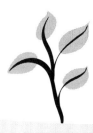

Imagine for a moment, just like that which may be a consequence of certain neurological conditions, what it would be like to have the ability to experience one or several of these feelings (or to notice these feelings in others) either diminished or exaggerated. Here are just a few examples on both sides of the coin.

Happiness

Without happiness life would be uninteresting, or just dull or sad. Hobbies or activities would be meaningless because you wouldn't have the capacity to enjoy them. You wouldn't be able to notice happiness in others, and therefore would fail to evaluate whether someone was satisfied or dissatisfied (with you). On the other hand, happiness in excess or extreme is possible as well in neurological conditions, in such cases taking the form of misplaced contentment (ie. denial of a very serious situation or disability), mania, or hedonism (ie. constantly seeking the fulfilment of pleasure at the expense of other activities or personal safety).

Anger

Without anger you could be taken advantage of and you wouldn't defend yourself or act appropriately when treated unjustly. You wouldn't know either how to 'read' anger in others, if you had done something to upset someone (and thus may not see reason to adjust your behaviour). Anyone who has worked with people with neurological conditions knows that unpleasant, if not downright destructive anger and irritation can be just below the surface at nearly all times, sometimes being expressed explosively and unpredictably.

Surprise

Without surprise every event in life would be experienced as the same, as routine, even perhaps as dull. A surprise gift or visit wouldn't elicit an appropriate corresponding reaction, such as excitement. Or events that should be noticed as unusual (such as toast burning) may not cause you to take sufficient and timely action to remedy the problem.

Fear

Without fear you would not know or be able to evaluate danger. Some fear is useful, as it provides the motivation to try to accomplish certain goals (because you need to survive) or to avoid failure or unpleasant consequences. On the other hand, in some neurological conditions, anxiety, fear, even paranoia are rife and often associated with decreased skills or confidence in social situations, or even an over-active perception of threat

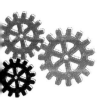

in the environment, meaning that they see the actions and behaviours of others as more dangerous or hostile than the person actually intended.

Sadness
Without sadness we would not appropriately appreciate and experience loss, or have compassion for someone else's grief. Too much sadness is an obvious problem though, leading to depression.

Disgust
Without disgust you wouldn't know what to avoid, or would not be sufficiently put off by something toxic (such as waste products, or even a bad relationship). Excessive experience of disgust, however, can lead to anxious avoidant symptoms or behaviours, such as obsessive compulsive-like rituals to avoid imagined toxic dangers in the environment.

Additional thought 1: E-Motion

Notice how closely emotions are linked to behaviours. It is as if emotion provides the motivation to take action in some way. People feel an emotion and they are either driven to do or to avoid something, based on how it feels. People might take a walk in the garden because it makes them feel happy, or they may avoid a certain person who makes them angry.

People are attracted to positive emotions in others (such as happiness or surprise) and repelled by negative emotions (such as rage). Being in the presence of someone else's laughter or rage can 'transfer' similar feelings to others, for example, consider being in a comedy club or the experience of 'road rage.' Fear or sadness in others may motivate people to want to reach out and help.

Emotions come or are experienced in a reaction to something, but they also possess a force to get people to act. The term 'E-Motion', meaning energy-in-motion is a useful way to think of emotion, as they motivate us to do things. They're like a creator of energy and thus cause us to be who we are and do what we do. Emotion is intrinsically linked with what is called, 'personality' so you might say, 'we are our emotions'. Just to put a finer point on it, there are attractive personalities and unattractive personalities, and people sense when they are in the presence of each. We are attracted to people who seem to know their own emotions and the emotions of others – it is truly an effective survival skill.

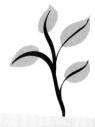

2. Emotional behaviours

Apart from feeling states, which are experienced internally and subjectively, emotional behaviours are the actions that are driven or come to be based on the feeling states. To some degree, all behaviours are driven (or powered) by emotion, just some more than others. Have a look at some examples of behaviours that are more or less powered by emotion:

Less emotional behaviours:	More emotional behaviours:
Opening a tin of soup	*Yelling at someone who cut you off*
Catching a bus	*Calling a friend whose mother just died*
Grocery shopping	*Tuning into a favourite television show*
Brushing your teeth	*Unwrapping a gift*
Taking a lift to the 3rd floor	*Avoiding a job interview*

The less emotional behaviours tend to occur as a matter of routine or need. They would not happen if not for necessity and people do not tend to feel overly emotional (either positively or negatively) about them. The more emotional behaviours on the other hand tend to be carried out because an emotional response drives it. Feeling anger might lead to an (unregulated) response of yelling. Sympathy may lead to calling a friend to offer condolences and so forth.

People with neurological conditions tend to either demonstrate excessively emotional behaviours for example, smashing plates, hitting or yelling or a diminished reaction such as failing to feel and act concerned in a traumatic situation, thus it may be said that their impaired emotional functioning has a direct negative impact on their behaviours and their personality. With this comes a host of 'social consequences', such as not being able to maintain a job or a relationship, finding oneself isolated, and so forth. A complete model then, to illustrate neurologically-based emotional impairments looks like:

Emotions/feeling states → emotional behaviours → social consequences

Keep this model in mind when reading about the brain structures that control emotion in the next section. What you'll find is that specific damage or disease to particular 'centres' in the brain lead to feelings and behaviours that (judge for yourself) can cause significant negative social consequences. This thought is expanded upon on the next page.

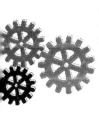

Additional thought 2: IQ vs. EQ

EQ, otherwise known as emotional intelligence, is a concept that has grown in understanding and favour in the last few decades. It used to be considered that IQ (abbreviation for 'intelligence quotient') was of significantly more importance than any other factor in 'success' (such as at school or in work). IQ is a score that represents a person's a) ability to learn and reason verbally and visuo-spatially, b) lifetime acquired knowledge, and c) ability to concentrate and work quickly. EQ has been noticed, however, as contributing equally (or more so) to success in life, such as getting and keeping jobs, maintaining relationships, being a person who is evaluated positively by others, and being happy. High EQ is a general ability that includes knowing and moderating what you feel, having empathy, recognising the feelings of others, using feelings to guide choices and judgments, being socially adept, and a long list of other attributes. Brain damage or disease can have a direct and negative impact on EQ as we'll see in the next section. In some people with neurological conditions, their IQ remains intact while their EQ is impaired, and their life may become a social disaster. Such people may achieve high scores on clinicians' tests of IQ, memory, and even what is broadly called 'executive functioning', but yet for some reason they are failing at life (ie. lost jobs, relationships, making unwise decisions) since the onset of their neurological condition or acquired brain injury.

Brain structures that play a role in emotion

The brain stem

The brain stem is like a power station supplying the higher (cortical) areas of the brain with the arousal that is needed to function at its optimum. Direct and severe damage or disease to the brain stem often causes coma or death because of its role in basic survival processes, such as breathing and keeping the heart beating, but it is possible that humans do survive with milder brain stem damage, though it follows that they are left with impairments of arousal and emotional control. It is like being tired or under the influence of a depressant, such as alcohol much of the time. Behaviourally, the processing of information is slower, inhibitions wane, and temper and irritability control may be compromised.

Problems associated with reduced 'arousal' (provided by the brain stem) means that the everyday mundane or routine activities are particularly vulnerable to meltdown and displays of irritability. Everyday existence does not add that extra 'boost' to maintain persons with brain stem damage

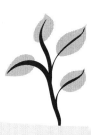

to control their emotional outbursts, to inhibit acting on impulses, or to control strong emotions and not let irritations get the better of them, for example. Something new or of interest to the person is needed as a boost, in order to see that person's best. It is usually the family member or the carer who sees the worst effects of reduced arousal caused by brain stem damage, the highest incidents of emotional lability, and the most challenging behaviour of a neurologically impaired person because they are with them through the dullest of times.

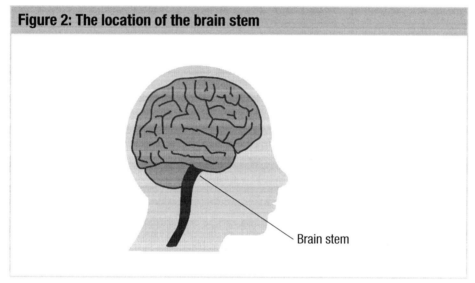

Figure 2: The location of the brain stem

Brain stem

The brain stem is like your brain's power station

Damage to or within the brain stem contributes to inconsistency in an individual's feeling states, emotional behaviour and social consequences. One statement that a family member or carer may express is, '*He remembers what he wants to remember*'. A translation of this could be, '*He remembers what sufficiently aroused his interest and attention*'. Another is, '*Others don't see him as I do. To others he is kind and engaging, making it look like he's just fine, but he's not*'. Again, it may be that the non-routine of being around 'others' that helps him to be and display his best, because the power supplied by the brain stem is turned up in situations of novelty.

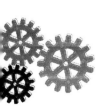

Case study 2

A 60-year-old factory foreman who had a haemorrhage on his brain stem slept around 10 hours a day. His wife tried often to get him up to do the dishes or DIY, or something other than lying in bed. This man seemed depressed to everyone around him but he denied feeling it, but he didn't feel happy either; he just reported feeling nothing but apathy. He could still walk, talk and work, but he just didn't have the energy to carry out the mundane tasks of life and would get very upset with any family member who challenged him on this. When he attended his doctor appointments, he was talkative and appeared to have nothing wrong with him as this was something new and therefore arousing, and he would convince the doctors that he was fine. He would even talk about jobs he had done around the house and how he hoped to get back to work soon. However, his wife and children knew differently and that they did not have their husband or father they knew before the haemorrhage.

The limbic system

The limbic system is composed of several structures of the mid-brain and medial temporal lobes, and in it contains the basic neural circuitry for primal or 'raw' feeling states. It plays a role in recognising rewards and dangers in the environment, it is concerned with self-preservation (and sexual interest and procreation), and is the origination point of many of human being's basic drives and impulses. The limbic system contains thousands of circuit connections with all the senses of the body and contributes to some of the 'early' interpretation of incoming sensations, whether through vision (eg. seeing a dangerous animal or an attractive potential partner), hearing (eg. the sound of screeching tires approaching or gentle waves lapping up on the beach), or olfactory/smell/taste (eg. toxic/poisonous substances or chocolate).

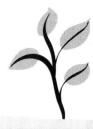

Figure 3: The location of the limbic system in the mid-brain

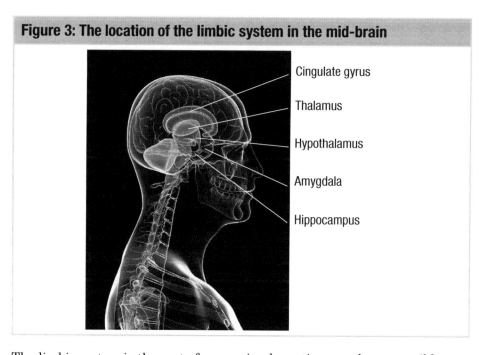

Cingulate gyrus

Thalamus

Hypothalamus

Amygdala

Hippocampus

The limbic system is the seat of raw, primal emotion, partly responsible for the feeling and expression of fear and anger, like 'animal' instinct. One of the most crucial structures in the limbic system relating to feeling states and behaviour is the amygdala, which is an almond-shaped structure located within the medial temporal lobes and is vulnerable to traumatic brain injury, viral infections, hypoxia, and other neurological conditions. The amygdala is particularly active in the analysis of danger or threat in the environment. In animal studies, electrical stimulation of the amygdala produces aggressive 'fighting' responses, as if the animal has to protect itself from a serious threat while removal of the amygdala causes the animal to become passive, fearless, and totally unaware of clear and present dangers. Persons with temporal lobe epilepsy may report feelings of excessive fear and anxiety during a seizure or fit, presumably due to the amygdala being over-stimulated. Space occupying lesions such as tumours or other intracranial pressure conditions may act similarly putting pressure on the amygdala, causing a near constant state of paranoia or anxiety and over-interpretation of even harmless comments or actions as threatening. On the other side of the coin, conditions that lead to bilateral destruction of the amygdala structures such as that which may occur from viral infections lead to passivity and unawareness of threats or danger (including inability to 'read' facial expressions or tone of voice that express fear, anger, or disgust).

Case study 3

A 32-year-old man with his own landscaping business, who was known to be mild mannered and an effective businessman severely beat one of his long-term female customers. The man punched the woman in the face and she fell backwards onto the ground, then he picked up stones and threw them at her for a further 45 seconds before he was satisfied she was no longer a threat to him. He then got in his van and drove back to his base seemingly unaware, or rather had forgotten that he had done anything wrong. Apparently, just before the attack the woman customer asked him not to spray the weed killer so close to the house. The man was arrested and later that evening while in police custody he collapsed and had a seizure. He was taken to the hospital and a brain scan revealed an aggressive tumour in his left medial temporal lobe had put pressure on the left amygdala structure and surrounding areas, and he died within the month.

The frontal lobes

The frontal lobes play a huge part in emotion and behaviour. Among other roles, the frontal lobes control emotion and behaviour like a traffic officer directing some emotions and behaviours to 'go' and some to 'stop' or 'proceed with caution'. In terms of volume, the frontal lobes account for approximately one-third of the brain's size. You can imagine that different disease or damaging processes to the frontal lobes produce potentially very different emotional and behavioural consequences, even though all would be considered 'frontal' emotional or behavioural change or dysfunction. Some of the key behavioural consequences or syndromes include:

A. orbito-frontal (ie. under surface of the frontal lobes) damage and *'problems with stopping'*
B. dorso-lateral and medial (ie. top and sides, and inner middle surface of the frontal lobes) and *'problems with starting'*
C. orbito-frontal damage and *'problems of social judgement'*.

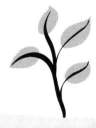

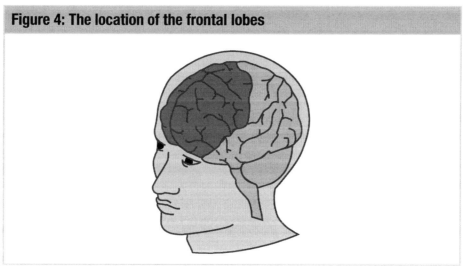

Figure 4: The location of the frontal lobes

Among the many roles of the frontal lobes is the 'executive' control over emotions and behaviours, deciding which impulses should 'go' and which should slow down or stop (ie. suppress).

Problems with excessive emotional expression

Some of the problems of 'stopping' emotional or behavioural impulses result from damage to the connections between the orbito-frontal lobes and the structures of the limbic system. As you recall, the limbic system is largely emotional and instinctive, and properly functioning frontal lobes exert control over these feeling states and instincts. The job of the frontal lobes is to try to satisfy the impulses of the limbic system by socially acceptable or measured means, or to suppress the impulses all together.

As a consequence of damage to the orbito-frontal lobes, or its connections with the limbic system, control of impulses may be absent or delayed. People may 'speak without thinking', joke inappropriately, tell inappropriate stories or ask inappropriate questions, or otherwise just say what is on their mind. They may have sudden or explosive displays of emotion and perhaps be particularly aggressive or abusive verbally; they may seem to act without thinking, impulsively and suddenly. Sound judgement may seem to be lacking in their actions and behaviours, and behaviours may be disinhibited, including sexual acting out, picking vegetables from the neighbour's garden, being too friendly or talking excessively and so on.

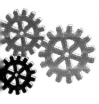

These effects may all be said to be characterised by an absence or delay in considering the potential consequences of certain actions, by not using past experience to inform the best way to respond, and by not considering socially sanctioned norms or expectations before acting. They are 'basic' almost primal emotional behaviours that get displayed, and it is not uncommon for persons with frontal lobe damage to seem immature or child-like, egocentric, excessively emotionally expressive, and socially inappropriate. On the other hand, it is not unheard of to have displayed positive features as well, such as expressions of 'heart-felt honesty', flirtation, or an emotional expressiveness that is attractive. This could be a possible change in anyone but perhaps most noticeably from a previously stoic individual.

Case study 4

A 42-year-old man who was a scooter enthusiast and shop assistant was involved in a scooter accident when a passenger in a parked car opened the car door into the scooter's path. This man was wearing a helmet and collided head first onto the road at about 25 mph. The injury he sustained involved his orbito-frontal cortex coming into speedy and sharp contact with the rough linings of his inner skull, causing contusions, as his brain bounced forwards and backwards in his skull. When he emerged from a coma it was clear to those that knew him well that he had changed. For example, he would often make comments to women about how pretty or ugly they were, for the sake of 'just being honest'. Any offence that he would cause by his comments he would just brush off as it being their problem and not his. He could fly into rages quickly, often leaving those around him stunned as to what he got so upset about. The expressed anger was intense when it came, but he could also be a lot more fun than he used to be, making people laugh at parties by his unconventional (often rude or brutally honest) jokes. He tried returning to work, but was disciplined and let go for various incidents with his customers, involving arguing with them or talking excessively, and making the customers feel uncomfortable.

Problems with starting and suppressing emotional experience

In most cases, in the majority of neurological conditions that affect the frontal lobes, problems of stopping or problems of starting will characterise the presentation to some degree. Problems with starting are characterised by apathy, inertia, lack of motivation, and lack of spontaneity. Cues in the environment that should produce sufficient anxiety and indicate that

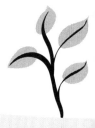

action is needed immediately (such as the toast burning example) may not even produce a response, and so again in extreme cases, a person may just watch the toast burn in the toaster. Such people are quite alright to sit around and do nothing, and are apathetic to the fact that they are not doing anything, or 'not making anything of themselves'. They are not likely to initiate a conversation or ask questions, and answer most questions themselves with a minimal utterance.

Alongside the motivation and initiation issues are often diminished emotional expression, apathy and indifference. Such persons may demonstrate a lack of emotional reaction to pleasant or unpleasant events, and thus may appear to feel the same (ie. nothing) about the death of a grandmother or winning the lottery. As mentioned earlier, emotion is intrinsically linked with motivation; we've got to feel something in order to know what to do about it, and indeed to start it. When actually, seemingly nothing is felt, there is no subsequent motivation to do anything but eat, drink, sleep and to use the toilet. There is often one exception to this lack of feeling and motivation and that is when a situation frustrates or angers people then they may react with aggression or verbal abuse, and perhaps this is due to such reactions having their origination point 'lower' than the frontal lobes, within the limbic system.

Case study 5

A 46-year-old man who was diabetic and unemployed took an intentional overdose of insulin causing him to go into a deep coma. Brain scans revealed severe hypoxic/ischaemic damage (ie. lack of oxygenated blood), largely to his medial frontal lobes bilaterally (ie. the inner area between the frontal left and right hemispheres). When he came round from the coma he learned to walk and talk again, although he mostly just seemed to stare with a smug, amused expression, and only answered questions with minimal utterances. He rarely initiated anything except to take himself to the toilet. His wife cared for him and brought him meals and drink and if she didn't she believed he wouldn't eat or drink. The only emotion he showed was anger especially when his teenage daughter taunted him. Since he was physically capable and could communicate clearly, many felt he was faking his disability, although he actually had a significant disease which could strongly feel and display anger. On a few occasions he smashed up the living room following an argument with his daughter and then went back to watching television amongst the mess. His wife would clean it up and while she did so he would just sit still and watch the television. He lacked empathy or appreciation for the help and sacrifices made by others on his behalf, and his wife had

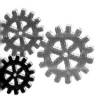

to pick up a second job. When she asked him if he would return to work, he would always say yes, but he never did try in the seven years that he lived post injury. While she cared for him, his wife described feeling like a servant to a non-emotional, non-sympathetic couch potato.

Social judgement

In the following descriptions, you will again notice familiar themes of the limbic system and frontal lobes working together (or not) to produce sound or ill-judged behaviour in the context of social relationships and interactions. By 'social judgment' what is meant is the ability to 'read' people and situations correctly, to be aware of potential rewards and dangers in the context of dealing with others, to know how you feel about various courses of action, and finally to use sound reasoning and previous experience to carry out a preferred (and wise) course of action.

People with this type of disorder seem not to be able to read warning signs or evaluate risk properly, and could make catastrophically poor decisions. In this syndrome their emotional evaluation may be flat, or emotions or feelings that are so important for making sound decisions do not seem accessible to them. Such people may 'give away' too much, such as private bank details or inappropriately discuss relationship difficulties, or enter bad business dealings. Like other frontal lobe syndromes, they may be unaware of the boredom or disinterest of the person they are speaking to, and have inadequate self-monitoring skills or lack a 'feedback loop' that could help them to consciously understand their behaviour's effect on others and adjust accordingly.

Case study 6

A 19-year-old university student majoring in business was attacked and repeatedly kicked in the head by a group of thugs while he was on his way home from a football match. Always having been a polite young man, after his injury he became very easily irritated with his parents. On two occasions he punched his father, something he had never done before and having also usually been a good 'older brother' he now regularly got into bitter, screaming arguments with his 12-year-old sister. When they fought, it was hard to tell which of them was younger as they both acted like 12 year olds. This young man's IQ and memory were relatively intact and to some health professionals

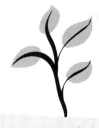

it seemed that he had no effects from the brain injury, only just that he was a 'spoiled, petulant child'. He acquired a new set of 'friends' since the injury and unlike his family, he never argued with his friends and, in fact, he gave away too much. Within a month, he had given away two mobile phones, his bicycle and £120 in cash. Amongst his peers, he was often made the object of jokes and ridicule but he didn't seem to notice and kept following this group of people, not able to see, as others did, how he was being taken advantage of. He failed to 'read' the ill intentions of others while he drove a wedge into the relationships with people who loved him his whole life.

The right and left hemispheres

Figure 5: The location, appearance and emotional functions of the left and right hemispheres

Left anterior (front)/right posterior (back) hemisphere

Understands language like a 'literal' transcript.

Sees facial expressions as non-integrated facial parts.

When damaged, people may be acutely aware of their own disabilities, even excessively so, and may react 'catastrophically' to minor problems.

When damaged, depression is often experienced.

When damaged, people may be pessimistic and underestimate their true abilities.

Right anterior (front)/left posterior (back) hemisphere

Understands the emotional meaning, jokes, or sarcasm in language.

Contributes to providing tone, pitch, volume, and emphasis (ie. prosody) in speech (giving speech an 'interest' factor).

Sees facial expressions as a whole and as conveying a particular meaning.

When damaged, people may not be aware of, or particularly concerned about disabilities they have.

When damaged, people may be optimistic and overestimate their true abilities.

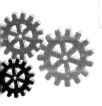

Right anterior and left posterior damage

Damage to the anterior (ie. towards the front) right hemisphere and the posterior (ie. towards the back) left hemisphere may be the cause of some similar types of emotional and behavioural disturbances. Both are generally associated with a denial or unawareness of an illness or condition, or reduced self-awareness of the severity of an illness or condition. The technical term for this phenomenon is 'anosognosia', meaning without knowledge (of a problem). Such persons may seem blasé about the fact that the left side of their body is paralytic, or that they are not able to understand what is being said to them, or something of a similar nature. They may seem blissfully unaware, even manic or happy. Their 'elevated' mood and actions are not congruent with the reality of their situation, and they may 'defend' or 'excuse' their predicament by proclaiming normality, or that everyone else is concerned but they are not. Motivating them to 'do something' or engage in rehabilitation can be a challenge, because to them, nothing is wrong. It is just other people who are 'hassling' them. On the other hand, they may at least give 'lip service' to lofty, unrealistic goals, given their state/condition and non-participation in planning or executing action plans. They may suffer from the problem of over-estimating their current levels of ability.

Left posterior damage may be associated with language comprehension deficits, and again is often accompanied by what would not seem to be an appropriate level of awareness of the existence or severity of deficits. Those who experience damage of the left posterior do not have a language feedback loop (ie. they can't monitor and adapt what they are saying because they can't even understand themselves) and they often talk in what seems gibberish to us, but feels perfectly sensible to them. They may still pick up on visual cues and have some ideas about the social context and talk or respond in kind, but alas it may have nothing to do with what you actually intended to communicate to them. Despite this, there is often the characteristic happy-go-lucky attitude among these patients, with only occasional upset. The seriousness of the situation takes a while to dawn on them, if it ever does fully. If their ability to pick up on context or social cues is also affected (such as through visual impairment), they may not have the ability to correctly perceive or understand situations that should (and normally would) produce an appropriate feeling response, such as feeling and expressing sadness to the news that a relative just died.

With both right anterior and left posterior damage, there may exist an emotional indifference or a lack of concern to a situation that should

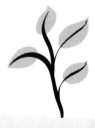

produce feelings of sadness, compassion, or anger. It is characterised by an underwhelming response/reaction to emotionally laden events, in the context of generally elevated (sometimes egocentric) mood.

Case study 7

A 58-year-old female school teacher developed a left posterior tumour and had it surgically removed. Her subsequent impairments included very poor comprehension of what was said to her and this was accompanied by a very poor general understanding of what was going on around her, for example, who the nurses were and what they were doing to care for her, and an apparent misunderstanding or apathy regarding the seriousness of her condition. She seemed 'happy-go-lucky' and often talked about the weather, her kids and so forth. Over time it became evident that her language comprehension and understanding of nonverbal communications improved, however. Her communication improved on topics of her choosing or initiation, but if any communication was directed at her regarding the weak right side of her body, brain damage, or poor prognosis, her comprehension was very poor indeed, and her light-hearted mood was incongruent to the seriousness of the conversation. The difference in her comprehension in the two situations was related to her inability to process negative emotions and some degree of not being attentive to any signs of disease, disability, or weakness.

Left anterior and right posterior damage

Damage to the anterior (towards the front) left hemisphere or the posterior (towards the back) right hemisphere produces rather an opposite picture than that described above. In such cases, agitated and anxious depression and heightened, even catastrophic, awareness of deficits may be present. Most people are right-handed and most people have their 'dominant' (inclusive of language) hemisphere in the left. Some types of damage to the left anterior hemisphere result in expressive language difficulties and paralysis on the dominant right side of the body. Therefore, an apparent 'neurological' emotional and behavioural deficit is coupled with a situation that is indeed very difficult to cope with.

In general, depression is associated with 'underactive' left frontal lobe activity. It is as if when damage is sustained in the left anterior area, our normal 'balance', sense of optimism, ability to moderate reactions to difficult situations and so forth are compromised. The 'catastrophic reaction' is associated with left anterior damage and to some extent with right posterior damage. The 'catastrophic reaction' is a situation in which

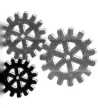

a person's coping resources are suddenly and rapidly depleted, and they may demonstrate a disproportionally negative and emotional response to a situation, which may include, crying, yelling, or aggressive behaviour towards oneself, others or property.

Damage to the left anterior (front) or right posterior (back) areas may be associated with, along with anxiety, difficulties in taking up or responding to challenges. For those things that are tried such damage may result in critical or even self-deprecating self-appraisal. Again, this is associated with a motivation problem, just of a different kind. Situations may be avoided and feelings of the ability to cope may be absent or very low. They may experience feelings of inadequacy or profound sense of embarrassment, and thus may have learned to cope by avoiding situations and seeing their self-esteem tumble.

Case study 8

A 46-year-old man who was a computer programmer had a spontaneous stroke in his left anterior communicating artery (ie. left frontal lobe). Before his stroke he rarely got depressed but following his stroke he became highly prone to depression and even battled with suicidal ideation. The stroke left him with the ability to understand what was said to him, but he couldn't express himself and his speech was not fluent. Furthermore, he was hemiplegic, ie. unable to move his right side, but he recovered some function through physiotherapy. His hobbies – woodworking and walking in the country – were compromised and although this may have given him reason to feel depressed, the location of his stroke exaggerated his depressive symptoms. He lost his coping skill and often felt like self-harming, and he often reacted catastrophically to small problems or disagreements. He lost his psychological or 'mood' balance and became pessimistic, gloomy and noticed the worst in everything.

Another emotional processing function of the right hemisphere

When the right hemisphere is not damaged and is functioning properly, it is largely responsible for communicating and receiving or comprehending tone (or prosody) and emotional meaning in what someone says to us and in what we see (such as analysis of facial expressions and gestures). This is where the phrase, 'It's not what you say, it's how you say it' becomes relevant. Sarcasm and the point of jokes are often interpreted and expressed within and through the right hemisphere (whereas the left hemisphere interprets language more like a written transcript), and people with damage to the right hemisphere may not seem to pick up on

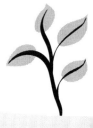

the point, the tone, the abstraction, or the joke in something that is said to them or seen by them. Similarly, their speech, expressions, and gestures may appear flat in tone and concrete in content. This is perhaps why people with right hemisphere damage may seem self-absorbed and indifferent to their surroundings or to the plight of others, and they may not get the point of a joke. Furthermore, a person who was previously very engaging and dynamic may seem to have had more of a personality change following a brain injury or neurological disease process, than someone who was naturally more reticent to start with. Similarly, right hemisphere damage may disproportionately affect the career prospects of a politician, an orator, or an actor, than it would to a computer data entry specialist.

Additional thought 3: Biological determinants of emotion and behaviour

Further evidence that emotions or emotional behaviours do indeed have a biological basis and could change with brain damage or disease can be seen in these examples that illustrate some biological influences of emotion and behaviour.

a) Lesion or brain tumour (such as on or near the amygdala or frontal lobes) case studies have shown that previously mild-mannered, upright citizens turn to slovenly behaviour and even murder over a minor dispute.

b) Identical twin case studies, which have shown that even twins who share the same genetic make-up but are raised separately in different families and environments, end up with very similar skills and abilities, interests and likes, even similar fashion sense and interest in a particular type of spouse.

c) There is evidence that biological agents such as psychotropic medication or alcohol affects thought patterns, moods, and behaviours of human beings. In short, people act and feel differently when under the influence of a powerful drug.

d) Human beings have a temperament, which may change with time and experience, but there seems to be something 'inherent' in personality. It is first evident in infancy, with 'easy' or 'difficult' temperaments. Just like if we were made of a base compound, such as baking flour. We could grow up to be many things, bread, crackers, matzo balls, brownies depending on our life experience.

On the other hand, following on that idea that people may become many things (ie. bread, crackers, matzo balls, or brownies) due to their biological endowment, it needs to be stated that environment, help, love, support, opportunity and culture also plays a huge role in shaping human beings.

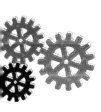

Similarly, rehabilitation and the quality of nursing care and other 'environmental' factors play an absolutely huge role in how persons with brain damage or disease will feel and experience life and behave. The eventual and ultimate presentation of people with brain damage or disease has so much to do with opportunities, family, carers, and the culture they live in and this is where carers may have the greatest influence to help. We're not doomed simply because emotion and behaviour are biological, in fact, environment and experience shapes our biology and vice versa. Consider all the experiences you've had and people you've known that have influenced who you became and how you behave. Similarly, think of someone born with a 'difficult' temperament (biological) and all the negative reactions such a person would elicit from the wider world. This person's experience of the world would be negative, feeling despised, alienated and so forth. Finally consider that there may be a feedback loop regarding difficult neurological patients; they're difficult and the world reacts negatively towards them because of this. The bad emotions and behaviours get reinforced, but we can try to break this cycle by providing our clients/patients with a positive and loving 'corrective' experience.

Take away message

Emotions and behaviours have a biological basis in the brain and changes happen when the brain is damaged or sustains disease, and therefore to some extent emotions and behaviours are going to be outside the conscious control or intention of the client/patient, so latitude for this should be given. On the other hand, environmental factors and experience could help to improve (relatively) or worsen an unpleasant or even unsafe emotional experience and behaviour, so therefore frontline staff working with neurological clients should try to respond in a way and create interventions that may not be what is 'naturally' elicited from the client's 'bad' emotions and behaviour, but try to help it turn around.

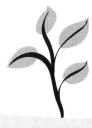

Quiz

1. What are the six 'universal' emotions?

2. Why is disease or damage to the brain's 'emotional centres' so often accompanied by social impairments?

3. The part of the brain that is usually associated with arousal, helping all other systems to function optimally is:
    a. the brain stem
    b. the frontal lobes
    c. located in the limbic system
    d. predominately a right hemisphere function.

4. The part of the brain that is the seat for most of our primal feeling:
    a. is the brain stem
    b. are the frontal lobes
    c. is located in the limbic system
    d. is predominately a right hemisphere function.

5. What is the main role of the amygdala?

6. What are the two main 'behavioural syndromes' associated with orbito-frontal lobe damage?

7. What is the main 'behavioural syndrome' associated with dorso-lateral or medial frontal lobe damage?

8. The human frontal lobes:
    a. are responsible for moderating 'instincts'
    b. play a role in correctly interpreting social situations
    c. play a role in motivation and executing plans
    d. do all of the above.

9. Accurate self-awareness of the extent of deficits following brain damage is more likely to be affected in cases of:
    a. left hemisphere damage
    b. right hemisphere damage
    c. both right and left hemisphere damage.

10. What are the main effects of right anterior or left posterior brain disease or damage?

11. What are the main effects of left anterior or right posterior brain disease or damage?

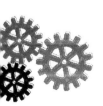

Bibliography

Damasio R (1994) *Descartes' Error: Emotion, reason, and the human brain*. New York: Putnam Publishing.

Gainotti G (2000) Neuropsychological theories of emotion. In: JC Borod (Ed) (2002) *The Neuropsychology of Emotion*. New York: Oxford University Press.

Goleman D (1996) *Emotional Intelligence: Why it can matter more than IQ*. New York: Bantam Books.

Heilman KM, Blonder LX, Bowers D & Crucian GP (2000) Neurological disorders and emotional dysfunction. In: JC Borod (Ed) (2002) *The Neuropsychology of Emotion*. New York: Oxford University Press.

LeDoux J (1996) *The Emotional Brain: The mysterious underpinnings of emotional life*. New York: Touchstone.

Lishman WA (1997) *Organic Psychiatry: The psychological consequences of cerebral disorder* (3rd edition). Oxford: Blackwell Publishing.

Prigatano GP (1998) *Principles of Neuropsychological Rehabilitation*. New York: Oxford University Press.

Raskin SA, Bloom RL & Borad JC (2000) Rehabilitation of emotional deficits in neurological populations: a multi-disciplinary perspective. In: JC Borod (Ed) (2002) *The Neuropsychology of Emotion*. New York: Oxford.

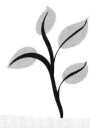

Chapter 5

Common neurological conditions

Robert Poppleton

Aims of the chapter

The chapter aims to:

1. define and describe the main types of cognitive disorders

2. highlight the occurrence rates of these different disorders

3. discuss some of the signs and symptoms shown by people who have these disorders

4. describe the disease process of these disorders and, if applicable, their different types

5. name and describe the treatment of these disorders.

Introduction

This chapter looks at cognitive disorders and the diseases and conditions that cause them and it also provides some information on how they affect the people who have them. Cognitive disorders are those which affect our basic cognitive functions including memory, attention, perception, problem-solving and language. It's these skills and functions that are primarily affected when the brain becomes damaged. A cognitive disorder is any disorder which affects the brain's abilities to function ie. to think, to problem solve or to learn information etc. The main type of cognitive disorder is called organic disorder which actually causes brain cells and nerves to die or be damaged, causing them to cease or to work less well. This damage can be caused by events such as a stroke and this will result in permanent brain damage, ie. damage that will not improve and will be life-long. These conditions have many causes such as infections through

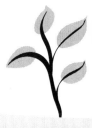

bacteria or viruses, for example, meningitis, or they are sometimes inherited from parents, such as Huntington's disease, or are related to the ageing process, for example Alzheimer's disease.

However, these are not the only consequences, there are also what is referred to as secondary consequences, which include the subsequent emotional and coping problems following brain injury, such as depression, anxiety and emotional changes, which not only affect the individual, but also their surrounding families and support workers (see chapters 4 and 11). These emotional reactions will cause the brain to function less effectively, for example, the speed of processing information may be reduced. This chapter will look at these factors in more detail and address how health professionals try to deal with their consequences to enable people to move on with their lives. The chapter will also focus on the more common neurological conditions, which include strokes, dementia, epilepsy, Huntington's disease, multiple sclerosis, motor neuron disease and traumatic brain injury.

Stroke

What is a stroke?

A stroke is usually apparent by a sudden appearance of physical symptoms such as a weakness on one side of the body or cognitive symptoms such as slurred speech due to a severe disruption in the blood flow within the brain (see chapter 2).

There are three main types of stroke and these are: ischemic (a blockage usually consisting of fatty material in a blood transport pipe, eg. a vein or an artery) haemorrhage (burst blood vessel, ie. an artery or a vein pipe) and transient ischemic attack (temporary interruption of the oxygen and food supply to a part of the brain). Strokes disrupt the blood supply to brain cells, which results in them being starved of oxygen and essential nutrients. If this occurs for longer than three to four minutes it will cause the brain cells to become distressed and if it continues they die causing permanent damage.

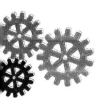

Ischemic 'blockage' stroke

An ischemic 'blockage' stroke is where a blockage occurs within a blood pipe that carries blood to the brain and this is the most common type of stroke. There are three main causes as follows.

1. A cerebral thrombosis, which is where a blockage occurs in a main artery to the brain.

2. A cerebral embolism is where a blood blockage, air bubble or fat globule forms somewhere else in the body and is carried to the brain through the blood supply.

3. A lacuna stroke, which is where there is a blockage in the small blood vessels deep within the brain.

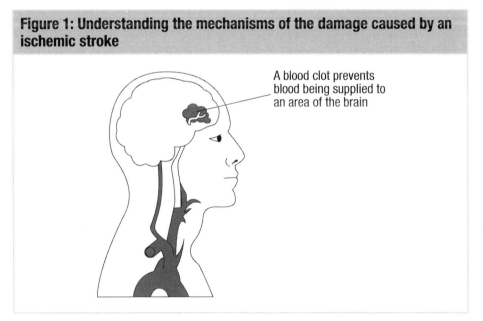

Figure 1: Understanding the mechanisms of the damage caused by an ischemic stroke

A blood clot prevents blood being supplied to an area of the brain

(Image courtesy of The Stroke Association: www.stroke.org.uk)

Haemorrhage 'burst pipe' stroke

A haemorrhage stroke is where a blood pipe in the brain bursts causing bleeding into the brain, and this causes damage by putting pressure on the brain as there is limited space in the skull. It also reduces the blood supply to other areas of the brain, and this can be caused by the following:

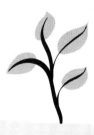

1. an intracranial bleed is where a blood pipe bursts within the brain.

2. a subarachnoid haemorrhage is where a blood vessel on the surface of the brain bleeds into the area between the brain and the skull causing a build up of pressure.

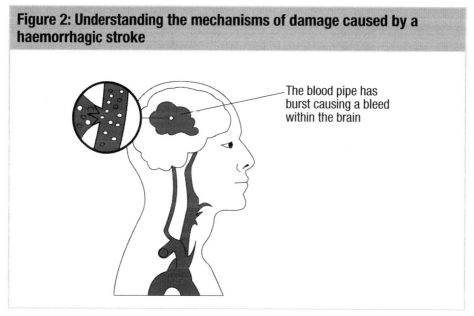

Figure 2: Understanding the mechanisms of damage caused by a haemorrhagic stroke

The blood pipe has burst causing a bleed within the brain

(Image courtesy of The Stroke Association: www.stroke.org.uk)

Transient ischemic attack (TIA)

Transient ischemic attack is where the blood supply is interrupted for only a brief amount of time (ie. less than 3–4 minutes so it does not tend to cause significant or permanent brain cell death) and is often referred to as a 'mini stroke'. The symptoms can be similar to those of a stroke such as slurred speech and weakness on one side of the body. However, with a mini stroke these symptoms normally only last for a few minutes to hours before completely disappearing by 24 hours. A TIA causes the brain to be without nutrients and oxygen at most for only a few minutes, but it is a sign showing that the brain may not be getting enough blood supply, so it should still be taken seriously.

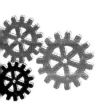

Prevalence

At least 450,000 people in United Kingdom are severely disabled as a result of a stroke and it is the third largest cause of death in the UK. A stroke also causes a greater range of disabilities than any other condition, from memory and concentration, to walking and speaking; this is why understanding and preventing strokes is so important. Each year in England and Wales over 130,000 people have a stroke and 25% of these are under 65. Those that have had a stroke have an 8% increased risk of another stroke over their lifespan.

Table 1: Age groups of people who suffer strokes			
Sex	**Age group**	**First stroke**	**Recurrent stroke**
Female	0-44	723	362
	45-64	6,814	3,163
	65-74	9,749	5,035
	75+	32,092	19,969
	Total	49,378	28,529
Male	0-44	994	389
	45-64	9,910	3,893
	65-74	11,195	9,139
	75+	16,262	11,758
	Total	38,361	25,188

(Taken from the Stroke Association: www.stroke.org.uk)

This table shows that even though people can suffer from a stroke at any age, the risk is dramatically increased when you reach 75. Females are also more likely to suffer a stroke than males, although males are more likely to have a stroke before the age of 75. Two of the main factors that contribute to this are that men on average have higher blood pressure and females live longer than males.

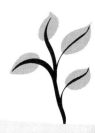

Different types of stroke

▶ 69% are blockage stroke

▶ 19% are a haemorrhage stroke

▶ 12% are other types of stroke.

Disease process

Depending on the type of stroke that the patient has suffered and the severity of it, the sooner a stroke is discovered and treatment is started the better the chances of recovery for the person. A stroke can have a variety of effects on individuals so it is important to address care based on their needs.

The injuries are dependent on the area of the brain affected. If the stroke occurs on the left side of the brain then it will most likely be the right side of the body that is affected, and if the stroke is on the right side of the brain then it is most likely the left side of the body that is affected (see also chapter 2). The brain can regain some of its functions by forming new connections between the cells that are not damaged. Furthermore, some parts of the undamaged brain may take over some functions for example, if language is damaged a person may use more visual stimuli as this uses a different part of the brain. However, this reorganisation can take a long time but intensive rehabilitation improves the chances of a better recovery.

Table 2: Possible consequences and effects a person may suffer after experiencing a stroke	
Physical	Patients: ▶ can lose the ability to walk or have any movement of the legs ▶ can lose the functioning of their upper limbs such as arms and hands ▶ can experience problems with their balance.
Speech	Some patients: ▶ can lose the ability to express or understand aspects of speech ▶ have problems with swallowing, presenting a higher risk of choking.

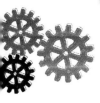

Cognitive	Some patients:
	▶ can experience memory problems; both short-term and long-term can be affected
	▶ can experience attention problems as patients can become more distractible
	▶ can experience problems with reasoning and planning skills (also see chapter 3, executive functions)
	▶ can experience emotional problems such as anger and depression/ tearfulness (mood swings are more common).

Risk factors

▶ **Smoking** – increases the risk 1.5–3 times

▶ **Family** – there is a genetic component of stroke, those who have family members who have suffered a stroke are more likely to have a stroke themselves. This is not the only factor though and is related to the lifestyle that the person leads

▶ **Diabetes** – increases the risk 1.5–2 times

▶ **Alcohol** – 1–4 times

▶ **Diet** – unhealthy diets of little fruit and vegetables, too much salt, and high cholesterol all increase the risk of strokes

▶ **Overweight (obesity)** – increases the risk

▶ **High blood pressure** – is the most important causal risk factor for stroke, causing about 50% of blockage strokes

▶ **Lack of exercise or being physically unfit** – even moderate physical activity can reduce the risk of stroke by up to 27%

Treatments

The damage caused by strokes can be reduced depending on how quickly the stroke is discovered and treated. There are four steps to help recognise symptoms and act quickly and these are:

F – Facial weakness, can the person smile, has the mouth or eye drooped?
A – Arm weakness, can the person raise both arms?

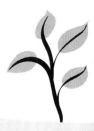

S – Speech problems, is the speech slurred, can the person speak clearly
   and can you understand what they are saying?

T – Test these symptoms/time to call 999

Stroke rehabilitation aims to aid the natural recovery of patients and it
also teaches them to cope with their new disabilities, and helps them to
work out new ways around their difficulties. Carers help clients with the
relearning of old skills, developing new skills and learning to adapt to some
of the limitations caused by the stroke. This is usually undertaken as part
of a multidisciplinary team approach.

To help improve outcomes, it is best to have a multidisciplinary team
involving doctors, physiotherapists, clinical psychologists, occupational
therapists, speech and language therapists and nutritionists. For example,
someone who suffers from memory difficulties may be given memory
exercises as well as a diary for aiding memory. For physical symptoms,
treatments involve relearning effected functions and building of muscle.
As the effects of stroke are so individual, every patient's rehabilitation
programme is made to their own individual needs.

Drug treatment

One treatment method for blockage strokes is to give patients a drug such
as Alteplase, which helps dissolve blood clots. However, this is only effective
if it is used within the first three hours of the stroke.

For haemorrhage strokes, vitamin K helps the clotting process; another
drug that can help to prevent strokes is asprin as this thins the blood
making it less likely to get caught on something and cause a blockage.
Doctors will also watch a patient's cholesterol and blood pressure levels as
if these are too high then there is an increased chance of a further stroke.

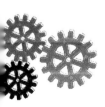

Case study 1

Mrs Jones is 53 years old and she has sustained a right-sided subarachnoid haemorrhage. She was in intensive care for three months and was finally transferred to a rehabilitation hospital six months after her stroke.

She had severe memory problems and on the ward she would frequently ask the same questions such as, '*when is my husband coming to see me?*' She needed a lot of prompting to write important information down and to look at it when she lacked insight, but she did not understand that she needed to compensate for her memory loss. Both formal assessment and informal observation showed that she had a left-sided inattention; she enjoyed walking to the shops with members of staff to buy sweets and chocolate, but would often walk past the hospital on the way back as the hospital was on her left-hand side. Once back in the hospital she would eat a lot of unhealthy snacks, forgetting she had eaten a snack not long before. Mrs Jones was highly disoriented and would often talk about how she had only got married six months ago, however, she had actually got married nine years before.

Case study 2

Mr Smith is 42 years old and was having dinner with his wife in a restaurant when he began to feel ill and weak on his left hand side. His wife noticed that his speech started to slur and his mouth was drooping on the left so she immediately called an ambulance and Mr Smith was taken into hospital where they discovered he had a stroke.

Mr Smith went on to make a good recovery and a few months later he returned to work, however, on returning to work he began to notice that he found certain things harder than he did before the stroke. He found it hard to concentrate on work and was easily distracted and he had some difficulties trying to keep organised and would often forget the details of conversations.

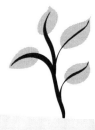

Dementia

What is dementia?

Dementia is the term used to describe the set of symptoms usually displayed when the brain cells die at a rate greater than the normal ageing process. It is usually a progressive disease meaning it gradually becomes worse over time, although this varies between individuals and is usually irreversible.

The main types and causes of dementia are as follows.

▶ **Alzheimer's disease** – during Alzheimer's the brain cells stop functioning normally due to chemical and structural brain changes. This can include nerves becoming tangled and small aluminium deposits within brain cells which can occur all over the brain.

▶ **Vascular dementia** – is caused by no or reduced blood circulation, resulting in parts of the brain not receiving enough oxygen and food to the brain cells, which may consequently cause them to die. This results in a patchy appearance of damage to the brain.

The main contributory causes for this are: high blood pressure, heart problems, high cholesterol, diabetes and excessive alcohol consumption and smoking.

▶ **Dementia with lewy bodies** – this is where abnormal structures called lewy bodies develop inside the nerve cells leading the brain cells to function abnormally.

▶ **Frontotemporal dementia** – this occurs when brain cells from two lobes of the brain (the frontal and the temporal lobes) start dying quicker than the normal process, which results in these areas shrinking. These are the areas responsible for our behaviour (eg. problem-solving or reasoning skills), emotional control (eg. anger control) and language skills.

There are several other rarer causes of dementia, including Korsakoffs syndrome (this related to prolonged poor diet or alcohol consumption), HIV and AIDS related dementias. Patients suffering with multiple sclerosis, Down's syndrome, Parkinson's and Huntington's disease are also more likely to develop dementia.

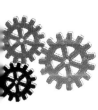

Prevalence

There are around 700,000 people in the UK currently with dementia and it is expected to double within the next 30 years or so. It is more prevalent in older people and is estimated that as many as half of those above 80 years old may be affected. However, there are an estimated 15,000 cases of people suffering from dementia who are under the age of 65.

Table 3: Demographics of males and females with dementia by age		
Age group	Female	Male
5–69	1.5%	1.4%
70–74	2.2%	3.1%
75–79	7.1%	5.6%
80–84	14.1%	10.2%
85 or over	27.5%	19.6%

Table 3 shows that even though you can suffer from dementia at any age, the risk dramatically increases with age. Females are also more likely to suffer with dementia than males but this may be due to the fact that women tend to live longer than men.

Disease process

Alzheimer's disease progresses with subtle advancement and this means that a person's cognitive abilities become damaged over a prolonged period of time eg. their memory gradually worsens. In the early stages of dementia, the symptoms are mild and often go undiagnosed. Loss of memory of recent events is usually one of the first signs and as the disease progresses the symptoms become more severe. Memory loss increases significantly and patients start repeating themselves or fail to recognise faces. Some become upset at this point and can become very frustrated or unconfident. In the later stages of dementia patients are no longer able to care for themselves and are often residing in nursing homes. Occasionally sufferers have sudden flashes of recognition but overall their loss of memory is very pronounced. Sufferers also become increasingly frail and less mobile, for example, they need help with transfers.

Figure 3: Progressive decline caused by Alzheimer's disease

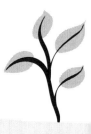

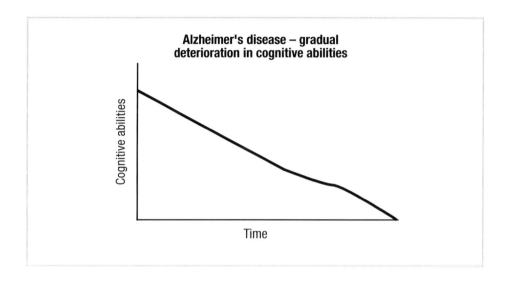

Alzheimer's disease causes a gradual progressive decline in a sufferer's cognitive abilities over time and this progressive deterioration is usually quicker in younger individuals.

In multi-infarct (vascular) dementia, which is commonly caused by a series of strokes, symptoms usually remain constant over time and suddenly decline as a result of another stroke. In other words, there is a stepped progression in vascular dementia where the symptoms level off before abruptly deteriorating.

Figure 4 on page 127 shows the deterioration in a multi-infarct dementia sufferer's cognitive and physical deterioration over time. Multi-infarct dementia causes a sudden deterioration in a sufferer's abilities before they stabilise for a while, and before further deterioration occurs again. This is a different deterioration pattern compared to Alzheimer's disease.

The most common symptoms of Alzheimer's disease are the loss of mental abilities such as thinking, memory, reasoning, language, understanding and judgement. As part of this process the person may also suffer from mood and personality changes and may have communication difficulties. These symptoms gradually get worse over time and become more generalised so that the sufferer is less able to function in everyday life. As the dementia progresses the sufferer will require more support in looking after their personal care needs ie. eating, drinking, using the toilet etc. Eventually they will become bed bound and require total nursing care, but

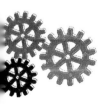

individuals are unique and therefore may experience dementia in different ways. A list of typical symptoms can be seen in **table 4** below.

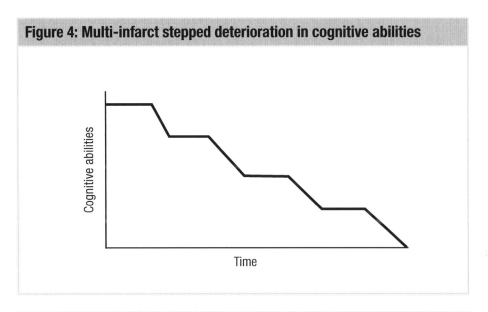

Figure 4: Multi-infarct stepped deterioration in cognitive abilities

Table 4: Typical symptoms of dementia	
Symptom	**Sensation**
Memory loss	Individuals may forget recent events, people's names and appointments more than normal.
Confusion	Patients may have problems working out where they are or what they are doing and be unable to cope with the demands of everyday life.
Mood swings	Patients can often feel sad, angry and frustrated by the uncertainty of what is happening to them.
Withdrawal	Due to loss of confidence and problems communicating.
Concentration/ attention span	Individuals may have a short attention span and find it difficult to complete tasks involving sustained attention skills. They become easily distracted.
Hallucinations	Seeing or hearing things that are not there.
Delusions	Believing in things that are not true (eg. believing that they have to feed their baby).
Aggression	Sometimes they display physical or verbal aggressions, as they may feel agitated because of misunderstandings (eg. when some unknown person comes to help them undress).

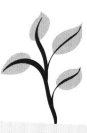

Some individuals may experience some of these symptoms such as memory loss and difficulty thinking clearly, however, they are usually not severe enough to be diagnosed as having Alzheimer's. Therefore, this has been termed mild cognitive impairment (MCI) and research suggests that they may have a higher risk of developing Alzheimer's although this may not be the case.

Risk factors

1. **Diet** – a low fat and high fibre diet is recommended to prevent vascular dementia. Diets with too much salt and saturated fat can raise blood pressure and cholesterol levels therefore increasing the risk of vascular dementia.

2. **Weight** – being overweight or obese increases blood pressure therefore increasing risk of vascular dementia.

3. **Exercise** – this can lower cholesterol, blood pressure, and improve blood circulation, lowering your risk of vascular dementia. The recommended amount of exercise is 30 minutes a day, at least five times a week.

4. **Alcohol** – excessive amounts will raise blood pressure and cholesterol increasing your risk of vascular dementia. The recommended daily level is 3–4 units of alcohol for men and 2–3 units of alcohol for women.

5. **Smoking** – causes narrowing of the arteries therefore increasing blood pressure. This will again increase the risk of vascular dementia.

6. **A medical history** – of stroke, high blood pressure, high cholesterol, diabetes, heart problems and sleep apnoea can increase the risk. Also having a family history of stroke or vascular dementia can also increase the risk.

7. **Ethnicity** – individuals with an Indian, Bangladeshi, Pakistani, Sri Lankan or African-Caribbean background have a higher risk of developing vascular dementia.

8. **Genetics** – research is ongoing in this area, so far it has shown that there may be a small inheritance factor of dementia.

Treatments

There is no treatment for Alzheimer's disease.

Interventions

There are ways to manage or reduce symptoms caused by Alzheimer's and other forms of dementia. Early diagnosis is a critical tool for the prevention of rapid memory loss and it can slow the progress of symptoms.

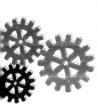

▶ It is very important to keep dementia sufferers fit and healthy.

▶ To prevent confused states a good diet and consistent hydration is important as it helps to prevent chest and urine infections.

▶ Blood samples must be monitored in order to keep vitamin intake, white blood cell count and iron etc. balanced. Imbalance can considerably worsen symptoms and increase confusion.

Drug treatment

▶ In the last few years drugs have been developed which can sometimes delay the progress of symptoms but these work better in mild to moderate forms of dementia since they help maintain memory functions for a short-term period.

▶ Aricept (or donepezil hydrochloride) is a common drug given to people suffering from mild to moderate dementia in Alzheimer's disease.

▶ In severe forms of dementia, drugs are not usually administered because memory problems are severe and permanent.

▶ Some daily practical routines are helpful in order to reduce confusion: keeping a diary or buying the daily newspaper to keep track of time, writing reminders and keeping a consistent environment and routine.

Psychological treatments

There are many psychological treatments that can be used to help a person to cope with the symptoms of dementia.

▶ **Cognitive stimulation** involves activities and exercises such as memory games or discussions.

▶ **Reality orientation therapy** helps a patient to process and retain information on the time, the place and the people around while also improving feelings of self-esteem.

▶ **Validation therapy** is a form of therapy specifically developed for dementia sufferers where the therapist acknowledges, respects and hears the patient's experience.

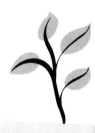

Case study 3

John is a 67-year-old man who has been diagnosed with Alzheimer's disease. He used to work as a foreman at a building site which he enjoyed, but although he has stopped working he wants to go out of the door to go to work and when staff refuse to let him go out he becomes very agitated. This is possibly due to the fact that he is reliving past experiences and is concerned that if he does not get to work on time he will get into trouble. When the staff started acknowledging that he must miss his work since he retired, his levels of agitation declined over time. This was a success because the staff members were helping to resolve the emotions behind the behaviours.

Epilepsy

What is epilepsy?

If a client is diagnosed with epilepsy it means that they have a tendency to have seizures (also known as fits), which start in the brain. The brain has millions of specialised nerve cells called neurons, which transmit messages via electrical impulses from the brain to the rest of the body (see **figure 5** below and also chapter 2) and these messages allow individuals to carry out everyday functions such as walking, talking and eating.

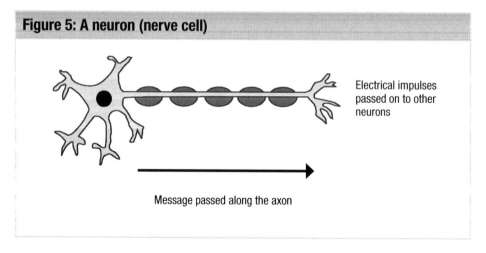

Figure 5: A neuron (nerve cell)

Electrical impulses passed on to other neurons

Message passed along the axon

A seizure happens when a group of these neurons suddenly fire excess electrical impulses uncontrollably. The excess electrical activity temporarily disrupts the normal passage of messages between brain cells, leaving the message mixed up or cut short. The resulting behaviour is largely dependent on where the abnormal electrical activity begins and whether it is confined to a single area or whether it spreads across the brain. For this reason there are many types of seizures, each unique to the person that experiences them.

Prevalence

Epilepsy is the most common neurological condition, or disorder of the nervous system in the UK affecting one in every 131 people. This means that there are at least 465,000 people in the UK that have been diagnosed with the condition, and 75 are being diagnosed daily. It is a condition that affects all age groups, but has been found to be more common in children and adults over 65. Only 52% of people with epilepsy in the UK are seizure free through treatment, it is estimated that this figure could increase to 70% if the right treatment was given to all individuals with the condition. (Epilepsy Action, 2010)

It is not always clear why an individual develops epilepsy and for most people (six out of 10) there is no known cause for their condition. However, in cases where there is a known cause it is usually via damage to the brain for a range of reasons and these can be seen in **figure 6** below.

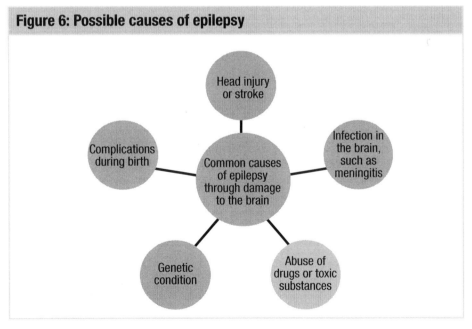

Figure 6: Possible causes of epilepsy

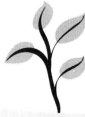

Disease process

Partial seizures – These seizures involve epileptic activity limited to one area of the brain, resulting in localised symptoms. These seizures can be split into two main types which are called partial or complex seizures as shown in **figure 7** below.

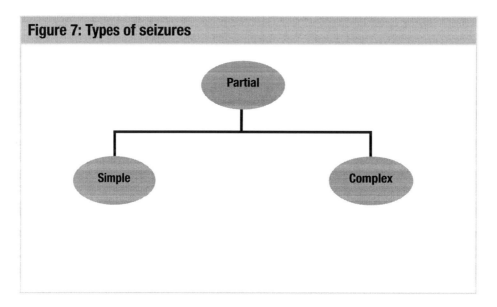

Figure 7: Types of seizures

Different parts of the brain control different functions, so symptoms that are displayed during both simple and complex partial seizures depend on the area of the brain where the epileptic activity begins. **Table 5** below summarises different areas of the brain and the symptoms displayed during seizures that begin in specific areas of the brain.

Table 5: Symptoms of seizures	
Area of the brain	**Common symptoms**
Temporal lobe	Flushing/sweating and going very pale. Feelings of fear or happiness, or feeling detached from one's surroundings. Chewing, fumbling with buttons or wandering off.
Frontal lobe	Head may turn to one side, hands and arms may become stiff or drawn upwards. Jerking or trembling movements beginning in the finger then the whole hand or arm. May scream or cry.
Occipital lobe	See flashing lights or balls of light. Experience brief loss of vision.
Parietal lobe	Tingling or warm sensations that run down the arms or legs.

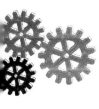

Generalised seizures – These seizures involve epileptic activity which spreads to both halves of the brain. There are a range of different types of generalised seizures, and these are summarised below.

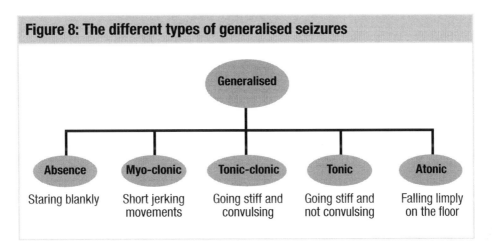

Figure 8: The different types of generalised seizures

In some types of generalised seizures a small part of the brain may not be affected, which means the symptoms displayed are less severe than when the whole brain is affected. For example, in absence seizures individuals do not fall onto the ground as they would during a tonic-clonic seizure. A list of typical symptoms/behaviours displayed by individuals experiencing different types of generalised seizures are summarised in the table below.

Table 6: Different types of presentation of epileptic seizures

Type of generalised seizure	Symptoms
Absence	An individual appears to be daydreaming or switched off.
Myo-clonic	This type of seizure can affect the whole body or individual limbs such as an arm. An individual loses consciousness and experiences jerk movements.
Tonic-clonic	This is the most common type of seizure and involves two phases. During the tonic phase the individual's body muscles contract causing them to lose consciousness and fall to the floor. During the clonic phase the individual's limbs begin to jerk as the muscles tighten and relax, they then slowly begin to regain consciousness.

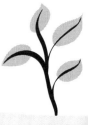

Type of generalised seizure	Symptoms
Tonic	The individual's body muscles tighten causing their body to stiffen and more than often (if their body is not supported) causing them to fall.
Atonic	All muscle tone in the body is lost causing the individual to fall forward, which increases the risk of banging their head.

Treatment

Epilepsy has no cure but can be controlled through a range of treatments such as the following.

Anti-epileptic drugs (AEDs) – This is the most common form of treatment for epilepsy and has been found to control seizures in seven out of 10 people who take the medication for the condition (BNF, 2010). The aim of AEDs is to prevent seizures by controlling the excitability (excess electrical impulses) in the brain.

The doctor will usually decide what drug is best for the individual depending on the type of seizures they have. It is preferred that only one type of drug is taken. However, if the seizures continue more than one drug may be used. Many AEDs have side effects and the time it takes for them to control seizures varies from person to person. Some of the most common AEDs include penytoin, sodium valporate and clonazepam.

Surgery – If an individual's epilepsy is so severe that it cannot be controlled by medication, they have the option of undergoing brain surgery. However, this option is only available to those whose epilepsy is the result of damaged tissue in a specific area of the brain.

Although a range of surgeries are available the most common one involves removing a small area of the brain that is responsible for the seizures; the more tissue that is removed the greater the risk for the patient. Surgery may or may not have an effect on the number of seizures an individual has.

Vagus nerve stimulation – This only tends to be used when medicines have failed to control seizures and brain surgery is not an option. Around 43,000 people worldwide have undergone this procedure (Epilepsy Action, 2010) and it involves an electrical device being implanted under the skin

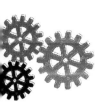

below the left collar bone. This is connected to a lead with coils and the coils are wrapped around the vagus nerve, which is in the neck. The electrical device is programmed to be stimulated at set times and it sends impulses from the vagus nerve in the neck to the brain.

Ketogenic diet – This is a carefully designed diet which consists of high levels of fat, sufficient protein and low carbohydrates to control seizures. This diet is most often used with children whose epilepsy has been found difficult to control using medication.

The diet mimics the effects of starvation. Normally the body converts carbohydrates into glucose which fuels the brain, however, when there is little carbohydrate (as in this diet) the liver converts fat into fatty acids and ketone bodies. The ketone bodies pass into the brain providing it with energy, and replacing the effects of glucose. It has been found that higher levels of ketone bodies in the blood reduces the number of epileptic seizures.

Complementary therapies – Some individuals find that complementary therapies help to control their condition and these health-related therapies fall outside conventional medical practice, therefore it is highly recommended that such treatment be used with AEDs. Common alternative therapies include acupuncture, homeopathy, herbal treatments, biofeedback and aromatherapy.

Aromatherapy involves using aromatic oils that have been taken from plants and include lavender, rosemary and sage. Research from Queen Elizabeth Hospital suggests that they can help to control epilepsy especially in individuals that experience warning signs before the onset of a seizure. The oils have been found to reduce the severity or the risk of having a seizure (Epilepsy Action, 2010).

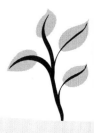

Case study 4

Sara was a 26-year-old professional who had been knocked off her bicycle by a car while she cycled to work. When she fell to the ground her head hit the pavement with great force, causing her to lose consciousness. When she was admitted to hospital doctors discovered that a small blood clot had developed in her brain and drugs were administered to disperse it. After six weeks Sara had made a good recovery and was discharged from hospital. She was told to continue a course of anti-epileptic drugs (AEDs) that she had been on since her injury to reduce her chances of having seizures. Three months later Sara was sitting at her desk talking to a colleague when she began to stare at her blankly before she fell to the floor. She lost consciousness and her limbs began to jerk, and it later became apparent that she suffered a tonic-clonic seizure. When Sara saw the doctor she was prescribed some AEDs, however, four months later she had suffered another three seizures. The doctor then changed Sara's medication and she has been seizure free for a year.

Case study 5

Jim has been suffering from seizures since he was 15 years old and the doctors put him on AEDs with the hope that his condition could be controlled. However, three years after his first seizure Jim's condition became worse and at times he had up to 15 seizures in a day. The AEDs he had been taking were frequently changed, however this had no affect on the number of seizures he experienced. The doctor became increasingly concerned about Jim as he became withdrawn from the outside world and the condition was heavily affecting his quality of life. After conducting some tests the doctor found that Jim's epileptic activity always started in his temporal lobes and Jim was told that he may be eligible for surgery to remove part of the temporal lobes where his epileptic activity usually starts from. Six months later, Jim went through with the surgery and it has dramatically reduced the number of seizures he experiences, in fact over the last year Jim has had no seizures.

Huntington's disease

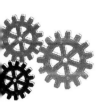

What is Huntington's disease?

Huntington's disease is a hereditary disease that affects the central nervous system, especially the basal ganglia (see chapter 2). Usually developing in adulthood although not exclusively, it can cause a wide variety of problems associated with our movement, communication, behaviour and cognitive skills.

Huntington's disease is an inherited illness caused by a faulty gene on chromosome 4 (a chromosome is genetic material made of protein which transfer certain traits from one generation to the next generation eg. eye colour). This gene produces the protein Huntington, a protein whose full purpose is currently unknown, but we know that it is essential for development as its absence causes death in animal studies. This gene is larger in those who have Huntington's disease, which in turn produces a larger version of this protein. This abnormal protein interacts with cells in the brain causing them to reduce functioning and eventually die, and the mechanisms behind why this is caused are still unclear and are being researched. **Figure 9** below shows the genetic possibilities if one parent is a carrier of the affected Huntington's gene, and there is a 50% probability of inheritance.

Figure 9: The genetic possibilities if one parent is a carrier of the affected Huntington's gene

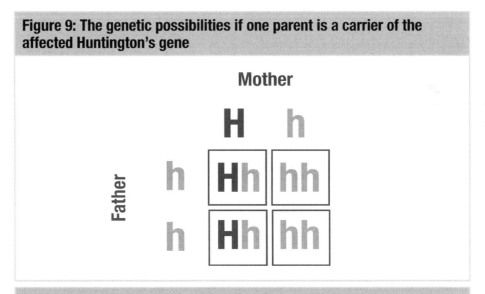

Figure 10: The genetic possibilities of inheriting Huntington's gene if both parents are a carrier

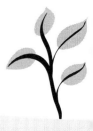

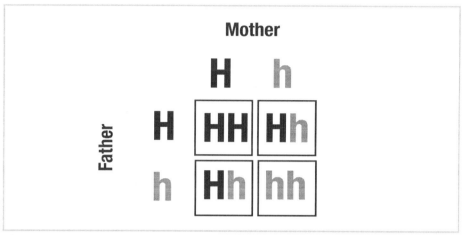

If both parents are a carrier of the affected Huntington's gene then there is a 75% probability of inheritance.

Prevalence

Huntington's disease affects approximately five to eight people per 100,000 in western countries. Whilst it can occur at almost any age, most people will develop problems between the ages of 35 and 55 years.

Disease progression

Early symptoms of the disease include small, uncontrollable movements (which may be misinterpreted as clumsiness), lack of concentration, short-term memory lapses, depression and sudden changes of mood, which may include aggressive behaviour. This can put great strain on relationships, especially in the early stages of the illness in which the diagnosis may be unknown.

Later on in the development of the disease symptoms become more serious, with patients experiencing a multitude of effects. These may include more severe involuntary movements, increasing difficulty in swallowing and speaking and increasing weight loss. There are also a wide range of psychological issues which become more prevalent as it progresses, with emotional problems that result in the continuation of mood swings and depression. Cognitive changes also occur, which results in difficulties relating to memory, concentration and a loss of initiation and organisational skills which may give the impression of laziness. **Table 7**

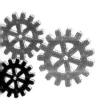

shows a list of typical symptoms below.

Table 7: Typical symptoms	
Symptom	**Sensation**
Movement disorder	Huntington's disease affects movement with early stages of the disease showing slight, uncontrollable movements, which become worse as the disease progresses.
Language	Usually know what they want to say, but due to poor muscle control they are often unable to effectively state what they want.
Executive skills	They by and large know what they would like to do but as the disease progresses they are less able to put these actions into action (which may be interpreted as laziness).
Memory	Learning and memory difficulties are a common complaint in Huntington's disease patients especially as it progresses, which can add to confusion.
Attention	Patients with Huntington's disease perform worse when having to divide their attention between tasks or shift attention, which can increase their frustrations.
Mood	Huntington's disease patients are liable to experience mood swings, with alternating periods of anger and depression, and may not be emotionally responsive to other members of their family. This is often added to by confusion from deficits in the areas covered above.
Sexual problems	Those with Huntington's disease may experience problems with sexual relationships, either through loss of interest or often making inappropriate remarks.
Eating/swallowing	As the disease progresses, those with the disease often lose weight, often finding eating tiring and frustrating due to lack of control. This can also lead to swallowing problems, which can increase the risk of choking.

Treatment

There is currently no cure for the progression of Huntington's disease, and current therapies are aimed at managing its symptoms. Drugs are used to alleviate the involuntary movement disturbances, as well as the psychiatric problems such as mood swings and depression. The problems associated with speech and swallowing can be managed with speech

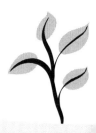

and language therapy, and a high calorie diet is used to try and prevent the weight loss associated with the disease. In helping to control the movement disorders associated with Huntington's disease, medications reduce the amount of dopamine affecting the nerves in the brain, reducing these involuntary movements.

Those who wish to have children and would like to have them free of risk have the option of some complex genetic testing, using pre-implantation genetic diagnosis (PGD – also known as embryo screening). PGD requires the parents to have in-vitro fertilisation (IVF) treatment, the embryo of which is then genetically tested to see whether or not it has the faulty gene, and will only be placed in the womb if this is not the case.

Case study 6

Martin was a 55-year-old man who had been diagnosed with Huntington's disease 10 years ago after he began to suffer from small movement ticks, which he felt he had no control over. During this time he had been supported and cared for by his wife, although their relationship had become strained. He often had alternating periods of aggression, depression and apathy, all of which were taken out on his wife. His memory was also affected, which meant he became easily confused and this often triggered mood swings because he was frustrated. His movement problems had also worsened with him often flicking his limbs out which had become dangerous for himself and those around him. He had also lost a lot of weight because eating had become difficult with the muscles in his mouth no longer working effectively.

Multiple sclerosis

What is multiple sclerosis?

Multiple sclerosis (MS) is the central nervous system that consists of the brain and the spinal cord and linked through a complex array of neurons it forms the body's communication network (as shown in **figure 11** below).

Figure 11: Major nerve pathways of the body

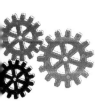

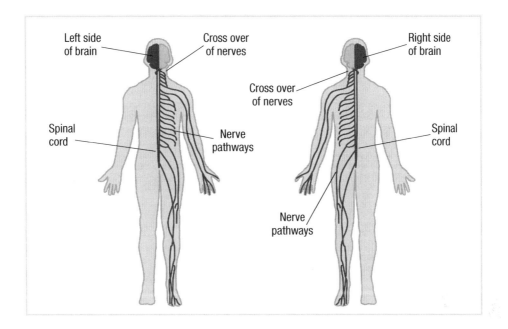

The brain acts as a command centre and controls bodily functions such as movement and emotions. The spinal cord is the central message pathway and it is made up of bundles of nerves that send messages (via electrical impulses) from the brain to the rest of the body, controlling conscious and unconscious behaviours. The structure of neurons can be seen below in **figure 12**.

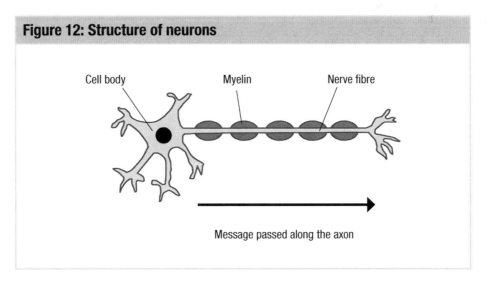

Figure 12: Structure of neurons

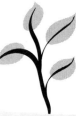

As shown in **figure 12**, nerve fibres are protected by a substance called myelin. Myelin is a fatty layer that allows messages to be transmitted quickly and smoothly between the brain and the rest of the body.

MS is an autoimmune disease, which means that the immune system mistakes healthy tissues as foreign bodies (such as infectious bacteria) and attacks it. In MS, the immune system attacks the myelin sheath around the nerves in the brain and spinal cord, and this process is called 'demyelination'.

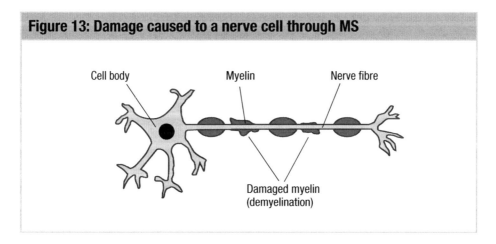

Figure 13: Damage caused to a nerve cell through MS

Cell body · Myelin · Nerve fibre

Damaged myelin (demyelination)

Demyelination, either partially or completely, damages the myelin leaving scars. This damage disrupts the flow of messages along nerve fibres and so they can become slower, distorted or do not get through at all. As these nerves are linked to different areas of the body, the symptoms that appear depend on the role of the damaged nerve.

To put it in a simpler way, imagine the brain as a power source and the rest of the body as electric goods such as fridges, lights or TVs. Your nerves link the power from the brain to the electrical appliances, they are like wires that are surrounded by a protective layer of plastic (ie. the nerves are coated with myelin). If the plastic is damaged in any way it may cause a problem within the circuit so that the appliance may not function properly (MS Society, 2010).

Prevalence

Multiple sclerosis (MS) is the most common disabling disease in young adults, affecting approximately 100,000 people in the UK. It is most often diagnosed between the ages of 20–40 and is two to three times more likely to develop in women than men. MS is both a chronic and highly unpredictable condition where the immune system attacks itself (MS Society, 2010).

Disease progression

It is not usually possible to determine the type of MS an individual has when they are diagnosed and this only becomes evident over time. There are four main types of MS as follows.

Benign
▶ Some patients that suffer from relapsing remitting MS find that 10–20 years after diagnosis their condition has not worsened and they do not develop secondary progressive MS.

▶ These individuals are known to have 'benign MS'.

▶ They tend to make good recoveries during remission and don't acquire significant disability.

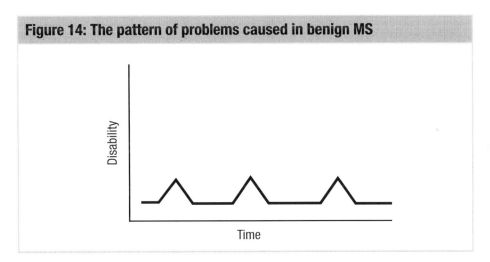

Figure 14: The pattern of problems caused in benign MS

Relapsing/remitting
▶ For most individuals this is the way in which their MS begins.

▶ Symptoms appear (a relapse) and then improve partially or completely (remission).

▶ A relapse (an attack or occurrence of old or new symptoms lasting more than 24 hours) can be mild or severe and last anywhere from a few days to a few months.

▶ Periods of remission (when symptoms become less severe or disappear)

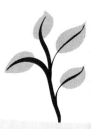

can also vary from a few days to a few months.

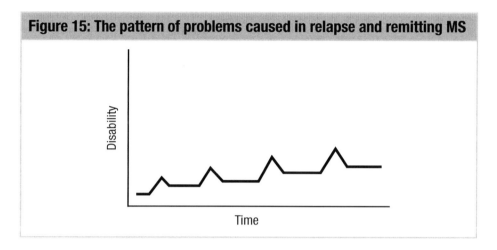

Figure 15: The pattern of problems caused in relapse and remitting MS

Secondary progressive

▶ Most individuals who have suffered from relapsing/remitting MS eventually develop secondary progressive.

▶ Approximately 65% of relapsing/remitting patients develop secondary progressive 15 years after diagnosis.

▶ Individuals experience a progressive increase in their symptoms, where the severity and occurrence of relapse decreases, but the level of disability increases.

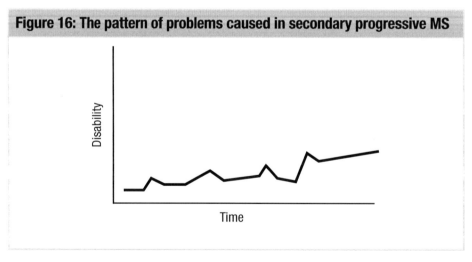

Figure 16: The pattern of problems caused in secondary progressive MS

Primary progressive

▶ Affects about 10–15% of MS patients.

▶ Symptoms are slow but persistent and become progressively worse.

▶ Approximately 85% of these individuals develop walking difficulties.

▶ MS related lesions are more frequently seen in the spinal cord than in the brain.

Figure 17: The pattern of problems caused in primary MS

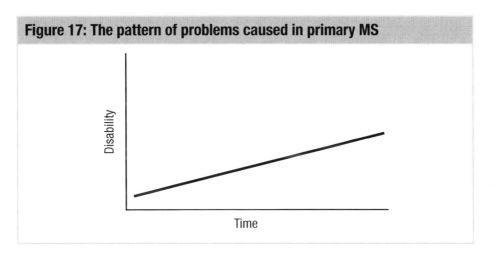

Due to the unpredictable nature of MS it is impossible to say how the condition will develop over time and it is different for everyone. A list of typical symptoms can be seen in the table below.

Table 8: Presentation of an MS sufferer with moderate symptoms

Symptom	Sensation
Fatigue	An overwhelming sense of tiredness making physical or mental activities overwhelming. One of the most common symptoms experienced.
Dizziness or loss of balance	Individuals may lose their balance and therefore need to take more care when moving. They may experience 'vertigo' a sensation where they feel dizzy, as though the world is spinning.
Visual problems	May begin to experience double or blurred vision, or loss of sight in one eye or both.
Numbness	Tingling sensation in limbs, almost like pins and needles which can come and go in short bursts or last longer.
Symptom	Sensation
Bladder problems	Loss of ability to feel if their bladder is empty or they may see an increase in frequency in the need to urinate.

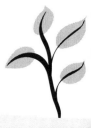

Mood changes	Individuals may find their mood and emotions change rapidly; they may experience feelings of depression.
Speech problems	Speech may become slower or slurred; one's voice may start to weaken with difficulty in controlling pitch.
Tremor	Most likely to affect individual's arms and hands but can also affect their legs or head. It can also affect everyday activities, making it difficult to eat, dress or co-ordinate movements.
Cognitive problems	Individuals may experience problems with concentration, problem-solving, learning and memory.

Treatment

Disease modifying drugs – These are usually prescribed to reduce the number and severity of relapses in relapsing/remitting MS and they are occasionally prescribed in secondary progressive MS (if relapses still occur). These drugs tend to be injected under the skin or into a muscle, depending on the drug that is prescribed.

An example of such a drug is Natalizumab, which prevents white blood cells crossing the blood brain barrier and entering the spinal cord and brain, which in MS causes inflammation and damage. This drug has shown to be very effective with an average of 67% of MS sufferers seeing a reduction in relapses over two years (MS Society, 2010).

Symptom relieving drugs – These drugs used to treat symptoms are widely available with some being more responsive to symptoms than others. Drugs are often prescribed to treat symptoms such as bladder weakness, muscle spasms, aches and pain.

An example of such a drug is Sativex, which is an oral spray that contains cannabis and is administered under the tongue or inside the cheeks. Clinical trials have shown that it helps relieve symptoms such as bladder problems, nerve pain and muscle spasms.

Alternative therapies – It is estimated that around 50–75% of MS sufferers use alternative therapies for relieving symptoms or improving their overall well-being. These health-related therapies outside of conventional medical practice include aromatherapy, homeopathy, acupuncture, herbal remedies and reflexology.

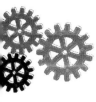

An example of how alternative therapy can be used is an MS sufferer who takes herbal medicine, such as cranberry to prevent urinary tract infections and psyllium for constipation. Some studies have reported the beneficial effects of using such alternative therapies in relieving certain symptoms (MS Society, 2010).

Case study 7

Sarah was a 29-year-old professional who had started to experience visual blackouts which left her with tunnel vision for up to a few hours. As a frequent migraine sufferer she ignored the symptoms and soon she noticed that sometimes she felt unsteady on her feet and had tingling sensations in her right hand. Her symptoms would come and go, often affecting her mood and leaving her tired and unable to complete her daily activities. One evening she went to dinner with her husband, when leaving she stumbled and fell hitting her head on the floor. Despite telling her husband that this might be due to drinking too much wine, she was taken to the hospital for a check up and there it was revealed that her symptoms were the result of multiple sclerosis.

Case study 8

John had been diagnosed with MS at the age of 27, having lived with the condition for the past 20 years he often experienced periods of relapse (onset of symptoms) and remissions. However, recently John found that his symptoms, such as the numbness he often experienced in his legs, were getting progressively worse and often when he went for walks he found it very difficult to lift his legs and they felt numb when he touched them. He also began to notice that he regularly forgot things which resulted in him leaving the gas on, revisiting the shops and buying things twice. His bladder problems became worse and the frequency in which he needed to urinate increased. As a result of his bladder problems John developed a urinary tract infection causing him to be hospitalised. It was in hospital that the doctor told John he had developed primary progressive MS.

Motor neuron disease

What is motor neuron disease (MND)?

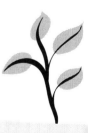

Motor neuron disease (MND) is a progressive degenerative disease that attacks the motor neurons of the upper and lower body. This degeneration leads to a weakness and wasting away of the muscles, causing loss of mobility in the limbs and a range of difficulties including speech, swallowing and breathing. There are four main types of MND with each one having its own specific affects on those who have it (Motor Neuron Disease Association, 2010).

Amyotrophic lateral sclerosis (ALS)

This is the most common form of MND, and involves the degeneration of both upper and lower motor neuron involvement. The main characteristics of this subset of the disease are weakness and wasting in the limbs (atrophy), followed by twitching, cramping or stiffness in the muscles that are affected. The average life expectancy in this type of MND is between two and five years from the onset of the illness.

Progressive bulbar palsy (PBP)

This form of MND can affect up to a quarter of those diagnosed with the disease and involves the degeneration of both the upper and lower motor neurons, and symptoms include difficulty swallowing and slurring of speech. Life expectancy is between six months and three years from the onset of symptoms.

Progressive muscular atrophy

This form of MND is much rarer, affecting only a small proportion of people, mainly causing damage to the lower motor neurons. Early symptoms of this type of MND can be mistaken for clumsiness and weakness of the hands and most of those diagnosed with this type of MND live on for more than five years after diagnosis.

Primary lateral sclerosis

This is the rarest form of MND, only attacking the upper motor neurons, resulting in weakness of the lower limbs, although people also experience speech and hand problems. Life span is generally unaffected in this type of MND although it may result in a limiting of what the person is able to do.

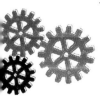

Prevalence

MND can affect all individuals at any ages, but it is most common in people over 40, with the highest occurrence in 50–70 year olds; it is almost twice as common in men. It is estimated that at any one time seven out of 100,000 people are living with MND and that two out of 100,000 people will be diagnosed every year. The prevalence of MND is rising, perhaps due to the fact that people are living longer and diagnostic tests are more accurate.

Disease process

Unfortunately, once diagnosed with MND there is certain to be a steady decline in the patient's condition. The progression of MND is often measured in terms of the severity and number of difficulties a patient is suffering from. **Table 9** below provides a range of presentations of people with MS.

Table 9: Presentation of MS sufferer with severe MS symptoms	
Symptom	**Sensation**
Pain	This is not caused directly by MND but is often an indirect symptom.
Muscle cramps and spasms	This can often be eased by changing position regularly.
Stiff joints	Gentle exercise can help stiff joints.
Incontinence	Occurs especially when there are difficulties with mobility and you cannot reach the toilet.
Bowel problems	Constipation is common due to poor mobility and dietary changes.
Saliva and mucous	May have excess saliva if swallowing becomes difficult, or it may become thick and sticky.
Coughing/choking	May occur when saliva or food becomes stuck in the airway.
Breathing	Eventually the muscles used to breathe may become affected.
Symptom	**Sensation**
Cognitive changes	Only 20% experience difficulty including memory, learning, language and concentration difficulties or personality changes, which may range from mild to severe. There is often no cognitive impairment in MND.
Dementia	10% are diagnosed with dementia.

All cases are individual and people can live between a few months and 30

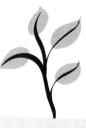

years when diagnosed with MND. The average life expectancy is between two–five years after the onset of symptoms and 40% live for five years and 8–16 % live for 10 years.

Treatment

Motor neuron disease currently has no cure, and treatment options are based around slowing the progression of the disease and managing the symptoms and discomfort associated with it. Issues surrounding respiratory and swallowing difficulties are addressed medically, using breathing equipment and alternative methods of feeding the patient. The main medication used with motor neuron disease is called Riluzole, which reduces the amount of the neurotransmitter glutamate in the body and can slow the progression of the disease. Communication difficulties do occur in people with motor neuron disease, and specialist intervention from a speech and language therapist can help to teach a number of techniques to either improve vocalisations or to introduce the use of communication aids (such as alphabet charts).

Emotional issues such as depression and anxiety can be addressed using medications designed to alleviate the symptoms involved in these. Alternatively, therapy input from mental health professionals such as clinical psychologists can help with these issues.

Case study 9

John initially felt that he was becoming increasingly clumsy in that he would drop things more often and trip over things. He worked as a carpenter and became aware that he was having difficulties in co-ordinating his movement to produce fine cuts and joints, which resulted in his bosses criticising the quality of his work. It was at this stage that he decided to visit his GP who referred him on to a neurologist who made the diagnosis.

Parkinson's disease

What is Parkinson's disease?

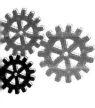

Parkinson's disease is a progressive neurological condition that affects the way in which an individual co-ordinates bodily movements. These difficulties include walking, talking and writing, or anything that requires muscle movement. It has been suggested that Parkinson's disease is caused by a deficiency in a brain chemical called dopamine because the parts of the brain that produce this chemical die. Dopamine is the chemical that allows messages to be carried to the brain to co-ordinate movement. This loss of brain cells and in turn the lack of dopamine causes the slowness in movement, which is experienced by Parkinson's disease. However, it is not the actual disease that causes people to die, it is the fact that their symptoms become worse over time. There has not yet been any discovery as to why people get Parkinson's disease and no cure has been discovered, however, there are many management strategies to help people cope as best as possible.

Prevalence

Parkinson's disease affects one in every 500 people, and that is 120,000 people in the UK alone. Statistics have shown that although both men and women can get the disease, more men are diagnosed with the disease than women, however, as of yet there is not scientific reason behind this coincidence. As we age, the likelihood of being diagnosed with Parkinson's disease increases as symptoms usually appear after 50 years of age. Though this is the usual case there are on some occasions when the disease becomes prevalent in individuals between the ages of 21 to 40, which is also known as young onset Parkinson's. On the very rare occasions and this only occurs to every one in 10,000 people, individuals are diagnosed under the age of 18, and this is referred to as juvenile Parkinson's. As discussed previously, the major cause of Parkinson's disease is this lack of dopamine being produced, which causes the symptoms of the disease. However, there have been suggestions into other causes such as genetic and environmental factors but they occur in very rare cases.

Disease progression

Parkinson's disease progression tends to be slow and gradual and symptoms appear over a period of time and in no particular order. Every individual case is different and symptoms vary greatly between individuals and people may experience more or fewer symptoms. As Parkinson's disease is very slow to develop, the earliest symptoms may be slight symptoms of feeling tired or weaker than normal. As more and more nerve cells die, less dopamine is produced causing symptoms to further develop and new

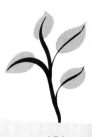

symptoms to appear as time goes on. As symptoms vary from person to person it may take a long time for the symptoms of Parkinson's disease to actually cause any problems. With the advanced treatment now available, research has shown that the life expectancy of individuals with the disease is only just below normal life expectancy. This is different to more rapid progressing neurological conditions such as Huntington's disease. There are many symptoms for Parkinson's disease and there is no specific order in which they occur as each individual case is different. However, the main three symptoms are bradykinesia, tremors and rigidity.

Table 10: Symptoms which may be present with someone who suffers from Parkinson's disease	
Bradykinesia	Bradykinesia is also known as slowness in movement. Those who have Parkinson's disease find that their movement becomes slow and everyday tasks such as getting out of a chair become very difficult. Some people will have bradykinesia in the way they walk and will tend to walk with a shuffle.
Tremor	Tremors also known as shaking are rhythmical movements that cannot be controlled by the individual. Tremors occur when an individual's muscles are at rest and the person is not doing anything. A tremor can usually improve as the individual starts to engage in activity using the affected limb. It also usually gets worse when the individual is stressed or anxious.
Rigidity	Rigidity also known as stiffness is where the muscles tighten up and the muscles feel tense. This can cause an individual cramps and can also be very painful as there is an inflexibility in movement. Individuals may find it difficult to swing their arms while walking as Parkinson's prevents the muscles stretching and relaxing.
Other	Other symptoms include incontinence and constipation, swallowing and saliva control which comes about because of the slowness in muscle movement, falls and dizziness. Another profound symptom which almost 50% of Parkinson's disease suffers experience is speech difficulty.

Treatment

As there is no current cure for Parkinson's disease the best way of managing it is through treatments to help control the symptoms as best as possible. The most common treatment is drug therapy, however, there are a number of other therapies that can make living with Parkinson's easier.

Drug therapy

There are a number of different drugs used to manage the symptoms of Parkinson's disease and each individual will react differently to different drugs meaning that a medication regime needs to be tailored to their own individual needs.

The main drugs fall into levodopa, dopamine agonists and monomine oxidase-B inhibitors and these are expanded upon below.

Levodopa – this medication is absorbed by the nerve cells in the brain and turn into dopamine. It can be a very effective drug at first instance, however, its effectiveness can be reduced over time due to the nerve cells in the brain dying and causing absorption to become difficult.

Dopamine agonists – these work by locking onto the dopamine receptors in the brain and act like a dopamine substitute. These are usually used in co-ordination with levodopa as a top-up drug.

Monomine oxidase-B inhibitors – this is another alternative medication and works by blocking the chemical called monomine oxidase-B, which prevents the breakdown of dopamine.

Other therapies

Other therapies include physiotherapy, speech and language therapy and occupational therapy.

Physiotherapy – physiotherapists are able to give advice on exercises that can help movement and make moving a lot easier. They can help to manage stiffness, restore muscle strength and help with muscle pain.

Speech and language therapy – as previously discussed over half of people with Parkinson's suffer with some kind of problem with communication and also swallowing. A speech therapist can give out exercises, advice and equipment, which can be used to help manage and improve speech and swallowing.

Occupational therapy – an occupational therapist works with people to help them attain their maximum functional ability and reach as much independence as possible. They can help with advice and equipment for activities of daily living such as getting in and out of the bath, making a cup of tea or getting dressed. They can provide adaptations and equipment for

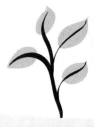

an individual to be able to manage in the home and outside.

> ### Case study 10
> Joe is a 52-year-old salesman who suddenly found walking more difficult and complained that it felt like he was trying to walk through water all the time. He also became aware that when he was driving his reaction times were slower and so he started to drive more slowly to compensate for his reduced reaction speed. As a result, his wife became very critical of his driving, which caused him to become very frustrated, and adding to his wife's irritation was the fact that he was becoming more forgetful especially of important dates and he would constantly lose his train of thought when talking to her.

Traumatic brain injury

What is traumatic brain injury?

There are two main types of brain injury.

1. Traumatic brain injury (TBI) is when a brain injury is caused by a sudden severe force being applied to the brain ie. your head hitting the windscreen in a road traffic accident, being hit or kicked in the face or accidents at home, eg. falling down the stairs etc.

2. Acquired brain injury (ABI) is a brain injury which develops gradually over time, ie. strokes such as brain bleeds, brain infections, brain tumours or strokes due to lack of oxygen to the brain.

Traumatic brain injuries have a number of stages.

The first stage
This can be different for different people depending on the type of injury.

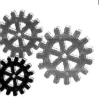

▶ **Closed head injuries** – this is where the skull is not broken and the brain is violently shaken because of, for example, rapid acceleration or deceleration forces such as when a car stops suddenly because it hits a wall at speed. This causes the nerve fibers throughout the brain to twist, stretch and tear, and this is known as diffuse brain injury. The violent shaking may also cause the brain's arteries and veins to leak reducing the oxygen supply to the brain.

▶ **Open or penetrating wounds** – this is where the skull is broken and the brain is exposed to the atmosphere.

▶ **Crushing injuries** – this is where the head is squeezed between two objects which may cause the skull to crack and nerves to be damaged.

Second stage
This is related to the secondary consequences of the trauma.

▶ The individual's breathing may be disrupted or there may be damage to their blood vessels supplying the brain with oxygen. This may result in the oxygen supply to the brain being reduced causing damage.

▶ There may be bruising and bleeding within the brain causing swelling, blood clots, pressure build up etc.

▶ Nerve damage causes neuro-transmitters (brain chemicals) to be released on mass causing cells to over stimulate and die.

▶ Brain cells die due to the impact forces and this is permanent brain damage.

Third stage
Initial treatment, for example, paramedics trying and stabilise the injured person's injuries and getting them to hospital as soon as possible.

Fourth stage
These treatments are usually undertaken when the injured person arrives at the accident and emergency unit. This is where further treatment is given to try and stabilise the patient if necessary and then to try and provide treatments to prevent further damage. This is usually undertaken in acute hospitals where fractures of bones are treated and bleeds into the brain may be treated to prevent further damage.

Fifth stage
Maybe undertaken if the patient is admitted to a rehabilitation hospital or unit, however, not all patients will receive rehabilitation. Rehabilitation focuses on trying to help the patient regain old skills ie. physiotherapy input to help someone to walk again or neuro-psychology input to help a patient's memory to recover. This may also include the teaching of

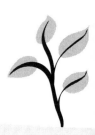

compensation techniques to overcome difficulties, which will not naturally recover, for example to overcome the permanent brain damage.

Sixth stage
To be returned to the community to try and be part of their families again and possibly return to previous social, leisure and occupational activities.

The severity of a TBI varies greatly on the following.

Minor brain injury

A minor TBI can occur from a small knock to the head and may result in a state of unconsciousness for a short time or post-concussion syndrome which includes minor symptoms such as dizziness, nausea, headaches, lack of concentration or memory, tiredness, an avoidance of light or noise, perhaps even anxiety or depression. Individuals can often be misdiagnosed or misunderstood as usually no scans are taken immediately after the incident and any subsequent scans do not show damage to the brain. It is important that friends and family understand the condition and act accordingly, for example keeping stress levels low and avoiding returning to work too soon especially at a mentally demanding job. A full recovery is usually made within three–four months, however a small minority of patients may never fully recover from this injury and it causes life-long difficulties. It is important that the individual is aware of any problems associated with their injuries and as a consequence adapt their life until they hopefully recover. This may involve not returning to work too soon after the injury, for example due to suffering a 'concussional injury'.

Moderate brain injury

This is when an individual remains unconscious after the initial injury for a few minutes up to six hours. As a result, an individual may have post-traumatic amnesia (an inability to learn new information and can be quite confused) for up to 24 hours. Symptoms experienced may be similar to those who have suffered a minor injury but can also include poor attention span, difficulty with sustained attention, slurred speech, loss of co-ordination and social agitation. Patients are also likely to suffer from cognitive difficulties, emotional and behavioural difficulties such as irritability. As a consequence, an individual's recovery time is longer, as the symptoms have a greater impact on their everyday functioning than that in minor brain injuries. They may be observed in hospital overnight before being discharged. It is important to be aware that a patient's symptoms may remain for up to nine months as they may become anxious, which can cause an exacerbation of their symptoms. In the early stages individuals often have difficulties returning to work and feel they are not functioning at their best.

Severe brain injury

In this case the individual remains unconscious for more that six hours and experiences post-traumatic amnesia for more than 24 hours. Patients are usually hospitalised and usually undergo intensive rehabilitation once they are able to. Their symptoms are usually much more severe. Usually the longer a patient is in a coma (in a reduced consciousness or unresponsive level) the poorer the recovery; however, this is not always the case.

The Glasgow coma scale is used in hospitals to monitor the level of unconsciousness by rating the patient's motor responses, their verbal responses and their ability to open their eyes. The scores range from 3–15 where individuals with more severe head injuries score lower.

Patients come out of a coma gradually, first by opening their eyes and then by slowly beginning to respond. A coma is often distressing for relatives but they are often advised by professionals to talk to the person in a coma even if they cannot respond. Coma arousal programmes may also be of benefit during periods of arousal and when rest is undertaken by the patient.

A very small number of people (usually less than 100 people at any given time) may be in a persistent vegetative state in which they remain unconscious for months or even years. They can breathe without mechanical assistance and show sleep-waking cycles but cannot speak or follow instructions. They usually score below 9 on the Glasgow coma scale, which may be diagnosed as irreversible after a period of 12 months.

Prevalence

One million people in the United Kingdom attend hospital every year as a result of a head injury. Every year out of 100,000 people:

▶ 10 to 15 people are likely to suffer a severe head injury

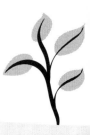

- ▶ 10 to 20 from a moderate head injury

- ▶ 250 to 300 with a mild head injury.

There are between 100–150 survivors per 100,000 of the population at any one time or more than 120,000 people in the UK suffering from long-term effects of a traumatic brain injury. Those figures are growing every year as those affected tend to be young and have a normal life expectancy. The age groups more at risk are 15–29 and over 65 years of age. Males are two to three times more likely to have a brain injury than females and in the age range of 15–29 males are five times more likely to suffer from TBI.

- ▶ 40–50% of all injuries, especially severe ones are due to road traffic accidents.

- ▶ 20–30% happens during domestic and industrial accidents.

- ▶ 10–15% during sports and recreational injuries.

- ▶ Assaults account for 10% of brain injuries.

- ▶ Cycling injuries account for approximately 20% of injuries in children but 85% of the risk can be reduced by wearing a helmet.

One family in 300 will be affected by a relative suffering a severe brain injury, however, 90% of people suffering from severe brain injuries make a good physical recovery. It is usually the cognitive difficulties such as having a poor memory, which causes the biggest difficulties over time. As the injury occurs within the brain and is not visible to people, this is called a hidden disability.

Presentation

The symptoms suffered will depend on the type, location and severity of the brain injury. For example, an acquired brain injury may affect a small localised area, whereas traumatic head injury usually causes more general damage as this damage is caused by forces usually affecting the whole brain. As different areas of the brain undertake different activities or have nerves passing through them to different areas, it often depends on what area of the brain has been injured, as to what symptoms the patient suffers from.

The symptoms can usually be broken down into the following.

Type	Symptoms
Cognitive	This can include: memory, reasoning skills, concentration, problem-solving and language.
Emotional and behavioural	This includes temper and mood swings, changes in emotional reactions and it can be difficult to stop. It may also be hard to cope with friends and family.
Physical	Problems with walking, co-ordination. Usually patients make a full physical recovery, although any physical problems can have a large impact on daily life.

The brain is connected to the spinal cord via the brain stem and consists of the brain stem, cerebellum and cerebral cortex (see **figure 18**).

The cerebral cortex has two hemispheres (the left and right) which join in the middle; the left hemisphere controls the right side of the body and vice versa. As a rule, the left hemisphere usually controls speech, whilst the right controls non-language, spatial and artistic skills.

Figure 18

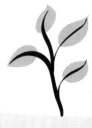

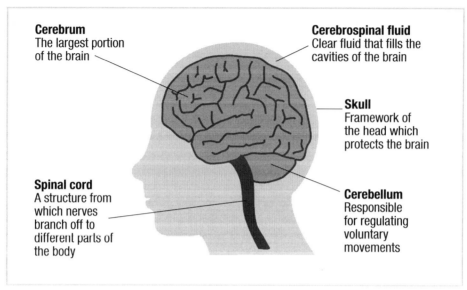

Cerebrum
The largest portion
of the brain

Cerebrospinal fluid
Clear fluid that fills the
cavities of the brain

Skull
Framework of
the head which
protects the brain

Spinal cord
A structure from
which nerves
branch off to
different parts of
the body

Cerebellum
Responsible
for regulating
voluntary
movements

(Adapted from Headway: www.headway.org.uk/About-the-brain.aspx)

The cerebral cortex has four main lobes and an injury to each of those has different symptoms accordingly (see also chapter 2).

Injury to...	Sensation
Frontal lobes (front of head)	This will affect executive functions such as planning and decision-making. A person affected by a frontal lobe injury may also have difficulty with their impulsivity, their problem-solving skills and may appear to be easily distractible and more emotional. Their personality may also be affected. The frontal lobes also contains the motor and sensory cortex, damage to these areas may cause loss of movement control and loss of sensation respectively.
Temporal lobes (behind the ear)	This will affect memory functions such as recognition and perception. It will also change a person's understanding and language skills.
Parietal lobes (above and behind the ears)	This will alter perception and sensory information. Knowledge of numbers and their relations and spelling may be impaired. The manipulation of objects and spatial relationships may also be affected.
Injury to...	**Sensation**

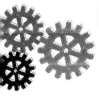

Occipital lobes (back of head)	This will strongly affect vision and may even cause partial or complete blindness. The individual may suffer from visual hallucinations, colour agnosia (where a person does not recognise colours), movement agnosia (where there is no perception of movement), and agraphia (the loss of the ability to write).
Hypothalamus	It is important to note that a TBI may affect more than one area.
Limbic system	Loss of control of appetite regulation, sexual arousal, thirst and temperature, and possibly memory.
Brain stem	Loss of control of emotion causing mood swings.
	Causes loss of consciousness and concussion.

Case study 11

Alice was a 24-year-old student when she fell on her head during a night out and suffered a traumatic brain injury. However, she did not lose consciousness but with the help of her friends went along to the local hospital for a check-up. The doctor who examined her told her she was fine so she carried on with her life as normal. She found, however, that she could not concentrate or remember things as she did before. She was more impulsive in her actions and would go on expensive shopping sprees using her student loan. She became increasingly upset and emotional with her inability to cope and was referred to a clinical psychologist who explained the nature of her brain injury. Alice learned new ways to reduce her stress levels and tried to get more sleep as she usually felt exhausted by the end of the day. She now feels back to her old self.

Case study 12

Steven, a 43-year-old accountant, had taken time off work when he fell down the stairs in his home and hit the front of his head. He was taken to hospital by his wife and was kept overnight for observation but was soon discharged since there were no obvious signs of him being injured. Steven quickly noticed some changes and realised he was not functioning as well as he did before the accident. He often felt tired and dizzy and had difficulty with his thinking. He was always a man who had enjoyed reading his paper but he described how he couldn't finish reading a whole article. His wife reported that he frequently forgot what he was saying in the middle of a sentence or couldn't

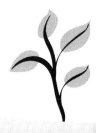

find his words. He often became worried and anxious about simple things like whether he had collected his post or checked his messages and he could rapidly become angry and annoyed. Steven was referred to a counsellor and a neuropsychologist.

Case study 13

Jane was a 30-year-old woman who was knocked off her bicycle by a car on her way to work. She was admitted to the hospital and was kept for a month, three weeks of which she spent in intensive care breathing and being nurtured by tubes. Due to the severity of her brain trauma, Jane was in a coma for the first week which was prolonged by sedation to prevent her from removing her life-supporting tubes. During her time at the hospital a craniotomy was also performed – this is a surgical operation to remove a bone flap from the skull to prevent pressure building up when the swelling of the brain pushes the brain against the skull. Jane was then admitted to a rehabilitation hospital where she received multidisciplinary care, with input from physiotherapists, occupational therapists and neuropsychologists.

Treatments

Firstly, quick medical intervention will try to reduce the extent of the brain injury and will try to prevent the build up of pressure. A lot of patients with a severe brain injury are put on a ventilator to ensure good oxygen supply and medical staff will also monitor the amount of water and salt in the body to reduce fluid in the brain.

After initial medical acute interventions, there is unfortunately no magic cure for repairing a head injury. Recovery is a combination of natural healing and rehabilitation. Rehabilitation can often greatly improve the patient's life.

'Rehabilitation is a process of change through which a brain injured person goes, seeking to regain former skills and to compensate for skills lost. Its aim is always to achieve the optimum levels of physical, cognitive and social competence followed by integration into the most suitable environment.'
(Headway, 2010)

Firstly, the individual will receive formal rehabilitation from professionals but it is very important that once discharged family and carers continue informal rehabilitation to maintain and continue improving their abilities. The most visible progress usually happens in the first six months, but less apparent improvements can continue over five and even 10 years.

Different members of the rehabilitation team can suggest exercises and strategies to improve patient difficulties.

Physical difficulties (see also chapters 9 and 10) – physiotherapists will usually provide exercise programmes and help the patient practise these to prevent muscle stiffness and improve balance. Speech therapists will help with speech and swallowing problems; medication may be provided for headaches and epilepsy and programmes may be developed to reduce incontinence.

Cognitive difficulties (see also chapters 3, 9 and 10) – external and internal strategies can be used to compensate for memory difficulties and breaking tasks down into stages can help with attentional difficulties. There are also a wide range of strategies that can be practised for executive functioning, such as visuo-spatial processing and language difficulties (see chapter 3).

Emotional and behavioural difficulties (see also chapters 4, 9 and 10) – programmes such as anger management classes may help with anger and irritability problems. Often the patient and family must learn coping strategies to help live with these difficulties. Patients that suffer from a lack of social skills may benefit from social skills training.

Quiz

1. Name the three different types of stroke, and what makes them different from each other?

2. Name some of the cognitive problems that are encountered by people who have had a stroke?

3. List some of the typical symptoms of dementia.

4. What risk factors are there which increase the chance of developing dementia?

5. What methods are used to help people control their epilepsy?

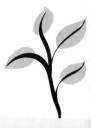

6. What are the probabilities of inheriting Huntington's if (i) one parent is a carrier of the gene (ii) both parents are carriers of the gene?

7. Name some of the symptoms associated with Huntington's disease.

8. What happens to the nerves in a person with multiple sclerosis?

9. What is motor neuron disease, and what part of the body does it affect?

10. Name five of the symptoms associated with motor neuron disease.

11. Parkinson's disease has been suggested to be the result of a deficiency of a particular brain chemical (neurotransmitter), what is this chemical?

12. A part from the use of drugs, what other therapies are used to help manage Parkinson's disease, and what are they used for?

13. What are the factors that determine the severity of a traumatic brain injury?

References

Epilepsy Action (2010) [online]. Available at: www.epilepsy.org.uk (accessed December 2010).

MS Society (2010) [online]. Available at: www.mssociety.org.uk/ (accessed January 2011).

Stroke Association (2010) [online]. Available at: www.stroke.org.uk/ (accessed January 2011).

Further reading

Alzheimer's Society [online]. Available at: www.alzheimers.org.uk/site/scripts/documents.php?categoryID=200120 (accessed December 2010).

AOL Health [online]. Available at: www.aolhealth.com/alzheimers/learn-about-it/how-the-brain-works/a-micro-view-of-the-brain (accessed December 2010).

Aphasia Alliance [online]. Available at: www.aphasiaalliance.org (accessed December 2010).

Appleton R & Marson T (2009) *Epilepsy: The facts*. Oxford: Oxford University Press.

Brooks DW, Taglaiti M, Guten G & Horne J (2007) *Parkinson's Disease for Dummies*. Chichester: John Wiley and Sons.

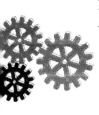

Coyle P (2008) *Living with Progressive MS: Overcoming the challenges.* Demos Medical Publishing: New York.

Department of Health [online]. Available at: www.doh.gov.uk (accessed December 2010).

Downs M & Bower B (2008) *Excellence in Dementia Care: Principles and practice.* Buckingham: Open University Press.

Heads Up [online]. Available at: www.headsup.co.uk (accessed December 2010).

Headway (2010) [online]. Available at: www.headway.org.uk/home.aspx (accessed January 2011).

Huntington's Disease Society [online]. Available at: www.hda.org.uk (accessed December 2010).

Kalb R (2008) *Multiple Sclerosis: The questions you have, the answers you need.* Demos Medical Publishing: New York.

Marler JR (2005) *Stroke for Dummies.* Chichester: John Wiley and Sons.

Motor Neuron Disease Association [online]. Available at: www. mndassociation.org (accessed December 2010).

Motor Neuron Disease Support Forum [online]. Available at: www. alsforums.com (accessed December 2010).

NHS Huntington's Disease [online]. Available at: www.nhs.uk/conditions/ Huntingtons-disease/Pages/Introduction.aspx (accessed December 2010).

NHS Motor Neuron Disease [online]. Available at: www.nhs.uk/conditions/ motor-neuron-disease/Pages/Introduction.aspx (accessed December 2010).

Orientation and Mobility [online]. Available at: www.orientationandmobility. org (accessed December 2010).

Parkinson's Disease Society [online]. Available at: www.parkinsons.org.uk (accessed December 2010).

Powell T (2004) *Head Injury: A practical guide.* London: Speechmark Publishing.

Quarrell OWJ (2008) *Huntington's Disease: The facts.* Oxford: Oxford University Press.

Sandy Sulaiman (2007) *Learning to Live with Huntington's Disease: One family's story.* London: Jessica Kingsley.

Talbot K & Marsden R (2008) *Motor Neuron Disease: The facts.* Oxford: Oxford University Press.

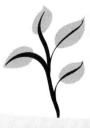

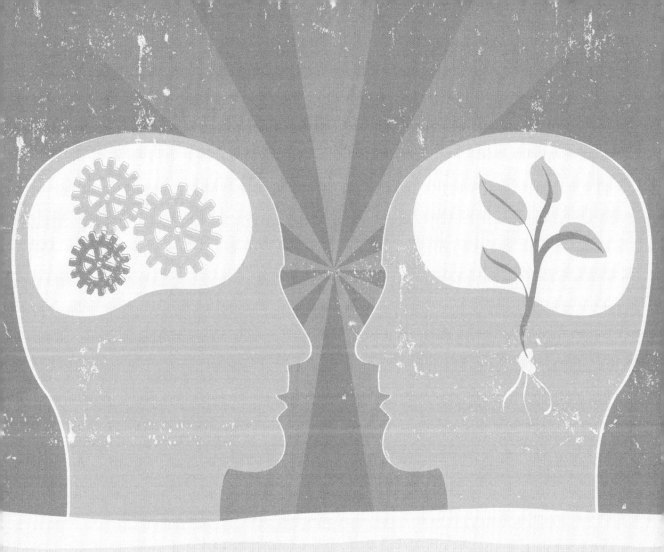

Part 2:
Getting into more detail

Chapter 6

Problems with fatigue and sleep

Nigel Schofield

Aims of the chapter

The chapter aims to:

▶ understand what is meant by fatigue in comparison to normal tiredness

▶ understand why people with neurological conditions are prone to fatigue

▶ look at ways people with neurological conditions can better manage their fatigue levels

▶ understand sleep and wakefulness, and the functions of sleep

▶ understand how neurological conditions can give rise to sleep difficulties

▶ look at practical ways of overcoming sleep problems.

Introduction

Fatigue
Everybody knows what it is like to feel tired, but it is very hard to define what that actually means and to differentiate tiredness from fatigue as the two words are so often used interchangeably. Various researchers have tried to define fatigue when they have been studying its causes and effects on people. They have found that it can have multiple causes, both physical and psychological, and is a component or consequence of many illnesses, and can be a side effect of many treatments. Most often recovery from those physical or psychiatric conditions, or completion of those treatments will lead to fatigue levels reducing but that is not always the case. We also know that fatigue is the primary presenting symptom in chronic fatigue syndrome (also known as myalgic encephalomyelitis) which some theorists think is caused by the body's immune system continuing to react as if the person is ill long after an initial triggering illness has disappeared.

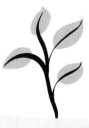

Traditional early medical approaches to fatigue saw it purely in terms of body parts (especially limbs) being, or progressively becoming, unable to maintain doing a task due to various physiological and mechanical processes. In other words they saw fatigue as something happening within the body rendering it less physically able to do a task. Subsequent researchers looking at fatigue have come at it more from additional cognitive or emotional directions. For example, central fatigue is defined as the failure to initiate or sustain attentional tasks and physical activities requiring self-motivation. Other researchers have described attentional fatigue as the tiredness that comes from having to think about and work hard at behaviours that used to be automatic and easy.

Many people with neurological conditions seem to show characteristics of all three types of fatigue described above, with physical, cognitive and motivational elements to their difficulties in various combinations at various times. It thus seems useful to approach our understanding of overall fatigue in any individual in terms of how they experience its impact on their ability to do things physically, mentally and in relation to their levels of motivation.

Tiredness versus fatigue

Tiredness comes on gradually the longer we do a single task or as we go through our day, and as it does so our limbs and eyelids can start feeling a bit heavy and it becomes increasingly difficult to concentrate, we begin to yawn and we have the urge to take a break, or even to have a nap. Fatigue feels slightly different to this, and can best be described as an individually experienced and personally defined set of symptoms most often encountered as a feeling of exhaustion, tiredness or weakness. However, patients with neurological conditions are usually well able to differentiate between normal tiredness and the fatigue they experience as a consequence of their condition in terms of their fatigue occurring:

▶ more suddenly and intensely

▶ with little warning

▶ immediately, rendering them unable to usefully carry on the task they were doing.

Indeed, many patients describe their fatigue as their most limiting, and consequently, disabling symptom. This is because it:

▶ is often accompanied by their other cognitive difficulties (for example, poor attention and concentration, reduced speed and accuracy of information processing, poor memory and difficulty problem-solving) becoming worse until they have rested

▶ can interfere with physical functioning such as hand-eye co-ordination, speed of doing things or gait

▶ can be unpredictable making planning day-to-day activities difficult

▶ can be very persistent and relative to their other neurologically associated difficulties

▶ can be worsened by heat

▶ comes on easily.

The following characteristics are shared by normal tiredness and this type of fatigue:

▶ worsens with exercise

▶ worsens with stress, anxiety or low mood

▶ worsens with prolonged activity

▶ is often worse as the day progresses

▶ improves with rest, sleep, positive experiences and sex.

Overall, addressing this issue in people with neurological conditions is vital because it:

▶ impacts on all areas of their quality of life

▶ exacerbates their other impairments and disabilities

▶ is intimately related to patients' sense of control over their condition and lifestyle

▶ impacts on mental health

▶ can often be their biggest barrier to taking up employment or education.

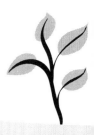

How common is fatigue?

Fatigue has long been associated with neurological conditions in research and literature. This has been especially so in traumatic brain injury studies, which have found that it is one of the most common problems even following mild injury, sometimes even severely so (Levin *et al*, 1987; Stulemeijer *et al*, 2006). In cases of more severe injury, researchers have shown it is commonly reported (in up to about 70% of patients in some research) by patients themselves and by relatives reporting on their head injured family members (McKinlay *et al*, 1981; Brooks *et al*, 1987; Kreutzer *et al*, 2001).

Similar findings have been found for fatigue following stroke, with one researcher (Stulemeijer *et al*, 2005) who reviewed the finding of a number of such studies showing that fatigue was a significant problem for 70% of people in the first year following stroke, decreasing to about 40% thereafter.

Fatigue is also recognised as the most common symptom of multiple sclerosis (MS). Surveys and case control studies indicate that 75 to 90% of individuals with MS experience fatigue, and 50 to 60% report it as one of their worst problems (Krupp *et al*, 2005).

Possible origins of fatigue problems in neurological conditions

There has been a plethora of studies trying to explain why fatigue is so common in patients with neurological conditions, and what the neurological mechanisms involved may be. The following possibilities are things to consider.

▶ Fatigue in traumatic brain injury (TBI) is due to failure in the integration of limbic input and motor functions affecting the functioning of the links between the basal ganglia, thalamus and frontal systems (see chapter 2).

▶ There is a correlation between fatigue and sleep disturbances in MS and brain injury patients, suggesting that alterations in normal sleep brainwave patterns and other sleep disruptions may play a role in the onset of fatigue in these conditions.

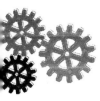

▶ Widespread cerebral axonal dysfunction, that is widespread lesions or damage particularly to the white matter in the brain (see chapters 2 and 3) is associated with fatigue in MS.

▶ Cytokines such as tumour necrosis factor and interleukins produced by the brain in response to tissue damage in TBI and MS may be associated with fatigue.

Steps to understanding fatigue in individuals

Clinicians involved in diagnosing and treating fatigue first need to take a detailed clinical history of the person's fatigue presentation, including as much qualitative and quantitative information as possible. The person will need a full physical examination to take into account other possible causes of fatigue, ie. other medical conditions and related neurologically based problems (for example, tinnitus, dizziness), pain and medications. Treatments may need to be changed or added as necessary. The person also needs to have any sleep disorder or mental health condition evaluated and treated via medication or other therapy. Finally, the person's cognitive and physical deficits due to their neurological condition need to be evaluated in relation to their impact upon the person's chosen or desired lifestyle, and particularly how these interlink with the person's fatigue complaints. The steps in this process are detailed below, and the acronym TUBE is useful in remembering what information needs to be collected, perhaps by a number of different professionals working with the person, and then collated by the most relevant clinician.

▶ **T**ake a full clinical history, not only one pertaining to the person's current neurological difficulty, but a full chronological history of the fatigue presentation.

▶ **U**se questionnaires if necessary.

▶ **B**asic blood evaluations – full blood count (FBC) and erythrocyte sedimentation rate (ESR), comprehensive metabolic panel, vitamin B12 and folate levels, thyroid function test.

▶ **E**xamine all records available. Speak to the GP if possible.

Other family members or support staff working with the person can help the process by being aware of the sorts of information clinicians will need and helping the person record this for them.

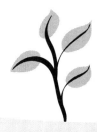

Key questions that should be asked are as follows.

▶ Have their levels of physical and mental functioning changed between pre and post onset?

▶ Are their sleep patterns and duration different pre and post injury?

▶ What is the type and severity of brain injury/damage?

▶ Have treatments been received since the onset?

▶ What is the alcohol and substance abuse history?

▶ What is the medical history, including chronic pain, dizziness etc?

▶ What is their current medication and dosages? (see **table 1** below)

▶ What is their past and current psychiatric history?

▶ What is the duration and description of their current problems?

Table 1: Medications known to sometimes be associated with fatigue	
Analgesics	Asthma drugs
Anticonvulsants	Cardiac drugs
Antidepressants	Diabetic treatments
Antihistamines	Gastrointestinal drugs
Antihypertensives	Hormone replacement treatments
Anti-inflammatories	Immune modulators
Antipsychotics	Muscle relaxants and antispasticity agents
Sedative hypnotic drugs	

Measuring fatigue

In order to gather more detailed information about the impact fatigue may be having on an individual, it may be useful to use questionnaires during this initial assessment process. They may also be useful when used serially to monitor any changes over time, or in response to treatment and rehabilitation. One possible questionnaire, the Fatigue Severity Scale, which is useful for this can be found in **figure 1** opposite. Another useful questionnaire is the Fatigue Impact Scale (Krupp *et al*, 1989), which is available on the internet as are a number of other possible measures. Alternatively, activity diaries and logs tailor made for each person's lifestyle can be useful tools, especially if the person is asked to rate their fatigue levels before and after activities of interest, or at particular times of the day on a 0 to 10 scale.

Figure 1: Fatigue Severity Scale

The FSS is a method of evaluating fatigue in multiple sclerosis and other conditions.

The fatigue severity scale (FSS) is designed to differentiate fatigue from clinical depression, since both share some of the same symptoms. Essentially, the FSS consists of answering a short questionnaire that requires the subject to rate his or her own level of fatigue but the obvious problem with this measure is its subjectivity.

Here is a sample FSS questionnaire containing nine statements that attempt to explore the severity of fatigue symptoms. The subject is asked to read each statement and circle a number from one to seven depending on how appropriate they felt the statement applied to them is over the preceding week. A low value indicates that the statement is not very appropriate whereas a high value indicates agreement.

FSS questionnaire

During the past week, I have found that:	Score						
1. My motivation is lower when I am fatigued.	1	2	3	4	5	6	7
2. Exercise brings on my fatigue.	1	2	3	4	5	6	7
3. I am easily fatigued.	1	2	3	4	5	6	7
4. Fatigue interferes with my physical functioning.	1	2	3	4	5	6	7
5. Fatigue causes frequent problems for me.	1	2	3	4	5	6	7
6. My fatigue prevents sustained physical functioning.	1	2	3	4	5	6	7
7. Fatigue interferes with carrying out certain duties and responsibilities.	1	2	3	4	5	6	7
8. Fatigue is among my three most disabling symptoms.	1	2	3	4	5	6	7
9. Fatigue interferes with my work, family or social life.	1	2	3	4	5	6	7

The scoring is done by calculating the average response to the questions (adding up all the answers and dividing by nine).

People with depression alone score about 4.5, but people with fatigue related to MS or other conditions average about 6.5.

Fatigue and sleep problems

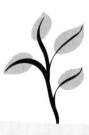

It is not surprising that people suffering from sleep difficulties also complain of constantly feeling tired and a propensity to fatigue in their everyday life. This will be looked at in more detail in the second part of this chapter. It may be that many people who initially present fatigue may need careful evaluation of their sleep patterns and treatment of sleep problems as part of the interventions for their fatigue.

Physical problems and fatigue

Many people with neurological conditions have physical problems affecting the strength, co-ordination and use of their limbs. This can include problems such as weakness or paralysis in a whole limb, several limbs or a whole side of the body, necessitating wheelchair use and physical assistance with activities of daily living. These problems make doing any task burdensome and tiring, contributing in turn to the onset of fatigue even if the person remains independent in such activities. The natural instinct is for a person to reduce physical activity to a minimum, but it has been well-established that decreased physical activity in itself can lead to tiredness and lack of energy. Research has shown that healthy people who are forced to spend lengthy periods doing very little physical activity often develop feelings of anxiety, low mood, bodily weakness, fatigue and nausea.

Good neurological physiotherapy rehabilitation, as well as focusing directly on any specific areas of physical disability, also tries to establish routines of regular moderate exercise within any boundaries imposed by a person's physical limitations. This can help the person to stay as active as possible for as long as possible in deteriorating conditions, and to gradually expand their repertoire of physical activities in those whose conditions are improving. This in turn leads to improving levels of stamina and energy (both physical and mental), allowing the person to make the optimal use of any other rehabilitation that may be available to them, as well as contributing to reduced levels of stress, anxiety and low mood. Useful therapy activities may include attending stamina groups run by therapists in health service settings, as well as assistance in joining fitness clubs, a gymnasia or social clubs offering appropriate physical recreational activities.

Alongside maintaining physical fitness and being as active as possible, it is also vital for people to maintain good levels of hydration and nutrition. Without adequate fluid intake and a well-balanced diet, anybody will be prone to feeling tired and lacking in energy.

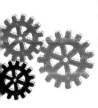

Cognitive problems and fatigue

Many people with neurological conditions, especially traumatic brain injury, experience cognitive difficulties that impact upon their everyday activities. These problems, which are covered in chapter 3 have the effect of making everyday activities more effortful and irksome, and thus probably considerably underpin the fatigue such individuals will experience. The most important of these are:

▶ slowed information processing

▶ difficulties sustaining attention and multi-tasking, especially in distracting environments

▶ difficulty learning and retaining new information

▶ difficulties co-ordinating other cognitive abilities in an integrated way to accurately problem-solve and complete tasks without errors.

It thus follows that providing good information, advice and rehabilitation for any identified cognitive problems will also have an impact upon any fatigue levels experienced by people with neurological conditions. Good neuro-rehabilitation should involve:

▶ providing information to enhance people's understanding of their problems in terms of why they occur

▶ planning and structured problem-solving

▶ pacing

▶ improving cognitive problems

▶ coping with anxiety and low mood.

Psychological problems and fatigue

It is entirely normal for people to show signs of psychological distress after developing a neurological condition or being brain injured in some way that interferes with their ability to lead their previously chosen lifestyle. As they undergo a psychological process to adjust to this new reality, they experience a complex set of losses in various areas (ie. social, occupational, recreational and familial), which they have to come to terms with, these

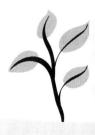

losses being experienced both serially and in conjunction with each other at various points over time. In many ways, this psychological adjustment shares many characteristics with grief, although it is more complicated since they are grieving for lost parts of themselves.

Core emotions involved in this process are guilt, anger and fear. Guilt often arises from people's worries about no longer being able to meet their responsibilities to other important people, as well as sometimes being related to a sense of being punished in some way for past misdemeanors or behaviour in their lives. Anger is primarily a consequence of frustration at no longer being able to do what they want, how they want, when they want, and from dashed hopes or dreams for the future. Fear arises from uncertainty regarding the situation they find themselves in, and whether or not they will be able to continue doing the activities they value in their lives.

Such emotions can contribute to a person developing frank anxiety, depression or other mental health difficulties. One sign of this being the case is a person consistently experiencing these emotions and mood variables over a period longer than a few days, and these problems sapping their motivation or ability to enter into therapeutic activities. At such times the person will also complain of being fatigued, or staff members working with them will notice that they seem to be less able or willing to do things than before. This may be a strong indication that the person requires a psychiatric or clinical psychological review to see if any treatments may be useful in altering their current mood state. Even if this is not so, the normal variation in mood state that people experience especially in the early aftermath of injury or illness onset, with bouts of tears, irritability or fear, may well underpin the variability seen in their propensity to fatigue.

It is important to note that psychiatrists do not have any medications that will make people feel happy and calm in response to such life situations, and psychologists do not have any counselling or psychotherapy techniques that will instantly help someone adjust to such a new life situation. This process of psychological adjustment, especially to a severely disabling condition, will take months or even years, and may well prove to be a lifelong process in many people as they age and have to meet new demands in their lifestyle, or as they experience either deterioration in their condition or other physical problems whether due to a different condition, injury or aging.

It is thus important for people with a neurological condition to learn ways of managing stress on a day-to-day basis as early as possible after its onset.

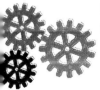

This may well include pacing themselves effectively, which will be dealt with later in this chapter. It will also undoubtedly be important for them to be as well informed about their condition and associated specific problems. This will not only allow them to benefit from rehabilitation, teaching them how to ameliorate and manage these, but will also help them adjust their expectations of themselves in all areas of their lives. If they can be taught or helped to communicate this understanding to other people around them, that will also help to reduce their stress levels when people become more supportive or less demanding. All of this will undoubtedly help to address some of the factors contributing to their fatigue levels.

Techniques or audiotapes that teach deep breathing, relaxation and visualisation techniques can help reduce stress, as can activities such as yoga or meditation. One note of caution here though is that techniques requiring the tensing and relaxing of muscles in various parts of the body coupled with breathing exercises should not be used early after diagnosis or condition onset with people who have weakness or paralysis in body parts. Trying to do so will instead cause them distress by focusing their attention on these symptoms rather than having the more desired effect of reducing their stress levels.

Participation in enjoyable activities that divert attention away from fatigue or other symptoms and difficulties will also be of benefit. For example, activities such as knitting, reading, watching television or listening to music require little physical energy but require attention as long as they are not impaired by a person's other neurologically based problems. If they are, the challenge will be to find other non-tiring recreational activities for a person to try.

Focused pacing

It is generally useful to provide all newly injured or diagnosed patients with advice regarding the likelihood of them experiencing fatigue. This may well need to be repeated many times during the rehabilitation process as very few people will accept the need to pace themselves until they have learned that their neurological condition prevents them from doing what they want, when they want and how they want as they used to. They will hopefully become more receptive to this advice as they begin to accept the reality of their new life situation. The sorts of things that are useful to say early in rehabilitation are, '*You have to listen to what your body and brain are telling you. If you*

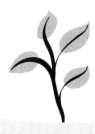

are doing something and suddenly feel tired or lose concentration, then have a break. You may even need to leave it to the next day to complete.' In terms of building up stamina and energy, you may tell them, *'Push yourself to gradually do more, but step this up in a planned way. Do things in a little and often way. Don't try to get things done all at once.'*

It is well-established that many people with fatigue difficulties tend to fall into a 'boom or bust' pattern of activity, trying to do as much as possible for as long as possible when they feel able to do so, and then when they consequently get fatigued, being able to do nothing at all for several hours, or even days thereafter. The need for pacing is thus particularly important for people who complain of fatigue. This is where keeping activity logs and diaries can be useful in helping them and people involved in their treatment learn how to best approach and organise their everyday activities. They also need to learn to grade and define activities across two dimensions, the first of these being 'must do', 'could do if I have the time and energy' and 'unnecessary' activities, and then rating the same activities as 'very tiring', 'tiring' or 'not tiring', so they can plan efficiently.

They then need to learn to juggle their commitments and desired activities so they can get the most done in a day without succumbing to fatigue after any single task that will interfere with other things they want to do. If they plan their activities and pace themselves more carefully they will find that their days and general lifestyle become more productive overall, even if on individual days they may not do quite as much as they would have on a 'boom' day. Such pacing will need to include having to plan around days when it is inevitable that they will need to do more than usual, for example, to attend a special event. They thus may need to plan a quieter day than usual, the days before and after, and try to plan as many ways as possible of breaking the busy day up into chunks with rest periods in between.

Some people find that they do not get as tired if they have a variety of activities to do in a day as each of these may tire them in a slightly different way, and so mixing them up allows them to actually get more done overall across the day. Thus instead of trying to complete whole tasks in a series, finishing one before they start another, they may well be better doing bits of each in conjunction, alternating between them during each day. However, some people find this approach demotivating if they need to see quick final results to feel they are achieving things, even if this approach means that overall more tasks get completed.

The goal-setting approach used in neurorehabilitation is a good model to teach people to apply in dealing with their fatigue on a day-to-day, week-to-week and month-to-month basis. Setting subgoals in tasks and activities can help people who have to take more time than they would like to fully complete things to see that they are indeed making progress and achieving things that are not immediately obvious when something has not been fully completed.

Case study 1

Tim was a 21-year-old university student about to start his final year of study when he was involved in a nasty road traffic accident and sustained a severe traumatic brain injury. After several days on the intensive treatment unit, and a few more on the neurology ward, he was transferred to the neurorehabilitation unit where he spent the next two months. At the start of his stay on that unit he was still disorientated not knowing where he was, why he was there, and who the people around him were (apart from recognising family visitors), nor did he know what day, month and year it was. He also had a right-sided body weakness making it impossible for him to walk or do self-care activities. His speech was extremely slurred so that he constantly sounded drunk. Within a few days he was fully orientated, and with a combined physiotherapy and occupational therapy treatment programme he was walking independently and was self-caring by the time of his discharge; his speech had also returned to normal. He had reluctantly but sensibly agreed that he would take a year out of his studies to allow him to both recover further, and to have outpatient rehabilitation focusing on a number of cognitive difficulties identified by the inpatient team, including slowed information processing, difficulty learning and retaining new information and problems with multi-tasking.

Having been very excited about being discharged home, Tim soon became very worried and annoyed by finding himself unable to do all the things he wanted to do each day such as play video games, read and socialise with his friends, especially on days when he had been to the hospital for rehabilitation, as he was prone to suddenly becoming very tired and unable to concentrate on anything. If he tried to ignore this and carry on with what he was doing he would find that his speech would become slurred like it had been early after his head injury and his right side would become mildly uncoordinated. He became worried that something was wrong, and that he was deteriorating neurologically in some way rather than recovering.

The outpatient rehabilitation team spent time with Tim helping him to understand how his fatigue and associated symptoms could be understood in terms of his other head injury related difficulties. He learned to plan his day-to-day activities carefully and

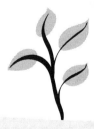

sensibly, building in rest periods, and counterbalancing rehabilitation and recreational activities. He was helped to build up his physical stamina initially in one-to-one physiotherapy sessions and then as part of a stamina group before he and his fellow group members were introduced to a local gym. The gym was able to offer the use of their facilities to continue self-directed fitness regimes with the advice of trainers who had some understanding of brain injury through their previous contact with the rehabilitation team and their patients.

Tim built up his mental stamina initially through activities with his therapists and the therapy assistant, as well as following their advice on how to approach doing things on his own, such as reading and playing computer games, gradually pushing himself to do more and more but taking breaks whenever he suddenly lost concentration or felt fatigued. He recognised that he was more prone to fatigue when he went out with his friends if they went into very busy or noisy places, so initially he restricted himself to only joining them on quieter activities, preferably with only a few other people in the group. As his stamina improved he found that he could cope with going into busier and noisier places, but he learned to recognise when he had had enough and would then excuse himself and leave.

Tim was encouraged to enrol in a community adult education IT course to see how he would cope in a classroom situation. This, alongside his clear progress in his rehabilitation, and the results of his detailed cognitive assessment by the clinical neuropsychologist, suggested that he would be able to go back to university to complete his degree. However, in discussion with the neuropsychologist and his university tutors and student support services, he agreed that his studies should be spread over two years rather than one. He successfully completed his degree, and was offered a job at the company where he had done a work placement in the second year. He was concerned how he would cope with this as he still found himself prone to fatigue on busy days and was honest with the prospective employer about this and his head injury history. He was instead offered a similar job on a jobshare basis with a young woman who was returning to work part-time after starting a family, which he accepted.

Why do we need to sleep?

The answer to this question is long, complicated and is still being scientifically debated. However, it is clear that it is part of what we need to do to stay alive, as bodily and neurological processes that go on whilst we are asleep are necessary for both our health, and ultimately, our survival.

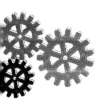

In short, these include processes that allow the body to replenish itself in order to equip it to physically deal with the next day. It is thought that bodily processes responsible for growth and healing are more active when people are asleep, and that our immune systems are not only more active then, but also bolster in the process. Neurologically, it is thought that processes happening in the brain during sleep help it to more effectively process and store information in long-term memory from the day before. In short, it seems that sleep allows our bodies and brains to recharge and restore themselves in preparation for the next day.

Perhaps a good way of understanding why humans need to sleep is to look at what happens when we don't get enough sleep. This will be more fully examined in the sections of the chapter below.

What happens neurologically when we sleep?

Although it may seem as if when we are asleep our bodies and brains totally shut down, that is not the case, and this can be seen when watching someone who is asleep and seeing them move and change position, clearly dreaming and reacting to what they are dreaming about. The body and brain go through phases of sleep in cycles through the night, which can be measured electrophysiologically using electroencephalogram (EEG) observation of brain waves, with different patterns being seen in each stage. There are up to five stages of sleep per cycle, the first four being known as NREM (non-rapid eye movement) sleep, and the fifth as REM (rapid eye movement) sleep, for reasons that will be discussed below.

If we have an EEG as we go to sleep, in the first stage as our attention to the outside world switches off so do our typical waking brain waves, and we slowly become unresponsive to noise and light. This is sometimes interrupted by brief dream-like thoughts or images, and sudden bodily jumps or jerks that some people describe as feeling like 'falling from a cliff'. These are known as hypnagogic phenomena, marking the transition from wakefulness to sleep, reflecting a brief 'switching on' of our brain again. In the next stage of sleep, a distinctive EEG pattern emerges showing that the person is now fully asleep. During these first two stages of sleep we are easily woken, and we tend to toss and turn a lot, mostly without waking.

This is followed by two further stages during which there is increasing prominence of a different distinctive kind of brain wave. These again

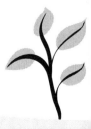

show that the brain is not totally switched off but is working in a different pattern to when we are awake. Stage four is the deepest stage of sleep in humans; it is the hardest time to be roused and there will be very little movement. If a person is woken from this stage of sleep then they will find it hard to 'switch on' and they will feel 'groggy' or confused for a while.

In the next stage, the human brain seems to switch on in an EEG pattern that closely resembles that of someone who is fully awake. It is at this time that we dream and experience rapid eye movements beneath our closed eyelids, hence the term REM sleep. Breathing and heart rate, which during the four stages of NREM sleep were slowed, now fluctuate in response to dream content. Generally also, below-neck body movement ceases as natural processes effectively paralyse the body to stop it from reacting to the dream content. Phenomena such as sleep walking or thrashing about in the bed during nightmares show that this is sometimes not fully effective.

After REM sleep the person most often returns to stage two, or even stage one, NREM sleep, and this is when we are most lightly asleep during the night, and we may wake briefly as we change position in bed to get comfortable; it may be that we become aware of having just had a dream before going to sleep again. People who have to get up during the night (for example to go to the toilet) most often do so at this point between sleep cycles and then to get back to sleep have to start at stage one NREM first again. A single sleep cycle of NREM followed by a REM period lasts about 90–100 minutes, and humans typically have between three and five REM periods per night. We often get as much deep sleep (stages three and four NREM) as we need in the first two or three sleep cycles, so we remain in lighter stages of sleep after that, alternating between stage two NREM and REM sleep, so the cycles become shorter. A diagram showing how these phases and stages of sleep typically occur is shown in **figure 2**.

Many people say that they do not dream, but that is not the case. Everyone dreams every night and the amount of dreaming depends upon how many phases of sleep the person goes through. However, dreaming is a primarily subconscious process so it is hard to remember everything about a dream, but often the vivid or distressing content of dreams such as that of a nightmare just before waking is memorable. This may be responsible for us fully waking after such dreams before getting back into stage two NREM sleep. If we are more fully awake, then trying to go back to stage one NREM may be difficult to do particularly if we are distressed.

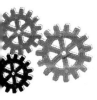

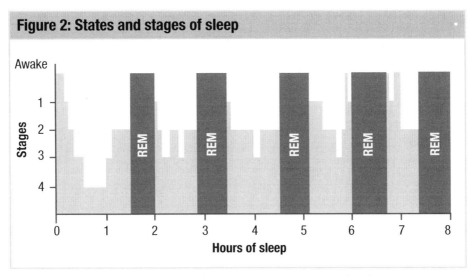

Figure 2: States and stages of sleep

(Adapted from www.sleep4health.com.au/wp-content/uploads/2009/08/
stages-of-sleep.png)

Figure 2 above shows the typical sleep stages and phases and it shows the typical cycle of five phases of sleep most people go through each night and the possible stages of NREM and REM in each.

How much sleep do we need?

We know that babies spend much of the day and night asleep, and as we grow older we generally need less sleep. Many theorists and researchers are investigating potential links between learning and behavioural problems in children and teenagers to them not getting sufficient sleep. Most adults talk about needing about eight hours per night to feel rested and healthy, but some people need less or more than that. On average, adults who get less than six hours sleep tend to feel out of sort, and few adults ever say they need more than 10. However, there are famous examples of people who claim to never need this much sleep, such as Margaret Thatcher who claimed never to need to sleep longer than five hours a night. There is also some recent research suggesting that consistently sleeping more than eight hours per night may actually be less healthy for many people than six or seven hours, but this is certainly not conclusive. *Typical hours spent sleeping at different times of life are shown* in **figure 3** below.

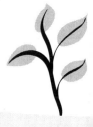

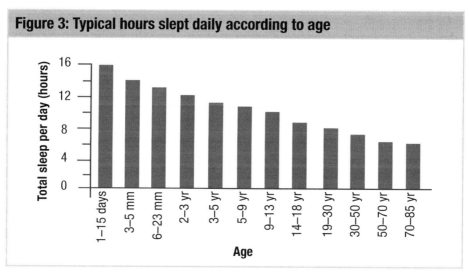

Figure 3: Typical hours slept daily according to age

(Adapted from www.patch4u.co.nz/blue/images/sn_graph.jpg)

What is insomnia?

Insomnia is simply a term used to describe having a sleep problem. Broadly speaking people who claim to have sleep problems describe one or more of three types of difficulty. These are difficulty getting to sleep in the first place, difficulty maintaining sleep (fully waking during the night and then struggling to get back to sleep) or early morning waking and total failure to get back to sleep. Specialist sleep clinics can recognise and treat a variety of sleep disorders, but all of these include one, two or all three of these types of sleep difficulty.

Sleep deprivation can:

▶ make a person prone to illness and infection, including ones that could be life threatening

▶ result in mood swings and irritability

▶ cause difficulty learning new information and being prone to forget what has been learned

▶ cause problems with concentration, problem-solving and decision-making

▶ demotivate

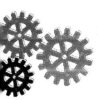

▶ increase the risk of accidents

▶ lead to the development of mental health difficulties

▶ enhance aging

▶ cause intrusive ruminative thoughts before and after going to bed that tend to make getting to sleep even more difficult

▶ increase the sensation of physical weariness, fatigue or tiredness

▶ increase bodily aches and pains, including headaches.

As many of these symptoms overlap with that of brain injury or neurological conditions, it is vital not to overlook the fact that sleep problems may exacerbate the very symptoms for which someone is referred to for treatment or rehabilitation.

Sleep problems in neurological conditions

Sometimes sleep problems can be directly caused by brain injury or neurological conditions as a result of damage to parts of the brain that are involved in sleep onset and waking. These are called primary sleep problems. Primary sleep problems by way of insomnia or excessive daytime sleepiness can occur especially with lesions in the midbrain, hypothalamus or thalamus. Broadly speaking, it is more likely to be a primary sleep problem with insomnia in the early aftermath of a brain injury that settles, or disturbed sleep that does not settle in severe brain damage cases.

However, sleep problems in brain injury and other neurological conditions are not necessarily the direct result of brain damage since a third of the general population report sleep disruption and studies have shown that between nine and 15% of people report daytime problems possibly associated with poor sleep. We also know that the prevalence of insomnia is higher in divorced, separated or widowed adults, and in those with lower income and education levels. Older people experience more awakenings during the night, lower sleep efficiency, less sleep, more variable sleep and lighter sleep than young adults. Thus, independent of any direct or indirect effects of neurological conditions, people may be experiencing sleep problems. If we then add in the distressing physical, cognitive and emotional consequences of having a neurological condition, quite often also associated with other injuries or illnesses causing discomfort, it is not surprising that the reported

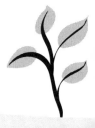

level of sleep problems in such patients is high. Thus, most often, people with brain injury or other neurological conditions have sleep problems connected with other problems from their brain injury or other injuries or conditions – as secondary rather than primary sleep problems.

A number of factors may underpin such secondary sleep problems. These could include:

▶ natural worry and anxiety about the neurological condition, its prognosis and its effects on the person's day-to-day life

▶ low mood in response to a negative life situation

▶ fatigue

▶ disturbed sleep secondary to other physical problems such as pain or other physical discomfort

▶ poor sleeping habit

▶ mental health problems – insomnia is commonly associated with anxiety disorders, attention deficit/hyperactivity disorder, depression, bipolar disorder, mania, post-traumatic stress disorder (PTSD) and schizophrenia

▶ other medical problems (see **table 2** below)

▶ drugs, both prescription and non-prescription (see **table 3** opposite).

Taking all of these factors into account, successful treatment of insomnia in a patient with a neurological condition may well have to include treatment of other medical conditions or alterations to treatments already in place, or involvement of mental health services. Such treatments may include drugs, counselling, psychotherapy or physical interventions such as continuous positive air pressure (CPAP) machines – the breathing machines used to treat obstructive sleep apnoea.

Table 2: Medical conditions known to be associated with insomnia

▶ Chronic pain

▶ Congestive heart failure

▶ Asthma

▶ Chronic obstructive pulmonary disease (COPD)

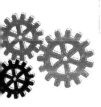

▶ Gastro-oesophageal reflux

▶ Nocturia

▶ Menopause

▶ Allergies such as hay fever

▶ Other primary sleep disorders, especially obstructive sleep apnoea

Table 3: Medications that may interfere with sleep

▶ Decongestants (including many common over the counter cold and flu remedies)

▶ Beta blockers and antihypertensives

▶ Selective seratonin reuptake inhibitors (SSRIs)

▶ Bronchodilators

▶ Analgesics with caffeine in the formula

▶ Stimulants

▶ Corticosteroids

▶ Thyroid hormone replacement

Steps to understanding a person's sleep problems

Just as in trying to understand fatigue, the starting point in trying to understand a person's insomnia is to take a detailed clinical history of the person's sleep problems, including as much qualitative and quantitative information as possible. The person may need a full physical examination to take into account other possible physical causes of sleep problems, and treatments may need to be changed or added as necessary. The full effects of the insomnia need to be evaluated in relation to their impact upon the person's chosen or desired lifestyle. Contrasts need to be made between the person's sleep before and after the onset of their neurological condition, focusing on all aspects of their sleep including their daily activities and their behaviour in the period leading up to going to bed. Differences in any of these could provide the key to resolving some of their difficulties with sleep.

Key questions to ask are as follows.

▶ What treatment are they receiving and for what problems?

▶ What medications are they taking, at what dosage, and have they noticed any side effects?

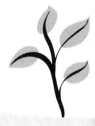

▶ Did their sleep patterns change when any medications were stopped, started or when the dosage changed?

▶ What about anything non-prescribed that they are taking for the same reasons?

▶ Are there any physical symptoms keeping them awake, or waking them in the night, such as pain or needing to get up to go to the toilet?

▶ How much are they eating and drinking during the day and in the evening, especially caffeinated drinks? Remember that many drinks other than coffee contain caffeine especially most brands of cola. It is also in many non-prescription medications such as cold remedies, as well as dietary supplements and so-called 'health drinks'; it is worth checking the contents labels of anything the person ingests.

▶ What types of physical and mental exertion are they doing each day, and at what times?

▶ Are they taking anything to help them sleep such as other substances ie. alcohol, over the counter medications, herbal preparations or illegal substances?

▶ Are they still sleeping in the same place as before? If so, are they in a different bed or different room, with different light and background noise levels or a softer or firmer mattress or pillows that are less comfortable? What about heating levels in the room? Is the bed and bedding too hard?

▶ Do they read, watch television, play computer games or do other activities in the bedroom or in bed? If so, for how long?

▶ Do they have a 'winding down' routine leading up to going to bed? If so, what is it, and over how long a period?

▶ Have they deliberately altered their sleeping pattern to go to bed later at night in order to sleep later into the next day?

▶ If they struggle to get to sleep, or wake up and struggle to get back to sleep, what happens? Do they lie there becoming increasingly worried or frustrated? Do they switch on the light and do something else like read or watch television, or do they get up and go elsewhere in the house to do something? If so, what do they do? Does this help them get tired and eventually fall asleep? If so, do they go back to bed to sleep or sleep on a chair or couch elsewhere?

▶ Does anything help them sleep better on some nights than others? Have they learned any 'tricks' to help them switch off thoughts that are keeping them awake?

Sleep diaries filled in every morning can be very useful in defining sleep problems, and then monitoring changes in response to advice or treatment. These can be found in a number of forms on the internet and in books on sleep disorders (for example, Hirshkowitz & Smith, 2004). Alternatively, they can be tailor made for each person to take into account their particular symptoms. They most often focus on issues such as what time they go to bed and get up, how long it takes to get to sleep, how many times a person wakes in the night, how many hours they actually slept, and how rested they feel in the morning. An example of one of these can be found in **figure 4** below.

Figure 4: A sample sleep diary						
	I went to bed at (time)	Last night I fell asleep in (mins)	During the night I woke at (time)	And stayed awake for (mins)	This morning I woke at (time)	Sleep rating (see key below)
Monday						
Tuesday						
Wednesday						
Thursday						
Friday						
Saturday						
Sunday						

Key to sleep rating
1 – Not at all rested
2 – Still tired
3 – Not rested, nor tired
4 – Quite rested
5 – Very rested. A good night's sleep

Interventions for sleep problems

Once you have a full understanding of the nature of a person's sleep difficulties, it is sometimes immediately obvious that some specific things could be altered or addressed to try to improve their sleep–wake patterns. This may mean that the person has to change or avoid patterns of behaviour around sleep and bedroom use, which did not have a negative impact on their sleep in the past but which now does. Some general

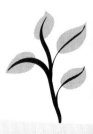

principles that most people find helpful are:

▶ increasing physical activity levels during the day

▶ preparation for sleep via a set of relaxing activities in the hour or two prior to going to bed

▶ regular meals with a balanced diet

▶ avoiding too much caffeine

▶ watching fluid intake in the evenings

▶ having regular sleep and wake times, whether or not they have to get up at a particular time

▶ time for a particular activity, and keeping this the same seven days a week

▶ avoiding day time naps

▶ thought-stopping techniques, relaxation training, meditation

▶ possible short-term use of the right medication to help re-establish a good sleep–wake cycle

▶ changing drug intake, especially drugs that have a stimulant property such as some medications prescribed for mental health issues, especially the SSRI's commonly prescribed for low mood. Sometimes a change in medication may be needed but often just taking the drugs at a different time of the day may be sufficient.

▶ Diuretic medications (water tablets) that lead to the person having to go to the toilet during the night may require review by the GP or hospital specialist who originally prescribed them, so different drugs, or different dosages that do not interfere with sleep can be tried. If the person is not on diuretics but is waking regularly to go to the toilet for other reasons, a urological review may be needed. They may even be able to be prescribed a medication to 'dry them up' at night.

A person who is having sleep problems needs to follow the principles of good sleep hygiene. These are as follows.

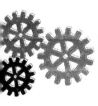

▶ No more than six caffeinated drinks per day, which includes coffee, tea, cola and energy drinks, and none within two hours of bedtime. (Preferably less than six a day and none at all after 6 pm if the person has a sleep problem.)

▶ No intense exercise within three hours of desired sleep time.

▶ No going to bed hungry.

▶ No heavy meals within three hours of bedtime.

▶ No drinking alcohol to excess at any time, and in particular any alcohol at all late in the evening within an hour or two of bedtime.

▶ No working, trying to solve problems or having intense discussions or arguments up to 1½ hours before bedtime.

▶ No watching exciting action-packed television or videos, playing video or computer games, or going on the internet until late in the evening.

▶ No using the bedroom to watch television or as an office, even at other times of the day.

▶ No reading stimulating books in bed.

▶ Not trying too hard to fall asleep.

▶ No lying in bed feeling angry.

The main thing a person needs to associate with being in bed is being asleep, and the only exception to that rule is using it to have sex, especially since sexual activity often helps someone to feel relaxed and sleepy afterwards. People with sleep problems need to develop a routine that helps their mind to slowly switch off in advance of bedtime, using calming and soothing activities such as having a hot bath, listening to relaxing music (or actually doing relaxation or meditation exercises) and having a hot, milky (non-caffeinated) drink.

Once in bed, the person should switch off the light and get as comfortable as they physically can. If they do not drift off to sleep within a few minutes because their head is full of thoughts then they should then try to use a relaxation exercise and focus on their slow deep breathing or visualise that they are in a peaceful and relaxing place.

If the person lies awake in bed for longer than 15 to 20 minutes after they switch the light off, and particularly if they progressively get more and more agitated, they should get up and go elsewhere to do a quiet, non-stimulating activity until they feel as if they are tired enough to fall asleep then going back to bed and following the steps detailed above. This should be repeated as many times as necessary each night until sleep is achieved.

If the person consistently follows this advice without any real improvement

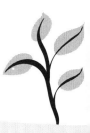

in their overall quantity or quality of sleep, they may well need a more formal medical examination from their GP or treating specialist clinician who can then decide if referral for even more specialist investigation and treatment at a sleep clinic may be necessary.

Some medications that may be tried to improve the person's sleep pattern are:

▶ benzodiazepines (the '–azepams') and hypnotics (the 'z' drugs such as Zopiclone and Zolpidem)

▶ antidepressants, especially the more sedating ones, often in lower than antidepressant dosages – the old antidepressant amitriptyline is now used in small doses to aid sleep, especially in pain clinics

▶ melatonin, a hormone naturally produced by the pineal gland in the brain is involved in regulating the sleep–wake cycle and is used to combat the symptoms of jetlag.

In prescribing such medications, doctors need to consider drug effects and side effects against the type of sleep problem. For example:

▶ quick acting drugs with a short half life will not help with difficulty maintaining sleep or early morning waking

▶ long-acting drugs can leave the patient tired, slowed and 'drugged' in the morning, thus exacerbating fatigue problems

▶ benzodiazepines exacerbate sleep-disordered breathing

▶ long-term use of most drugs usually produces more problems than it solves.

Case study 2

Theo is a 35-year-old man who had been diagnosed with multiple sclerosis 10 years ago and was forced to give up his job as a self-employed builder because he could no longer physically cope with its demands. He had never been academically interested at school and had been a poor attendee, leaving school with no formal qualifications. However, he had always wanted to be a builder and did well at college when completing a City and Guilds bricklaying and plastering course.

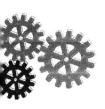

He had always enjoyed tinkering with computers and playing electronic games, but since giving up his business he filled his time up by going online or by playing these games often into the early hours of the morning. After several months he found himself struggling to get to sleep at night, often tossing and turning for several hours before eventually falling asleep, and then waking five or six hours later feeling very tired but being unable to get back to sleep. He would then get up and go on his computer or play some games but found he needed to have naps several times a day as he got so tired doing these activities he would make mistakes and then start losing games he ususally would have won, or take twice as long to do something on the computer. He began to worry that these difficulties were due to a different sort of MS relapse (all of his previous relapses had involved motor problems with his arms and legs), or his condition had become progressive rather than relapsing and remitting, and sought an appointment with his neurologist.

The neurologist did a detailed examination of Theo, which included a repeat MRI scan that ruled out a relapse or that Theo's MS had become progressive. He referred Theo to the outpatient rehabilitation team, knowing that the team had previously successfully worked with other patients complaining of fatigue and sleep problems without resorting to the use of medication. Having met Theo and taken down his full history, the team started by suggesting that his sleep problems were most likely related to his altered lifestyle, including his worries about the future. He was encouraged to follow sleep hygiene advice in the first instance, including regularising his bedtimes and getting up in the morning, particularly avoiding playing electronic games right up to bedtime. He agreed to start going swimming or to the gym daily so he would have some more physical outlets for his energy. He was also taught some relaxation exercises and thought-stopping techniques to try if his thoughts were keeping him awake at night. Theo noticed that his sleep improved within a few weeks with accompanying increases in his energy levels and abilities to concentrate, although he still had several nights a week when he struggled to get to sleep due to ruminative thinking about his very restricted lifestyle.

Having assessed him physically and cognitively, it was clear to the team that he would cope with further education or employment in a non-physically demanding job. A meeting was arranged with a disability employment advisor and when Theo's interest in computers and gaming was mentioned it was suggested that he enrol to do a part-time course at a local college to learn computer maintenance and repair, which would be funded for him. Theo enrolled on the course and just before it started the disability employment advisor told him that a local single-handed computer repair business had approached the Job Centre about taking on a trainee staff member. Theo applied for the job and got it. His sleep pattern returned to normal at about that time and has remained so since.

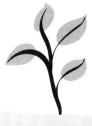

Quiz

1. What are the links between somebody's complaint of fatigue and their neurological condition?

2. What are the most important factors to consider if someone is complaining of severe fatigue?

3. What is the single most important thing to focus on in dealing with fatigue?

4. What is my starting point in trying to help someone with a sleep problem?

5. What do I need to try to assess when I'm looking at sleep hygiene with someone?

6. What environmental factors may be important in sleep difficulties?

7. What are the keys to intervening in sleep problems?

References

Brooks N, Campsie L, Symington C, Beattie A & McKinlay W (1987) The effects of severe head injury on patient and relative within seven years of injury. *Journal of Head Trauma Rehabilitation* **2** (3) 1–13.

Hirshkowitz M & Smith PB (2004) *Sleep Disorders For Dummies*. Indianapolis: John Wiley & Sons.

Kreutzer JS, Seel RT & Gourley E (2001) The prevalence and symptom rates of depression after traumatic brain injury: a comprehensive examination. *Brain Injury* **15** (7) 563–576.

Krupp LB, Christodoulou C & Scombert H (2005) Multiple sclerosis and fatigue. In: De Luca J (Ed) *Fatigue as a Window to the Brain*. Cambridge: Massachusetts Institute of Technology.

Krupp LB, LaRocca NG, Muir-Nash J & Steinberg AD (1989) The Fatigue Severity Scale – application to patients with multiple sclerosis and systemic lupus erythematosus. *Archives of Neurology* **46** 1121–1123.

Levin HS, Mattis S, Ruff RM, Eisenberg HM, Marshall LF, Tabaddor K, High WH & Jr Frankowski RF (1987) Neurobehavioral outcome following minor head injury: a three-center study. *Journal of Neurosurgery* **66** (2) 706–713.

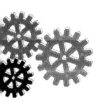

McKinlay WW, Brooks DN, Bond MR, Martinage DP & Marshall MM (1981) The short-term outcome of severe blunt head injury as reported by relatives of the injured persons. *Journal of Neurology, Neurosurgery & Psychiatry* **44** 527–533.

Stulemeijer M, Fasotti L & Bleijenberg G (2005) *Fatigue After Stroke.* In: De J Luca (Ed) (2005) *Fatigue as a Window to the Brain.* Cambridge: Massachusetts Institute of Technology.

Stulemeijer M, van der Werf S, Bleijenberg G, Biert J, Brauer J & Vos PE (2006) Recovery from mild traumatic brain injury: a focus on fatigue. *Brain Injury* **253** (8) 1041–7.

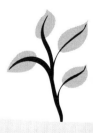

Chapter 7

How psychologists assess cognitive functions

Karen Treece

Aims of the chapter

The chapter aims to:

▶ understand what is a cognitive assessment

▶ appreciate the importance of information gathering and history taking

▶ understand how a psychologist would conduct an assessment.

Assessing cognitive functions: an introduction

Many of the important cognitive functions have been described and explained in Chapter 3, but this chapter explains how psychologists measure these functions and place them in the wider context of the person. There are many reasons why an assessment of cognitive function may be performed, and these include measurements of changes in ability, formal recognition of the person's symptoms, assistance with diagnosis, planning rehabilitation and treatment, joint goal setting with the patient, research, and medico-legal claims for compensation following injury.

In clinical practice a good cognitive assessment is one which comprehensively answers a clinical question. The psychologist must take into account the clinical question, the appropriateness of the referral, all available information from different sources, results of medical and clinical investigations, Glasgow coma scale (GCS) scores and post traumatic amnesia (PTA) duration. The psychologist must also consider the patient's

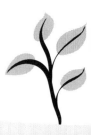

ability to be tested and attitude towards testing, the correct choice of test materials, the results of the assessment, and the validity of the results. The results must be interpreted taking into consideration all the other influences on patient performance, not just the scores of the cognitive tests.

Following the assessment a report will be written which will be shared with the referrer, and all the clinicians who will be involved in the rehabilitation of the patient, with the patient's permission. This report will contain details of strengths, preserved abilities, weaknesses and areas of difficulty. It may be possible to state which difficulties have arisen due to the recent injury or illness, and to estimate how the patient functioned before that event. An explanation of the report should be shared with the patient, and with permission, their partner or carers.

Step-by-step cognitive assessment

Preparation for the cognitive assessment

In terms of undertaking a cognitive assessment the first factor to consider is whether the referral is appropriate or not.

▶ Is the referral appropriate?

▶ Is it in the person's interest to be assessed?

▶ Is it in the interest of the wider population for an assessment to take place?

▶ Would a cognitive assessment answer the clinical question?

▶ How will the assessment results be used?

Before the first meeting with the person, information should be gathered from the referral letter or from the referrer, if the letter is not clear. Information about the nature of the referral, the purpose of the assessment, details of the current condition, any reported difficulties, any current or previous medico-legal claims and the appropriateness of a cognitive assessment need to be considered.

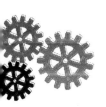

Information relating to medical condition, current and past medication and current or previous psychiatric opinion should be obtained from the medical notes. Details of diagnoses, brain scans and previous injuries or illnesses should also be collected as well as results of any earlier cognitive assessments.

First interview

At the first interview with the person, the purpose and content of the assessment would be fully explained. The person would be encouraged to ask questions about the process and full informed consent would be requested from the person.

The first interview with the person for a cognitive assessment should consist of a full psychological assessment including:

▶ demographics (age, gender, handedness, cultural background)

▶ educational history and qualifications

▶ occupational history and current socio-economic group

▶ social history and current social situation

▶ medical history (including details of current condition and medication, and any sensory impairment)

▶ psychological history

▶ smoking, drug and alcohol use (past and present)

▶ medico-legal history

▶ forensic history.

Following the completion of the full psychological assessment, the cognitive assessment would start and the entire process could take a number of sessions.

Observations

When first meeting with the person, the psychologist would make a series of observations. The psychologist would observe the way the person entered the room, greeted the psychologist or other professionals and interacted with any accompanying carer or partner.

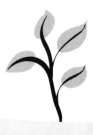

Observations would continue throughout the first interview and cognitive assessments, and these would include:

▶ orientation (to person, place, date, companion and reason for appointment)

▶ physical appearance (significant body features, dysmorphic features, asymmetries)

▶ level of arousal (drowsy, alert, hyper vigilant, easily startled, overwhelmed)

▶ attention (short span, easily distracted, neglects one side of body or space)

▶ executive control (behavioural regulation, poorly or excessively motivated, impulsive)

▶ language comprehension (requests repetition of instructions, needs simplification of instructions, loses attention if language is speeded up or slowed down)

▶ language expression (fluency, grammar, sound substitutions, naming difficulties)

▶ speech and voice quality (hoarse, volume, breath control, articulation, rate, prosody)

▶ social interactions (turn taking, eye contact, gaze aversion, aggressive or passive, personal boundaries, takes instructions well, understands roles of self and psychologist)

▶ motor control (hemiparesis, gait, tremor, excessive body movements, slumps in chair)

▶ emotionality (mood swings, anxiousness, response to failure, response to praise).

Questions to ask

It is most important to find out how the patient views the current situation. It is useful to ask the following.

▶ How is the person currently functioning and how did they use to function?

▶ What aspects of life have changed and what has remained the same?

▶ What did the person use to enjoy doing and whether or not they are still able to enjoy the same activities?

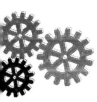

▶ What difficulties they have noticed and if these appeared suddenly or slowly over time?

▶ Have there been any changes to their employment status?

▶ Has there been any additional help and support received from family, partner or other carers?

Occasionally people report that they are not experiencing any difficulties and that they are functioning just as they always have.

What friends and family say

If the psychologist is unsure of the accuracy of the information provided by the individual then it is appropriate to ask the opinion of family or carers, provided the individual has given consent. Occasionally this information will be given spontaneously during the interview by accompanying persons, especially if that person views the situation as more serious than the person being assessed. The difference in views may be due to the person's condition being associated with loss of insight and under reporting of symptoms.

Differences to be aware of

It is important to note that the views of the person or carer may not agree with the referrer and this may be due to the time constraints of the consultation with the referrer, or the person's difficulty in expressing the effects of the injury or illness, or even down to person and carer reporter bias. In addition to this, the person and carer's opinions may not agree with each other, and again this may be due to reporter bias or the condition being associated with loss of insight and a tendency to under-report the severity of symptoms. Frequently, carers appear to be far more troubled by the difficulties than the person themselves; this can be due to carer strain following an enormous change in roles.

Nonetheless, there are various reasons why the information supplied by an individual or carers may not be completely dependable. A person and carers may not remember the course of events, or may not have fully understood or remembered conversations with doctors. They may not realise the level of importance that some factors have. On the other hand, they may be motivated to exaggerate the seriousness of the difficulties and the impact of disability. This may come about due to external factors such as a compensation claim, or the hope of being prescribed particular medications

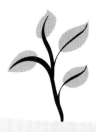

which the person or carer may think of as being beneficial to them. It is important to gather as much supporting information as possible, and to make qualitative observations during interviews and assessment sessions.

Choice of assessments

Following the first appointment, an initial formulation would be generated, including hypotheses about the potential cognitive deficits (see chapters 3 and 8). The assessments chosen must be those most appropriate for testing that person, taking into account demographics, fatigue and motivational levels, the illness or injury and the stage of recovery. Using tests with the strongest properties is essential; the tests should be both valid to measure what they are supposed to be measuring, and reliable and consistently good at measuring that difficulty. The test should have been developed and tried out on large populations with sufficient numbers in each age band. The tests should be good at picking out particular cognitive difficulties, and should not fail people without those difficulties, that is to be specific and sensitive. The inclusion of norms (results tables) for specific groups of people is also very useful, although these are not always available for older tests.

Some traditional cognitive assessments have been criticised for being too artificial and unlike real day-to-day tasks. In order to assess people on more realistic tasks, many assessments have been designed to be more ecologically valid, using familiar stimuli and tasks that reflect activities of everyday living. It is important that the psychologist carefully considers the clinical question, and the person's attitude towards testing in order to decide which tests would be most appropriate. It is useful and common to use a combination of traditional and more ecologically valid tests.

Questionnaires and other paper-based measures

Self-rated measures of mood and symptoms related to the condition should be gathered as well as partner or carer ratings. If a person is in a hospital setting, a rehabilitation unit or a nursing/care home then the professionals involved with their care may also be asked to complete questionnaires. It is essential to use standardised measures, which have been normalised or specifically designed for the current condition, and the person's age.

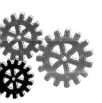

Questionnaires can be used as a quick way of gathering a great deal of information about the patient and the effect of their condition on everyday life. These can include measures of the following.

▶ Mood
  - ▶ Hospital Anxiety and Depression Scale   (Zigmond & Snaith, 1983)
  - ▶ Beck Depression Inventory   (Beck *et al*, 1996)
  - ▶ Beck Anxiety Inventory   (Beck & Steer, 1993)

▶ Health-related quality of life
  - ▶ Short Form Health Questionnaire (SF36)   (Ware *et al*, 1993)
  - ▶ EuroQol (EQ-5D)   (The EuroQol Group, 1990)
  - ▶ General Well-Being Schedule   (Dupuy, 1977)

▶ Activities of daily living
  - ▶ Nottingham Activities of Daily Living Test   (Nouri & Lincoln, 1987)
  - ▶ Barthel Index of Activities of Daily Living (Mahoney & Barthel, 1965)

▶ Health status
  - ▶ General Health Questionnaire   (Goldberg, 1978)
  - ▶ Short Form Health Questionnaire (SF36)   (Ware *et al*, 1993)

▶ Impact of illness
  - ▶ Impact of Illness Scale
    (Klimidis *et al*, 2001)
  - ▶ Expanded Disability Status Scale   (Kurtzke, 1983)
  - ▶ Carer Strain Index   (Robinson, 1983)

▶ Subjective measures of cognition
  - ▶ Everyday Memory Questionnaire – Revised   (Royle & Lincoln, 2008)
  - ▶ Cognitive Risk Profile for Pain   (Cook & Degood, 2006)
  - ▶ Dysexecutive Functioning Questionnaire   (Wilson *et al*, 1996)

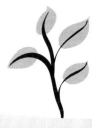

Checklists and the use of diary charts can also be useful when collecting information about the person's strengths and weaknesses. If a person complains of memory difficulties then asking them to keep a diary of the types of difficulties encountered can be very useful. The diary may show that the greatest difficulty is with prospective memory, which could lead to missing appointments, with word finding difficulties, getting lost, or not recognising familiar people. Diary charts that detail the frequency of difficulties may also be kept by family members or carers, this could be a more accurate way of evaluating the problem rather than just trying to estimate how often difficulties occur. It may, in fact, demonstrate that the difficulties occur far less often than previously thought.

Cognitive assessment tools

The next consideration is the selection of appropriate cognitive assessment tools. Generally it is necessary to perform pre-injury (or pre-illness) intellectual functioning measurements, then to assess each cognitive domain including current general intelligence, memory, executive functioning, language, attention/concentration and perceptual/visuo-spatial abilities (see chapter 3 for a full explanation of these cognitive domains). Full standardised batteries for most cognitive areas are available, however, it would be too time consuming for the psychologist, too tiring for the person being assessed, and unethical to complete full batteries for each. It is necessary to decide which core batteries would be used (if any) and which supplementary tests would then be appropriate. The assessment must also include measures of orientation (a person's awareness of their self, of current events, what time it is and where they are). Finally, symptom validity tests should be used to measure the accuracy or truthfulness of the individual's symptoms, behavioural presentation, and their performance on cognitive tests.

Orientation

There are a number of standardised measures of orientation available, including the Galveston Orientation and Amnesia Test (GOAT) (Levin *et al*, 1979). There are also tests of information and orientation embedded within batteries of tests such as the Repeatable Battery for the Assessment of Neuropsychological Status (RBANS) (Randolph, 1998), which is a test of general intelligence, and; the Wechsler Memory Scale (WMS) (Wechsler, 1997 & 2008a), which is a battery of memory tests.

In order to informally measure a patient's orientation, you could ask them their name, address, age and date of birth. You could also ask which day, date, month and year it is and where they are at the moment and who is with them. You could also ask about recent news events.

Pre-injury measures

The majority of measures of pre-injury ability are reading tests. Reading ability is thought to be resistant to the effects of ageing, dementia or acquired impairment through illness or injury (Crawford *et al*, 2001; Sharpe & O'Carroll, 1991; Green *et al*, 2008, Mathias *et al*, 2007). When choosing a pre-injury measure of ability a number of factors need to be considered. Is there a person-centred reason why performance on a reading test would not be representative of pre-injury ability? Is the patient: aphasic, dysarthric, dyslexic, visually impaired, a non-native speaker of English, or someone who has never learnt to read? Is there a test-centred reason for not using a particular measure? Does the test have adequate norms for people similar to the current patient (age, culture, socio-economic group, condition)? Can the results of the test predict performance on measures of current ability?

In general, within the UK the tests of choice for measuring pre-injury ability are the National Adult Reading Test (NART) (Nelson & Willison, 1991) and the Wechsler Test of Adult Reading (WTAR) (Wechsler, 2001), which are both well established reading tests and rely on pronunciation of irregular words. The NART score or the WTAR score can be used to predict performance on the Wechsler Adult Intelligence Scale (WAIS) (Wechsler, 1997). The NART has been shown to be a useful measure in patients with traumatic brain injury except in the acute phase of severe traumatic brain injury (Riley & Simmonds, 2003).

If a patient is unable to complete a reading test, then estimates of pre-injury ability can be made using educational history and occupational history. The estimate can be quite accurate if a person has reached their full potential during their schooling and working life, however, estimates can be artificially low for those people who did not engage at school, or spent many years unemployed.

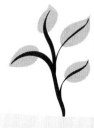

General intellectual functioning

It is important to have a measure of current general intellectual functioning because this forms the baseline for comparing the assessments of other cognitive functions. Current general intellectual functioning can be measured by using either batteries of tests, or a combination of individual tests. Some of the most commonly used tests are the Wechsler Adult Intelligence Scale (WAIS), the Repeatable Battery for the Assessment of Neuropsychological Status (RBANS) and the Raven's Progressive Matrices (Raven *et al*, 2003).

Until very recently the 'gold standard' for measuring general intelligence was the WAIS III (Wechsler, 1997) and you may come across many reports that have assessed intelligence using this measure. The new WAIS IV (Wechsler, 2008a) became available in the UK in 2010, so this will become the standard assessment for measuring general intelligence in the future. It is very important to use up-to-date tests in order to cancel out the Flynn effect, which describes an increase in the average IQ test scores over generations.

The WAIS battery measures verbal comprehension, working memory, perceptual reasoning and processing speed. These four measures can be combined to give a full-scale IQ score. A general ability index, which is free of working memory and speed measures can also be calculated by combining six of the subtest scores.

The Repeatable Battery for the Assessment of Neuropsychological Status (RBANS) is another measure of general intellectual functioning. It is shorter and quicker to administer than the WAIS but it will not provide as much information about intellectual functioning as the WAIS. Therefore, it is frequently used as a screening measure, or as a quick measurement of current general intelligence in services where clinical time for each patient is limited.

The RBANS consists of 12 subtests and measures four cognitive areas: language, attention, visuo-spatial abilities and memory (immediate, delayed and recognition). In addition to the subtests, there is an optional measure of information and orientation. This test is very quick to administer and is often used as a general screening measure. It is frequently used with patients following illness or injury because most patients can tolerate the length taken to administer the test.

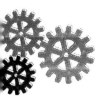

Some psychologists use shortened forms of the WAIS to provide a brief assessment of general intelligence. There are other short batteries of general intelligence available, however, these will not be discussed here.

A quick, stand alone measure of general intelligence is the Raven's Progressive Matrices test; it is a measure of non-verbal reasoning where on each page presented the person is asked to choose from a selection of six items, and which item would complete the pattern or series. The items become progressively more difficult over the course of the assessment and the score can be used to predict performance on the WAIS.

For a quick paper-based measure of cognitive function the Addenbrooke's Cognitive Examination–Revised (ACE-R) (Mioshi *et al*, 2006) is frequently used, which covers more areas of cognition than the Mini Mental State Examination (Folstein *et al*, 2000) that is frequently used by GPs and hospital doctors. The ACE-R is often used as a screening measure for cognitive decline following injury or illness.

It is insufficient to only administer a test of intelligence when deciding whether or not a patient's cognitive abilities have worsened. The WAIS is a reliable and comprehensive measure but it does not include assessment of memory functioning or executive functioning, and these should also be assessed.

Memory

The Wechsler Memory Scale (WMS) (Wechsler, 1997 & 2008b) is considered to be a core component of any thorough cognitive assessment (Groth-Marnat, 2003). It was designed to examine working memory, immediate memory and delayed memory in both visual and verbal areas; it also examined recognition memory. In addition to measuring memory, the WMS IV begins with a brief cognitive status exam, which includes a measure orientation and is quite similar to traditional measures of cognitive status used by psychiatrists, neurologists and GPs.

Traditional memory tests such as the WMS have been criticised for measuring the available memory capacity and how memory works, rather than how effectively a person uses their memory (Kinsella *et al*, 1996). To overcome this, the Rivermead Behavioural Memory Test (RBMT–3) (Wilson *et al*, 2008) was designed to be an ecological measure of everyday memory. It is used to predict everyday memory difficulties in patients and to monitor change in function over time.

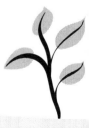

For a quick measure of everyday memory, the Everyday Memory Questionnaire (Royle & Lincoln, 2008) is a useful tool. It can be answered by either the person or their carer. For a quick measure of remembering to carry out planned actions (prospective memory) and remembering about the past (retrospective memory) the Prospective and Retrospective Memory Questionnaire (Crawford *et al*, 2003) can be used. It is completed by the patient's carer or close associate to report on the patient's difficulties.

If you wished to informally measure memory in a person you could:

▶ read the person a telephone number and ask them to give it back to you

▶ read the person a five item shopping list and then ask what was on the list

▶ ask the person what they had for breakfast or who had visited the day before

▶ ask the person the names of any staff who regularly work with them

▶ ask the person to close their eyes and describe the room they are in

▶ ask the person to describe some significant recent event from the news

▶ ask the person how frequently they miss appointments or forget arrangements.

Executive functioning

Executive functions refer to abilities to plan, organise, initiate and monitor our own cognition and behaviour (Burgess & Alderman, 2004). The frontal lobes play a crucial role in these functions and are particularly vulnerable to damage in road traffic accidents, therefore, a thorough assessment of executive functioning would form a cornerstone of the assessment of people following head injury.

The test battery of choice for measuring executive functioning is the Delis Kaplan Executive Function System (D-KEFS) (Delis *et al*, 2001). It measures a wide range of higher level executive functions (planning, decision-making, judgement, cognitive flexibility, self-regulation, self-monitoring and hypothesis generation) and draws upon underlying cognitions such as memory, attention, perception and information processing (Strauss *et al*, 2006).

Traditional neuropsychological tests of executive functioning have been criticised for measuring particular functions in isolation, when everyday life executive functioning requires a complex mix of skills and abilities. While it is useful to have measures of individual executive functions, it is also useful to measure how a patient functions on more familiar tasks that require executive functioning abilities, this type of assessment would be able to predict more accurately everyday activity performance (Wilson *et al*, 1996).

Many psychologists use the Behavioural Assessment of the Dysexecutive Syndrome (BADS) (Wilson *et al*, 1996) for a more ecologically valid measure of executive functioning. The BADS consists of six tests and two questionnaires. The tests measure mental flexibility, rule learning and following, planning, problem-solving, and abstract thinking. An overall profile score is generated from the results of the six tests and this is converted to a standardised score. This battery would appear to be more ecologically valid than other tests of executive functioning, and patients tend to engage well with the tests (Chamberlain, 2003).

Psychologists often combine some tests from the D-KEFS with others from the BADS in order to measure both individual executive functions, and performance on tests which more closely reflect everyday activities and challenges.

There is a wide variety of additional tests of executive functioning, including:

▶ the Hayling and Brixton Test Battery (Burgess & Shallice, 1997). The Hayling is a sentence completion test, which measures verbal flexibility and rule following. The Brixton is a spatial anticipation test, which measures visual and spatial cognitive flexibility

▶ the Controlled Oral Word Association Test (COWAT) (Benton *et al*, 1994) which measures verbal fluency and is associated with executive functioning

▶ the Stroop Neuropsychological Screening Test (SNST) (Trenerry *et al*, 1989), which is often just referred to as the Stroop, it measures cognitive flexibility and the ability to shift set.

Questionnaire measures are very useful when trying to assess everyday effects of problems with executive functioning. The Dysexecutive Questionnaire (DEX) (Burgess *et al*, 1996) was designed to sample

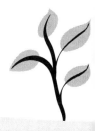

everyday problems associated with executive functioning difficulties and it targets those problems that are seen frequently following frontal lobe injury. There are two versions, one to be completed by the people and the other to be completed by the carer or close associate. The Behaviour Rating Inventory of Executive Function (BRIEF-A) (Roth *et al*, 2005) is frequently used to measure behaviour in the home and the work environment. There are two versions, one self-report questionnaire to be completed by the person, and one to be completed by an informant, normally a carer or employer. Together these two measures capture information which is not readily available through traditional cognitive measures of executive functioning.

Language

An assessment of language would need to be included in a good cognitive assessment and clinical observations during the initial interview and cognitive testing could indicate whether or not further language testing was necessary. The person's reading ability would have been established using the WTAR, and their word generation would have been evaluated using the verbal fluency test in the D-KEFS, and the naming ability could be measured by the RBANS naming subtest. The information and similarities subtests from the WAIS would give a broad picture of language use, but if a person performed very poorly on tests of general intelligence and executive functioning the Token Test (Benton *et al*, 1994) may be used to further assess language functioning.

The Token Test measures comprehension of verbal commands of increasing complexity. It is sensitive to minor impairments of receptive language even when much of the person's communication behaviour has remained intact, making it an extremely useful test (Strauss *et al*, 2006; Lezak *et al*, 2004).

The Frenchay Aphasia Screening Test (FAST) (Enderby *et al*, 2006) is a quick, easy to administer test to help identify and gauge language deficits. It measures language comprehension, language expression (output), reading and writing. If language deficits are observed on any of the above tests it may be useful to refer the patient to a speech and language therapist for a full language assessment.

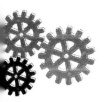

If you wished to informally test a person's language abilities you could:

▶ engage the person in a general conversation and observe any difficulties they might have finding the right words, or if they use incorrect words

▶ ask the person to name objects from a magazine

▶ ask the person to write their name and address

▶ ask the person to read out loud the titles of articles in a magazine

▶ ask the person to look at the ceiling and then point to the door

▶ describe an object to the person and ask them to name it.

Attention

If the referral letter or the initial interview with the patient has revealed concerns about the patient's attentional abilities then the Test of Everyday Attention (TEA) (Robertson *et al,* 1996) would be useful to examine attention. The TEA is a battery of subtests designed to measure selective attention, sustained attention, attentional switching and divided attention (see chapter 3 for an explanation of each). It is able to differentiate which attentional abilities are preserved and which ones are associated with difficulties. This measurement of strengths and weaknesses is very useful for planning rehabilitation. The TEA is regarded as an ecologically valid test, using familiar tasks such as map searching, telephone directory searching and the lottery.

If you wished to informally measure attention and concentration you could ask the patient if they have difficulty following conversations since their illness or accident, also if they have stopped watching favourite television programmes or have difficulty following the plot of soap operas and films. Additionally, you could ask the patient to spell the word 'world' backwards, or ask them if they can count backwards from 100 in steps of three.

Visuo-spatial perception

In order to assess visuo-spatial ability, the copy condition that is copying a complex figure from the Rey Complex Figure Test (Meyers & Meyers, 1995) is frequently used. The immediate recall and delayed recall elements also measure visual memory. If a more in-depth measure of visual perception is

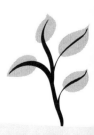

required then items from the Visual Object and Space Perception (VOSP) (Warrington & James, 1991) battery would be used. The VOSP battery was designed to explore visual object perception and space perception and consists of eight tests divided into those two categories. The individual tests were designed to require very simple responses, they do not rely on specific motor skills. Therefore, this test is suitable for use with people with motor difficulties. The TEA battery starts with a screening measure to establish whether or not the person's vision is sufficiently intact to permit further examination (Lezak *et al*, 2004; Strauss *et al*, 2006).

Included in the Addenbrooke's Cognitive Examination – Revised (ACE-R) are three short tests of visuo-spatial perception and ability – copying diagrams, counting dots without pointing to them, and identification of partially complete letters. These could be used as a very quick screen of visuo-spatial perception, prior to conducting a full assessment if needed.

Effort testing

People being assessed by psychiatrists may not always give their full effort during assessment. This can happen for a wide range of reasons, including emotional distress and lack of motivation. Therefore, psychiatrists will often endeavour to assess levels of effort by giving specific tests or looking at the pattern of tests performance. That is why it is important for anyone who is completing such assessments to make their best efforts when doing so.

Caution

There are many tests of cognition which have not been mentioned in this chapter; this does not imply that other tests are not useful. The tests mentioned are those which are most frequently encountered in clinical practice. For an almost complete list of neuropsychological and cognitive tests see Lezak *et al* (2004), Strauss *et al* (2006), Groth-Marnat (2009) and Tate (2010). For more details relating to questionnaire and paper-based measures please see Bowling (2001 & 2005) and Tate (2010).

Take away message

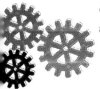

Cognitive assessments can be very useful in measuring a person's strengths, abilities and weaknesses and they can be used to help design rehabilitation programmes, to set realistic goals and to measure improvements or deteriorations. They can help differentiate between normal age-related losses, and those which are associated with acquired brain injuries and disease processes. Many other factors need to be taken into consideration when assessing and interpreting cognitive assessments. Reports frequently detail a person's strengths, abilities and weaknesses within each cognitive domain measured and they are unable to comment on those areas not examined.

Quiz

1. What is the aim of a cognitive assessment?

2. The two things which must be given and obtained when first meeting with a person are:
   a. the hospital address and telephone number
   b. the reason for the current assessment
   c. informed consent
   d. the GP address and telephone number.

3. Where would background information be gathered from?
   a. The person with a neurological disorder
   b. Carers and family members
   c. Referrer and medical notes
   d. Staff and support workers
   e. All of the above

4. What could be measured using questionnaires?

5. Who may be asked to complete these questionnaires?

6. Can you name four cognitive domains that could be assessed?

7. Why is it important to measure pre-injury ability?
   a. To assess and monitor changes in functioning
   b. To identify loss of ability
   c. To set targets for rehabilitation
   d. All of the above

8. How could you informally test a person's language abilities?

9. Why is it important to measure orientation?

10. What are the reasons for measuring effort during a cognitive assessment?

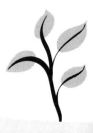

References

Beck AT & Steer RA (1993) *Beck Anxiety Inventory. Manual.* San Antonio: Psychological Corporation.

Beck AT, Steer RA & Brown GK (1996) *Beck Depression Inventory-II Manual.* San Antonio: Psychological Corporation.

Benton AL, Hamsher K & Sivan AB (1994) *Multilingual Aphasia Examination* (3rd edition). Iowa City: AJA Associates.

Bowling A (2001) *Measuring Disease: A review of disease-specific quality of life measurement scales* (2nd edition). Buckingham: Open University Press.

Bowling A (2005) *Measuring Health: A review of quality of life measurement scales* (3rd edition). Buckingham: Open University Press.

Burgess PW & Alderman N (2004) Executive dysfunction. In: LH Goldstein & JE McNeil (Eds) (2005) *Clinical Neuropsychology: A practical guide to assessment and management for clinicians.* Chichester: Wiley.

Burgess PW, Alderman N, Evans J, Emslie H & Wilson BA (1996) *The Dysexecutive Questionnaire.* In: BA Wilson, N Alderman, PW Burgess, H Emslie & JJ Evans (1996) *BADS. Behavioural Assessment of the Dysexecutive Syndrome.* Bury St. Edmunds: Thames Valley Test Company.

Burgess P & Shallice T (1997) *The Hayling and Brixton Tests. Test manual.* Bury St. Edmunds: Thames Valley Test Company.

Chamberlain E (2003) Behavioural Assessment of the Dysexecutive Syndrome – test review. *Journal of Occupational Psychology, Employment and Disability* **5** (20) 33–35.

Cook AJ & Degood DE (2006) The cognitive risk profile for pain: development of a self-report inventory for identifying beliefs and attitudes that interfere with pain management. *Clinical Journal of Pain* **22** (4) 332–345.

Crawford JR, Deary IJ, Starr J & Whalley LP (2001) The NART as an index of prior intellectual functioning: a retrospective validity study covering a 66 year interval. *Psychological Medicine* **31** (3) 451–458.

Crawford J, Smith G, Maylor E, Della Sala S & Logie R (2003) The Prospective and Retrospective Memory Questionnaire (PRMQ): Normative data and latent structure in a large non-clinical sample. *Memory* **11** (3) 261–275.

Delis D, Kaplan E & Kramer J (2001) *Delis-Kaplan Executive Function Scale.* San Antonio: Psychological Corporation.

Dupuy HJ (1977) *The General Well-being Schedule.* In: McDowell I (1996) *Measuring Health: A guide to rating scales and questionnaires* (2nd edition). New York: Oxford University Press.

Enderby P, Wood V, Wade W (2006) *Frenchay Aphasia Screening Test.* London: Witey.

Folstein MF, Folsein SE, McHugh PR & Fanjiang G (2000) *Mini-mental State Examination: User's guide.* Odessa: Psychological Assessment Resources.

Goldberg DP (1978) *Manual of the General Health Questionnaire.* Windsor: NFER Publishing.

Green RE, Melo B, Christensen B, Ngo LA, Monette G & Bradbury C (2008) Measuring premorbid IQ in traumatic brain injury: an examination of the validity of the Wechsler Test of Adult Reading (WTAR). *Journal of Experimental Neuropsychology* **30** (2) 163–172.

Groth-Marnat G (2009) *Handbook of Psychological Assessment* (5th edition). New Jersey: John Wiley & Sons.

Kinsella G, Murtagh D, Landry A, Homfray K, Hammond M, O'Beirne L, Dwyer L, Lamont M & Ponsford J (1996) Everyday memory following traumatic brain injury. *Brain Injury* **10** (7) 499–07.

Kurtzke JF (1983) Rating neurological impairment in multiple sclerosis: an expanded disability status scale (EDSS). *Neurology* **33** (11) 1444–1452.

Levin HS O'Donnell VM & Grossman RG (1979) The Galveston Orientation and Amnesia Test. A practical scale to assess cognition after head injury. *Journal of Nervous and Mental Disease* **167** (11) 675–684.

Lezak MD, Howieson DB & Loring DW (2004) *Neuropsychological Assessment* (4th edition). Oxford: Oxford University Press.

Mahoney FI & Barthel DW (1965) Functional evaluation: the Barthel Index. *Medical Journal* **14** 61–61.

Mathias JL, Bowden SC, Bigler BD & Rosenfield JV (2007) Is performance on the Wechsler test of adult reading affected by traumatic brain injury? *British Journal of Clinical Psychology* **46** 457–466.

Meyers JE & Meyers KR (1995) *Rey Complex Figure Test and Recognition Trial: Professional manual.* Odessa: Psychological Assessment Resources.

Mioshi E, Dawson K, Mitchell J, Arnold R & Hodges JR (2006) The Addenbrooke's Cognitive Examination Revised (ACE-R): A brief cognitive test battery for dementia screening. *International Journal of Geriatric Psychiatry* **21** 1078–1085.

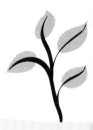

Nelson HE & Willison J (1991) *National Adult Reading Test Manual* (2nd edition). Windsor: NFER-Nelson.

Nouri FM & Lincoln NB (1987) An extended activities of daily living scale for stroke patients. *Clinical Rehabilitation* 301–305.

Raven J, Raven JC & Court JH (2003) *Manual for Raven's Progressive Matrices and Vocabulary Scales*. Section 1: General Overview. San Antonio: Harcourt Assessment.

Randolph C (1998) *RBANS Manual: Repeatable Battery for the Assessment of Neuropsychological Status*. San Antonio: The Psychological Corporation.

Riley GA & Simmonds LV (2003) How robust is performance on the National Adult Reading Test following traumatic brain injury? *British Journal of Clinical Psychology* **42** 319–328.

Robertson IH, Ward T, Ridgeway V & Nimmo-Smith I (1996) The structure of normal human attention: the Test of Everyday Attention. *Journal of International Neuropsychological Society* **2** (6) 525–534.

Robinson B (1983) Validation of a caregiver strain index. *Journal of Gerontology* **38** 344–348.

Roth RM, Isquith PK & Gioia GA (2005) *BRIEF-A Behaviour Rating Inventory of Executive Function – Adult Version*. Lutz: Psychological Assessment Resources.

Royle J & Lincoln NB (2008) The Everyday Memory Questionnaire-revised: development of a 13-item scale. *Disability Rehabilitation* **30** (2) 114–121.

Sharpe K & O'Carroll R (1991) Estimating premorbid intellectual level in dementia using the National Adult Reading Test: a Canadian study. *British Journal of Clinical Psychology* **30** 381–384.

Strauss R, Sherman EMS & Spreen O (2006) *A Compendium of Neuropsychological Tests* (3rd edition). Oxford: Oxford University Press.

Tate RL (2010) *A Compendium of Tests, Scales and Questionnaires. The practitioners guide to measuring outcomes after acquired brain impairment*. Hove: Psychology Press.

The EuroQol Group (1990) EuroQol-a new facility for the measurement of health-related quality of life. *Health Policy* **16** (3) 199–208.

Trenerry MR, Crosson B, DeBoe J & Leber WR (1989) *The Stroop Neurological Screening Test*. Odessa: Psychological Assessment Resources.

Ware JE, Snow KK, Kosinski M & Gandek B (1993) *SF-36 Health Survey: Manual and Interpretation Guide*. Boston: The Health Institute, New England Medical Centre.

Warrington EK & James M (1991) *Visual Object and Space Perception Battery*. Bury St. Edmunds: Thames Valley Test Company.

Wechsler D (1997) *Wechsler Adult Intelligence Scale-III*. London: The Psychological Corporation.

Wechsler D (1998) *Wechsler Memory Scale-III*. London: The Psychological Corporation.

Wechsler D (2001) *Wechsler Test of Adult Reading*. San Antonio: The Psychological Corporation.

Wechsler D (2008a) *Wechsler Adult Intelligence Scale-IV*. London: The Psychological Corporation.

Wechsler D (2008b) *Wechsler Memory Scale-IV*. San Antonio: The Psychological Corporation.

Wilson BA, Alderman N, Burgess PW, Emslie H & Evans JJ (1996) *Behavioral Assessment of the Dysexecutive Syndrome*. Bury St. Edmunds: Thames Valley Test Company.

Wilson BA, Greenfield E, Clare L, Baddeley A, Cockburn J, Watson P, Tate R, Sopena S & Nannery R (2008) *Rivermead Behavioural Memory Test* (3rd edition). San Antonio: The Psychological Corporation.

Zigmond AS & Snaith RP (1983) The Hospital Anxiety and Depression Scale. *Acta Psychiatrica Scandinavica* **67** 361–370.

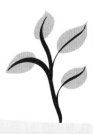

Chapter 8

Formulation – putting all the information together

Patrick Vesey

Aims of the chapter

This chapter aims to:

▶ define formulation

▶ examine how formulation can be helpful to a member of staff, the carer or patient

▶ consider how to reach a formulation

▶ look at the information needed to make a formulation

▶ show that a formulation might change over time.

Introduction

What is a formulation?
To provide good support to a person with a neurological condition or injury (eg. acquired brain injury, stroke, multiple sclerosis) you need a good idea and understanding of their difficulties, and this will help you to help them. A formulation gives an account of the difficulties facing the person, including their circumstances, relationships, abilities, disabilities, and the challenges that they (and significant others) face. It describes where the person has come from in their life and the influences and circumstances that make up their complete condition and well-being at the time they come to you.

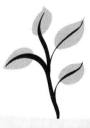

Helping people with neurological illnesses or injuries is sometimes straightforward, but often this is not the case. How do you put together all the information you have about a case, such as the person's medical condition; their activity, recreation or employment; what disabilities they have; their behaviour; their memory problems; their problems with organisation; their social life and relationships; why they are sometimes well, but other times not? In supporting a person with long-term or complex needs it can be difficult to know where to start.

Imagine the following person has been referred to your service for support.

Case study

Simon, a 31-year-old man, comes for help to the service you work in. He has epilepsy and a brain tumour, which was diagnosed when he was 14. For several years the brain tumour was only monitored because of the risks of an operation and until the diagnosis of his brain tumour Simon had had a normal life. His health and development in childhood had been good and he had grown up in a happy and caring environment. He was a bright boy who was popular at school. He developed epilepsy at the age of 12 and the tumour was diagnosed two years later when he had a brain scan.

However, his epilepsy worsened during his teens and began to have a bigger and bigger effect on his life. It interfered with his school-leaving exams, the job he had when he left school, and his social life. In his early 20s his specialists became more concerned about the tumour, and he eventually had a long operation at the age of 24. The surgery was proceeding well but towards the end of the operation he suffered a haemorrhage deep in his brain. He became critically ill and unresponsive. He gradually emerged from a nine-week coma. He had neuro-rehabilitation in two different specialist units (one NHS, one independent sector) lasting many months, but he had been left with severe neuropsychological and psycho-social disabilities.

The current situation is that he lives with his ageing parents in the family home with input from support workers during the day. He is closely supported by his family who remain very involved in his care. His activity consists of attending a local day centre once a week, going to his local shops, and listening to music.

Simon needs close supervision because of the medical risks caused by his epilepsy, and also because he cannot independently carry out many activities of daily living such as preparing food, doing the laundry, and paying bills. He has a mild and pleasant temperament but has difficulty judging personal space and knowing when to stop talking. He can be over-enthusiastic in his interactions, with undue familiarity and

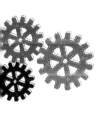

touching. Occasionally his behaviour can be very difficult. He tends to get on well with his carers but has intense verbal and occasionally physical altercations with members of the family, which have sometimes occurred in public places and caused other people to become involved to try and help. These events have been enormously distressing to all concerned, including Simon's family.

You want to help Simon and you need to work out if you can, but how do you begin to understand his difficulties; how do you decide what is causing them; how do you describe them; how do you explain them? Where do you start and, importantly, when do you finish?

This is where a formulation comes in. A formulation helps put together all this information in a way that permits a better understanding of what is happening to a person with a neurological condition and how you might go about helping them.

A brief history

Psychological formulation evolved within the practice of psychology partly as a response to the practice of psychiatric diagnosis. Both approaches have their strengths but psychological formulation developed as an alternative to the overly short descriptions that patients had about their condition when receiving a psychiatric diagnosis. Psychological formulation was seen as offering a richer and more human conceptualisation of psychological difficulty.

Psychological formulation is practised by professional psychologists and some other mental health specialists. It requires formal training and the continual updating of relevant knowledge and skills; there are different types of formulation according to the clinical orientation of the psychologist. This chapter has been prepared to give a general overview of formulation in recognition of the fact that a wide range of support, care, and therapy staff working with people with neurological conditions do not occupy roles requiring the construction of formal psychological formulations. Nevertheless, many staff attempt to understand the psychological aspects of a case to facilitate their own work and support of a client. They do this to strengthen their rapport and relationship with the client and enhance and further the benefit of their therapeutic, support, or care work.

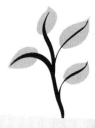

Formulation is one part of a systematic approach to helping a person with neurological difficulties

A formulation gives a meaningful summary of all the information gathered about a person in the early stages of contact with a professional such as psychologist, and it is usually put together after the first few contact sessions with them. It provides the necessary basis for building a plan of intervention or support, following which an evaluation can be undertaken of the help provided and the formulation revised. Formulation is one of four important stages of systematic help:

1. Assessment (see also chapter 5 and 7)
   ↓
2. Formulation
   ↓
3. Intervention (see chapters 9, 10 and 11)
   ↓
4. Evaluation (see chapters 9 and 10).

A formulation tells a story of a person's case

At its simplest level, a formulation is a person's 'story'. It puts together the information you know about a person in a way that tells an informed story of where they are in their life, what difficulties they face and how they can be helped. It offers direction on how to support a person, how to help them overcome the challenges they face, cope with their difficulties, maximise their autonomy and dignity, and progress to a better quality of life. It helps you pay proper attention to all the things that are impinging on a person's well-being.

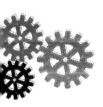

A formulation will:

▶ guide your thinking about the causes of a person's difficulties

▶ help you get a better idea of a person

▶ guide other questions you might want to ask

▶ help you get an overall view

▶ help you link their difficulties with what is going on in their life

▶ help you work out how to prioritise a person's difficulties

▶ help you plan your own involvement with a client

▶ help you decide who else could help

▶ help you think about successful outcomes

▶ help you be realistic about what you can achieve

▶ help you predict stumbling blocks and find ways around them

▶ help you to keep 'grounded' in the help or support you offer.

What information is needed in building a formulation?

A formulation uses two sources of information to build an informed story of a person's case.

1. It uses information about the person specifically.

2. It uses information from theories and models of psychological functioning.

Formulations use information from psychological theories and models and apply it flexibly to information about the person that comes from an assessment of them and their circumstances. The two sources of information go together to give an understanding of the client's difficulties and how they might be helped.

Non-psychologists are less likely to be familiar with the spectrum of theories and models of psychological functioning relevant to understanding the psychology of people with neurological conditions, but it is essential to the process of formulating to have an understanding of these.

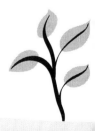

Theories and models of relevance to psychological functioning

Some of the important models are outlined here. They each provide a cornerstone, alongside client-specific information, for constructing a good case formulation. They offer a different perspective on the nature, cause, and remedy of the psychological issues facing people with a neurological condition (see also chapter 1).

Biological/medical model

Biological models of disease and disability are fundamental to reaching an understanding of a case, and therefore a case formulation. Biological models concern the actual physical injury or damage that can occur in the neurological system and the potential for recovery thereafter. They also refer to the injuries and recovery that may occur in relation to other aspects of a person's physical and medical well-being, such as any orthopaedic difficulties. This is important in some cases (such as traumatic brain injury) where multiple injury types can occur as a result of high speed impacts resulting from road traffic accidents, high elevation falls, or severe assaults.

Biological models orientate expectations as to the kind of disabilities and prognosis that might be expected with different conditions. They inform a sense of what is known about the scope for a person's neurological and physical recovery; whether the underlying condition is expected to worsen, remain the same or improve; and what physical disabilities may be associated with the condition. Importantly, they also have the potential to provide valuable information on a person's own understanding of their condition.

In a sense, the biological models constitute essential background knowledge about a person's neurological condition or injury. Such background knowledge can be found in the very accessible information provided by the charitable organisations and associations supporting people with various neurological conditions (such as Headway, the Multiple Sclerosis Society, the Parkinson's Disease Society, and Epilepsy Action).

Neuropsychological model

The neuropsychological models concern those aspects of psychological functioning thought to be directly and biologically associated with brain function. It is useful to consider two main aspects of neuropsychological functioning.

Cognitive functioning: Cognitive functioning (see also chapter 3) refers to the basic human mental functions of language, attention, memory, perception and executive functioning (eg. planning and self-organising). It also includes social-cognitive functions of self and other awareness, the ability to read and express emotions. In neurological conditions, these functions can be individually or severally affected. Many clients with neurological conditions experience problems with one or more cognitive functions; memory and concentration complaints are common. An awareness of these different functions is important in understanding how their impairment in neurological conditions can contribute to a client's difficulties.

Emotional and behavioural functioning (see also chapter 4): Emotional functioning concerns the emotional aspects of neurological conditions that are directly, biologically associated with changes in the neurological system. This might include changes in the ability of people with neurological conditions to self-regulate their own emotional states, responses, or behaviour. This is perhaps most clearly exemplified in cases of emotional/behavioural under-responsiveness or over-responsiveness after frontal lobe injuries in the context of traumatic brain injury, or some fronto-temporal dementias where such clients show emotional changes involving loss of warmth or empathy.

Psychological model

The psychological model offers a way of understanding the psychological challenges facing people with neurological conditions. These concern the psychological processes of potential relevance to all people regardless of whether or not they have a background neurological condition.

Psychological adjustment to significant life events: Rudimentary theories of psychological adjustment hold that adjustment to major life events is a process characterised by numerous psychological stages including disbelief, numbness, anger, insight, adaptation and acceptance, all of which people with medical conditions may experience in different times and in different orders. The model characterises the different ways that clients can react to neurological diagnosis such as their psychological response to the diagnosis, the process of coming to terms with the diagnosis, and the challenge of maintaining a good quality of life in the context of it. The model is particularly useful for considering the psychological impact of a neurological condition because:

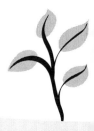

▶ many neurological conditions have a severe, sudden onset (such as a traumatic brain injury)

▶ many neurological conditions are progressive (such as some forms of multiple sclerosis, movement disorder or motor neuron disease)

▶ many neurological conditions have life-long implications (by virtue of the long-term disability they cause).

Adjustment models hold that psychological difficulties arise from a person's becoming stuck in certain (sometimes earlier) stages of adjustment such as denial and anger, and insufficiently progressing towards successful adjustment to their condition. The models suggest that progress can be made by processing, coming to terms with, or learning to effectively manage the set of challenges associated with each stage in a supportive and safe environment.

While the adjustment models can be helpful, they also have limitations in how relevant they are to understanding neurological cases. It is useful to bear in mind that the neurological condition itself may impinge directly on a person's experience of the kind of psychological response associated with other (non-neurological) medical conditions. For example, processes of insight–acquisition and anger–resolution/management may be compromised by damage to certain brain areas in neurological conditions. Additionally, models of adjustment assume a fixed set of circumstances to which a person might possibly adjust. However, this is not necessarily the case in neurological conditions where the person's underlying condition may deteriorate, improve, or even markedly fluctuate over time. As such, the overall process of adjustment, rarely straightforward anyway in chronic medical conditions, may become quite complicated in neurological conditions.

Cognitive-behavioural models: Cognitive behavioural therapy (CBT) models hold that a client's psychological well-being is influenced by how they see themselves, their condition, and the wider world. Examining the relationship between three essential components (thoughts, feelings, and behaviour) is said to reveal some of the roots of certain negative psychological patterns as well as some of the solutions. CBT models maintain that there is a pattern of cross-influence between feelings, thoughts, and behaviour, where each influences the other to either positive or negative effect.

For example, a person experiencing negative thoughts about themselves, their condition, and the wider world (thoughts) may become more withdrawn from social activities and networks (behaviour), will feel more dispirited and self-critical (feelings), and will pay more attention to negative thoughts and self-talk (cognitive). In this way a negative circle is maintained until the client is able to change one or more aspects of the thought/behaviour/feelings pattern, until a more positive circle of functioning is achieved.

Cognitive behavioural models are valuable for understanding how a client can be helped to change because they tend to articulate potential change in terms of specific goals that can be clearly targeted and worked towards as part of a rehabilitation, care or support package.

Family and systems models (see chapters 1 and 10): Family and systems models emphasise the importance of the wider family and care environment in understanding the challenges and solutions facing a client. Unlike the 'adjustment' or CBT models which focus on 'within-the-client' psychological processes, these models consider the person's emotional and behavioural well-being to be strongly and inevitably influenced by those around them. Some family and systems models go so far as to say that a person's difficulty is not actually a person's difficulty but a difficulty of the family or system. These models can offer powerful solutions for addressing a person's psychological difficulty but they can also be challenging for the family (or system) to hear without feeling threatened or criticised.

Psychological recovery is said to be principally achieved by changing one or more parts of the person's environment. Often, this means changing the behaviour of a family member or care giver so that, as a result, the influence upon the person changes and psychological progress is achieved.

Life span development: Life span models emphasise the different stages in people's lives such as childhood, adolescence, adulthood, and the different issues and challenges that people face at these times, such as securing important attachments in early life; making social relationships; developing autonomy and independence; becoming an adult; having a sexual partner(s); raising children; making sense and meaning of one's life. Life span models hold that a proper understanding of a person's difficulties can only occur when consideration is given to what life stage they are at, and how they have negotiated other life stages.

Psychological difficulty is thought to result from a difficult experience at one or more life stages. Progress is thought to depend on the successful

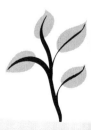

resolution of the challenges and complexities associated with each life stage. For example, learning to build successful social relationships, learning to separate from early care givers (both physically and emotionally), becoming an independent adult occupationally and domestically.

Social model (see chapters 1 and 10): Social models hold that psychological well-being is closely bound up with the accessibility of society to its members. For a person with a neurological condition, this includes the readiness of society to accept such persons as full members of society, and the readiness to adapt facilities and infrastructures for the needs and contributions of a person with neurological conditions, and any physical and psycho-social disabilities they have. Such social enablement will permit full community integration and enhance the quality of life of such persons.

Summary: None of these models are exclusively correct. Over several decades each model has accumulated a body of research that has investigated and enhanced the power of the models to explain and understand human psychology. The models are complementary and can be used at the same time to explain, alongside case specific information, one or more aspects of a case and build an informed case formulation.

Collaboration in formulation building

Formulations are for people with a neurological difficulty and are conducted with the person. They are for the person's benefit to help them overcome difficulties and improve their quality of life. Occasionally when psychologists formulate, for a variety of reasons it may not be possible to work with the person and engage them directly in the process of formulation building. In these circumstances psychologists will use formulations done with a family member or care team. As with most types of support, intervention formulations can only be undertaken with the person's agreement, and their engagement and participation. The quality of the formulation depends directly on the extent to which the person has provided information and input to the process of formulating and the extent to which they see it as relevant and applicable to them. This does not mean that the information they contribute has to be absolutely accurate or comprehensive, it just means that they have to be active partners in the process of using this approach, so that the story is meaningful to them and gives rise to a plan of intervention and support that they feel has a possibility of helping them.

The pre-formulation assessment

A formulation summarises all the relevant background information on a person from the assessment. The assessment covers many different factors that might have contributed to the development of a person's difficulties, such as the person's previous personality, or other stressful or significant life events such as financial difficulties or bereavements. Assessment is not the subject of this particular chapter (see chapter 7 for more information) so the detail will not be explored exhaustively, but a good assessment should include the following questions.

Assessment questions

The main complaints

When did the problems start (ie. the psycho-social difficulties prompting contact with your service); was the onset gradual or sudden; have they worsened or improved; are they the same all the time; who else is around when they happen and who else do they involve; what makes them better or worse; how the person sees the problem and how others see the problem; how the person copes with the difficulties; how others cope with the difficulties?

The person's psychological condition, if not already specified

Are there any problems with the person's various cognitive functions including memory, concentration, organisation, writing, spelling, reading; are there any other current or past psychological difficulties such as emotional/behavioural/personality; is there any past or present self-harm?

Person's condition on meeting

How is the person's appearance, behaviour, speech, mood, insight?

Activity

How the person passes the time; does the person work; what hobbies or interest does the person have?

Domestic and family circumstances

Who does the person live with; what is the person's marital and relationship status; are there any dependents; what is the social network like?

Day-to-day personal functional activities

Does the person have any difficulty with dressing, washing, bathing, using the toilet, handling money, driving, and mobility?

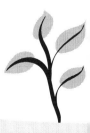

Early health and developmental
Were there any early problems with the person's in utero development, birth, or milestones?

Education and employment
Did the person attend mainstream schooling; did the person achieve any school leaving qualifications; what is the person's employment history?

General health
How is the person's general health; are there any other medical conditions; have there been any other serious illnesses or accidents (especially of neurological relevance); does the person have any pain or sleep disturbance; how is the person's appetite and diet; is there any relevant family history?

Medication and substances
Is the person taking any medication; does the person drink alcohol and if so is there a history of drinking to excess; does the person take any non-prescription substances?

Significant life events
Have there been any other recent or distant significant life events, either connected or unconnected to their present well-being (eg. bereavements, violence, abuse)?

Risk
Are there any factors of relevance to risk the well-being of the person or others (eg. violence or self-harm not previously identified)?

Treatment and support
What other support the person has had to date?

The formulation

The formulation summarises the assessment information, gives relevance to it with reference to psychological theories and models, and gives direction about things that might help. The formulation should include biological, psychological, and social factors – this is called a bio-psycho-socially based formulation. It is a formulation of the person's psychological difficulties taking into account all the relevant biological, psychological and social influences and aspects of their condition. It should consider the relevant

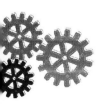

background information, the reasons why the person's difficulty has recently become significant, any particularly intense occurrences of the difficulties and the factors that set them off, and what keeps the difficulties going and what stops them getting worse. As such, the following framework is helpful for separating out the various categories of information in a formulation.

Tip: it is useful to write down the information and structure it using the following headings when building a formulation.

Presenting problem: This should be a clear summary of the person's psychological difficulties at the time of presentation or referral to the service. It should include a list of all the cognitive, emotional, and behavioural difficulties regarded as being problematic for the person or their family or carers.

Vulnerability factors: These are the factors in the person's history that made the person vulnerable to having developed the current difficulties.

Precipitating factors: These are the immediate experiences, events or circumstances that have caused the person to come to the attention of your service at this particular time.

Triggering factors: These factors 'set-off' any particularly intense difficulties in the immediate time building up to them (ie. minutes or hours).

Perpetuating factors: These are the factors causing the person's symptoms to continue to occur rather than get better.

Protective factors: These are factors that contain the difficulties in their present state and stop the situation from getting any worse.

Formulating Simon's difficulties

It might be useful to illustrate a formulation using the earlier example of Simon.

Following Simon's referral, there follows a period of assessment involving the collection of information, from Simon and his carers, about his difficulties (with his agreement).

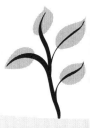

Putting all the information together permits the construction of a provisional formulation of Simon's case. A possible formulation is presented below along with the various theoretical models that potentially inform the various parts of the formulation. (For the purpose of formulating Simon's case it is assumed that the relevant information has been collected during the assessment and is now included in the formulation.)

Presenting problem: The clear summary of the person's psychological difficulties.

Simon currently has anger outbursts. These occur almost exclusively with his family; he becomes verbally, and sometimes physically aggressive towards them. Often this happens at home, but sometimes also in public places. Occasionally, members of the public have intervened to try and help out.

Vulnerability factors: The factors in the person's history that made the person vulnerable to having developed the current difficulties.

Simon developed a complex neurological condition involving epilepsy, brain tumour and haemorrhage. His rehabilitation specialists feel that his physical recovery will not progress any further (relevance of biological/medical model). He needs continuing support from family and formal carers.

Associated with his neurological condition, Simon has multiple cognitive difficulties such as problems with memory, concentration and self-organisation. He has been assessed by a neuropsychologist and the assessment has confirmed the cognitive, emotional and behavioural difficulties are likely to be associated with direct damage to areas of the brain associated with these functions. This suggests that his ability to monitor and control his emotions and behaviour has been affected by his neurological condition. It is also possible that his insight and awareness of his circumstances and abilities has been compromised (relevance of neuropsychological model).

As a result of his disabilities there will probably be disruption to many of the life events and achievements he would otherwise have encountered, and there may be a loss of meaning and purpose in his life (relevance of life span model). He may have some hidden frustration about this, although actually this is not obvious in discussions with him.

Precipitating factors: The immediate experiences, events or circumstances that have caused the client to come to the attention of the service.

During his rehabilitation years ago, Simon's family were advised to assist in his recovery by supervising him closely and giving him encouragement, prompting and instruction. The purpose of this was to help him self-monitor and self-regulate his behaviour and activity.

Now, years later, they think he no longer accepts the prompting and instruction they offer and that as a result he will make mistakes and not have the quality of life he has the potential of having. However, they persist in monitoring him closely and providing him with the same directive instructions in the way they were advised. They are puzzled about why his behaviour has deteriorated (relevance of family and systems model).

Things came to a head on a recent holiday after Simon became agitated and angry towards his parents. He started hitting his father, and his father had to try and restrain him. The police attended and there were lots of onlookers. Everyone was very shaken by this incident and it was this that prompted Simon's referral to your service.

Perpetuating factors: The factors causing the patient's symptoms to continue to occur rather than get better.

Simon's family now feel they are at the end of their tether. They are despondent and disillusioned and cannot cope with his aggression and do not feel they can manage him at home much longer. They are holding on to what they have always done since he became disabled, which is monitor him closely and give him clear instructions about what to do.

Triggering factors: These factors 'set-off' any particularly intense difficulties in the immediate time building up to them (ie. minutes or hours).

Information from the assessment suggests that Simon becomes angry in situations in which he is alone with his parents (ie. without his support workers) and when his parents instruct him to do something that he doesn't feel is necessary. Closer analysis suggests that these are generally not situations where instructions are given to him for risk or safety reasons, but just where Simon's parents think that it is better for him to do things in a certain way (there is no dispute that they believe it is for his benefit). Notably, the difficulties do not occur when he is with his support workers.

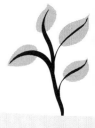

Protective factors: These are factors that contain the difficulties in their present state and stop the situation from getting any worse.

Simon seems happy in his day-to-day activities and enjoys attending the day centre, and generally there is a feeling of mutual affection between him and his family. They do spend quite a lot of time apart from each other; when he is at the day centre and when he is otherwise occupied with his support workers, and this sustains the current arrangements and allows Simon and his family to have space from each other.

Plan of intervention

Based on the formulation, some or all of the following tasks of support/ intervention might be indicated (there may be additional or alternative things you can think of):

1. Acknowledge everyone's efforts in supporting Simon and the difficult aspects of the current circumstances. It is important that nobody feels at fault for the current difficulties because it will be necessary to maintain a good working relationship for the other aspects of the support plan.

2. Emphasise that it is important for everyone's well-being for Simon and his parents to have a good relationship and for these altercations between Simon and his parents to be minimised as far as possible.

3. Encourage his family to consider that the valuable monitoring and instruction that they used to offer to Simon used to be very helpful but may no longer be so, and that they should consider employing a less intense form of support in recognition that his period of active rehabilitation and recovery is now over.

4. Encourage his parents to enjoy more 'quality time' where they do not feel a pressure to be his informal rehabilitation workers.

5. Plan to have some more time with Simon to explore whether he has any distress about his life circumstances that has not been apparent so far.

6. Consider whether a formal neuropsychological or neurorehabilitation review would offer Simon's family further clarity on how best to help him with monitoring and instruction.

7. Arrange for a social work review to consider domestic and respite arrangements.

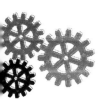

Revising formulations after a period of intervention or support

It is not possible to say in Simon's hypothetical case what might have happened next. Perhaps the difficulties would have improved and the quality of life for Simon and his family would have been enhanced. Perhaps the support and intervention would have been only partially or minimally successful and needed to have been substantially revised or radically changed.

For the case formulation, the important thing to remember is that whatever happens in the intervention should feed back into, and revise, the initial provisional formulation. The initial formulation is not static, fixed, or final. It is only provisional, to be refined by further information that becomes available as the case progresses, including information and experience from the support or intervention plan. A formulation is a live account of a person's story, the psychological processes and challenges the person faces, the person's needs, and the things that might help. This process of formulation and reformulation can potentially continue until such time as the parties relevant to it conclude that benefit from the person's contact with the service has been maximised. In this respect, the formulation is like a care plan that is devised and reviewed at intervals.

Take away message

Building a case formulation allows you to have an evolving and informed story of a person's difficulties by way of reference to psychological theories and models. It helps explain what has brought a person to your service and how you can go about helping them.

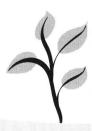

Quiz

1. Which one of the following best describes what a formulation is?
   a. A mixture of ideas about a person's disorder
   b. A fixed diagnosis
   c. A theory-informed 'story' of a person's case that leads to ideas about what can help
   d. Making decisions for the person

2. The purpose of a formulation is primarily to do with which one of the following?
   a. Decide which organisation should care for the person
   b. Establish what medication the person should be taking
   c. Check if they have capacity
   d. To help you provide good support to a person you need a good idea and understanding of their difficulties

3. A formulation is one part of a systematic approach to helping a person. Which of the following are the other parts?
   a. Doing an interview
   b. Assessment
   c. Making an activity plan
   d. Intervention
   e. Evaluation
   f. Decision-making
   g. Sending out letters to all professionals involved in the person's care

4. Formulations use two main sources of information to build an informed story of a person's case. Which two are they?
   a. How long the person has been disabled
   b. Person-specific information
   c. How often the person's problems occur
   d. Information from theories and models of psychological functioning
   e. How motivated the person is

5. Which two of the following theories and models are not of special relevance to building a psychological formulation in the context of a neurological condition?
   a. Biological/medical models
   b. Financial models
   c. Models of cognitive functioning
   d. Models of emotional and behavioural functioning
   e. Psychological adjustment models
   f. Family systems models
   g. Life span development models
   h. Social models
   i. Clay models

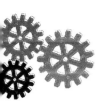

6. Who is the formulation for (it could be any or all of the following)?
   a. The carer
   b. The person with the neurological disorder
   c. The person's support team
   d. The person's family

7. Once a formulation is made:
   a. it is fixed and finalised indefinitely
   b. it is possible to amend and revise it after a period of intervention or when further information becomes available.

Further reading

The following organisations provide further information on various neurological conditions.

Alzheimer's Society [online]. Available at: www.alzheimers.org.uk (accessed January 2011).

Association for Spina Bifida and Hydrocephalus (ASBAH) [online]. www.asbah.org (accessed January 2011).

Child Brain Injury Trust [online]. Available at: www.cbituk.org (accessed January 2011).

Encephalitis Society [online]. Available at: www.encephalitis.info (accessed January 2011).

Epilepsy Action [online]. Available at: www.epilepsy.org.uk (accessed January 2011).

Headway –The Brain Injury Association [online]. Available at: www.headway.org.uk (accessed January 2011).

Huntington's Disease Association [online]. Available at: www.hda.org.uk (accessed January 2011).

Mind [online]. Available at: www.mind.org.uk (accessed January 2011).

Motor Neuron Disease Association [online]. Available at: www.mndassociation.org (accessed January 2011).

Multiple Sclerosis Society [online]. Available at: www.mssociety.org.uk (accessed January 2011).

National Society for Epilepsy [online]. Available at: www.epilepsysociety.org.uk (accessed January 2011).

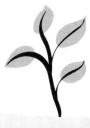

The Neurological Alliance [online]. Available at: www.neural.org.uk (accessed January 2011). This organisation provides contact details for a wide range of neurological associations and societies including, but not restricted to, the ones below.

Parkinson's Disease Society [online]. Available at: www.parkinsons.org.uk (accessed January 2011).

SCOPE [online]. Available at: www.scope.org.uk (accessed January 2011).

The Stroke Association [online]. Available at: www.stroke.org.uk (accessed January 2011).

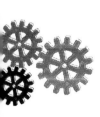

Chapter 9

What can be done I: restitution or compensation?

Melanie Stevens

Aims of the chapter

This chapter aims to:

▶ explain what is meant by 'restitution' and 'compensation'

▶ identify some of the core strategies used in cognitive rehabilitation

▶ appreciate what can be done for cognitive difficulties following an injury to the brain

▶ analyse what the evidence says with regard to the restitution and compensation of cognitive difficulties.

Introduction

When someone experiences an event that causes disease or damage to the brain it causes distress to all those involved; the person suffering the event, and their family, carers, friends and work colleagues (see also chapter 1 and 11). Any disease or damage to the brain can cause physical, cognitive, social, occupational and psychological changes. Once the areas of weakness are identified the question of whether to attempt to restore or to compensate occurs, and the decision is determined by a thorough assessment and research findings. Restitution is also referred to as restoration, and compensation is also referred to as substitution.

Neuropsychological rehabilitation is an over-arching term to describe the process of recovery and can be defined as the remediation or recovery from

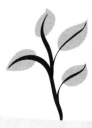

the cognitive, behavioural, emotional and motor consequences of brain injury. Its aim is to help the client recover to the best level of functioning possible. The aim is to help the individual return to their previous life as best they can in their own environment. This process is the focus of the chapter.

Background

The history of neuropsychological rehabilitation goes back as far as ancient Egypt (Walsh, 1987). Modern day rehabilitation began in the First World War due to a need for the rehabilitation of soldiers, many more of whom were surviving due to medical advances (Goldstein, 1942). Ever more sophisticated medical interventions, response units and intensive care units have led to improvements in survival rates for a range of events, for example, road traffic accidents and cardiac arrests. This has made it increasingly necessary to work with those who may have recovered physically, but are left with a range of cognitive and psychological difficulties. Therefore, neuropsychological rehabilitation has also developed, along with specialist occupational therapists, job coaches, case managers, physiotherapists, nurses, consultants and rehabilitation assistants.

The modern development of neuropsychological rehabilitation has taken place over a relatively short period of time and rehabilitation specialists have rapidly evolved new management strategies as a result. They have learnt it is imperative to work in partnership with the friends, relatives and work colleagues of those with injury to the brain. Increasingly, employers, colleagues, teachers, partners, children, parents and others are becoming part of the rehabilitation team's strategy to help the person affected by the injury to achieve their goals.

Neuro-rehabilitation has developed a goal setting approach (also called goal planning). Indeed goal setting is central to neuro-rehabilitation and typically serves as a cornerstone for the programme of recovery. Goals however, must be SMART (specific, measurable, achievable, realistic/relevant and time-bound). Thus goals should be well-defined, with a well developed plan for achieving them. Goals should always be developed on the aims and ambitions of the client, often with the family or carer's input and support. The rehabilitation team should also ensure that goals are a mixture of short-term and long-term to encourage the client to see some success in the short term, and thus help them to remain motivated despite the difficulties they now face. This is especially important for neuro-rehabilitation with children and adolescents who often struggle to remain motivated if only given long-term goals.

SMART goals have to take into account the links between the cognitive, emotional, social and behavioural consequences of brain injury and these goals then lead to specific interventions with a clearly defined path. Interventions are measured against the goal to see if they are effective. The kind of things SMART goals address include a return to social participation, ideally with the inclusion of some form of vocational activity, paid or voluntary, restoration of the ability to self-care, reduction of physical difficulties and improvement of cognitive functioning. An example of a SMART goal is being able to sit up in bed for 30 minutes without physical support and to achieve this within two weeks.

Theories of cognitive functioning

There are a number of theories and models of cognitive functioning which have proved exceptionally helpful in the field of rehabilitation. Coltheart (1985) for instance, suggests that cognitive rehabilitation should always be based on theories devised from cognitive neuropsychology. Caramazza (1989), on the other hand, argues that models contribute and are necessary, but are not enough by themselves.

When working with any psychological issue it is necessary to work out what problems there are and how these are related to an individual's past and current functioning. This is a process clinical psychologists call formulation (see chapter 8 for more information). This helps in the understanding of the meaning of the problem, how it fits into previous levels of functioning, social circumstances and the function of any behaviour. Neuropsychological rehabilitation also relies on all the members of the multidisciplinary team, involving family and carers as additional members of the team to collaborate in making a good formulation and SMART goals. Multidisciplinary rehabilitation can be defined as any intervention where two or more disciplines are working in a co-ordinated way. This could be an inpatient, outpatient, day patient or community service. Moreover, neuropsychological rehabilitation should focus on improving everyday functioning and should also promote the use of any strategies learnt to be used in the client's environment.

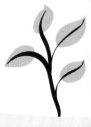

What we mean by recovery

This section will address what we mean by restitution and compensation. Where the part of the brain that is damaged recovers fully, this is called 'restitution' or 'reinstatement' (LeVere, 1980). 'Compensation', on the other hand, happens when restitution does not happen or is not possible, and refers to looking at ways that a person can do a task differently, for example, lift a kettle with their left hand if they have a weakness in their right hand, or provide aids and supports, for example, utensils with larger and/or shaped handles for someone with grip difficulties, or a diary/electronic organiser for someone with memory problems. Compensation involves enabling persons with neurological difficulties to manage their deficits.

Robertson (1999) suggests that a full restitution to previous functioning and abilities is possible for relatively small areas of damage, especially in more serious injuries, while compensation is more useful for larger areas of damage. The effectiveness of compensation varies from one person to the next and this will be further explored later in this chapter. Plaut (1996) also argues that lesion location and size predict the ability of a person to recover and relearn.

Cognitive rehabilitation often involves the following:

▶ endeavouring to achieve restoration or partial restoration of functioning via neuro-plasticity (the ability of the brain to reorganise itself around the damaged area and find a new route: a bit like using the A roads when the M1 is blocked)

▶ helping the client compensate for any deficit

▶ helping the client to learn more efficiently

▶ exercises to improve performance.

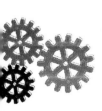

Case study 1
A 45-year-old man fell down a flight of stairs, resulting in multiple skull fractures sustaining damage to the frontal and occipital lobes in addition to a range of other serious physical injuries. He spent six weeks in the intensive care unit of the hospital before he was stabilised physically. Once he was medically stable he was transferred to the rehabilitation unit for treatment.

The treatment on the rehabilitation ward involved a detailed assessment of his current level of function, work with his family to identify his previous levels of functioning, as well as working with family members and friends to develop a detailed formulation. Before his accident he worked in his own business and had no previous physical injuries or notable illnesses and no mental health difficulties. Part of the formulation included previous personality traits of pride, the importance of not hurting others and good manners.

The rehabilitation programme also included family support, physiotherapy, occupational therapy, neuropsychological input and nursing. The patient displayed behavioural problems consistent with an injury to the frontal lobes; yielding low mood and behavioural issues, which included shouting abuse at nursing staff. From the formulation the team knew this behaviour was due to the injury and at odds with the previous personality of the man. The man was helped to manage this behaviour with a behavioural programme and the family members were also assisted with the behavioural plan until the man's behaviour improved so that he stopped shouting abuse at the staff on the ward. The man also reported being much happier by not shouting at others.

Different kinds of recovery

Recovery can be defined in a variety of ways and can mean different things to different people. Recovery is classified in the following ways.

▶ A complete recovery and return to previous level of functioning with no difficulties or differences (Almli & Finger, 1988). This is often not possible for people with a brain injury.

▶ A return to a normal or near-normal level of previous performance (Laurence & Stein, 1978).

▶ Resumption of a near normal life with some deficits (Jennett & Bond, 1975), which is sometimes possible.

▶ A reduction of deficits (Braun, 1978) or a partial recovery of function but with some compensation (Kolb, 1995), which is most frequently the aim of rehabilitation programmes.

Recognising and accepting the limitations of possible recovery can be difficult for some people with brain injury. Any recovery occurs over a long period of time and self-understanding can be affected by the brain injury itself, plus loss of intellectual functioning is difficult to adjust to. For example, Susan

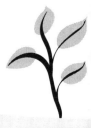

had an expectation that she would recover within weeks following her injury and found the time it took in reality very difficult to accept. She had a belief that rehabilitation should only last for a few weeks and then she should be able to return to her former life with no difficulties. Whereas another patient, Mark, had damaged his right frontal lobes and this injury affected his awareness of his difficulties. Although he demonstrated a range of difficulties, such as impulsive behaviour and memory problems, he could not appreciate these problems and so did not recognise the need for rehabilitation or see the need to change any aspect of his life.

The main task of rehabilitation is to allow the person to gain the best recovery they can (optimal functioning) in their usual environment. This may require ensuring that rehabilitation takes place in the area where the person lives and within their own home. For example, the person's own shower may have a completely different sized step or controls to master compared to one at a hospital unit. The person may need to learn to cook again in their own kitchen, using their own appliances. If a person is returning to work, then rehabilitation specialists, typically job coaches, will go into the place of work to help the person compensate and develop ways of managing their jobs, often in negotiation with managers and HR professionals (ie. place and train, not train and place). Rehabilitation should always occur in the same environment as where the person will stay later on, as this ensures the transferability of skills and compensatory strategies. Environmental modifications may be required, for example, hand rails in the home, written prompts and labels on cupboards in the kitchen to aid memory, medical dispensing boxes stored in seven compartments with each day of the week listed to aid memory etc.

Neuro-rehabilitation should also always consider the vocational aims of the person (see also chapter 11). Ben-Yishay (1978) initially argued for the use of vocational placements for those with a brain injury; the idea of involvement in meaningful activity as essential to our psychological well-being goes back to Freud. Whether the individual returns to paid employment or voluntary work is often determined by various factors such as degree of impairment, financial circumstances and the current job market.

How can we judge the effectiveness of rehabilitation?

There are major difficulties with strict research design when attempting to identify which method of rehabilitation is the most effective. The 'gold standard' for research is the randomised control trial (RCT) in double-blind conditions (client and clinician are unaware of whether they are in a treatment condition or control condition group). RCTs may not always be possible or ideal – rehabilitation programmes by their very nature are complex. The decision to exclude a group of clients and thus not provide rehabilitation so they can act as a control group is against the core ethical principles of rehabilitation. Thus RCTs in rehabilitation settings are practically very difficult and ethically complex.

Chesnut *et al* (1999) conducted a meta-analysis of a total of 114 research studies that explored the effectiveness of compensatory rehabilitation. They concluded that the RCTs reviewed did not answer the question clearly due to research design difficulties. Alternative ways to assess whether rehabilitation is effective include single case and small group experiments or studies. Rehabilitation programmes should be tailored to the individual and thus these research methods can prove very informative.

There is now more published evidence demonstrating the cost-effectiveness of neuro-rehabilitation. It can superficially look expensive to provide rehabilitation for someone with a brain injury due to the range of physical, social and cognitive aspects, as it is estimated that cognitive rehabilitation can take up to 400 hours (Leon-Carrion *et al*, 2004). This input is typically provided by a highly specialist team and could be viewed as expensive, although the evidence for the cost-effectiveness of rehabilitation is now increasing (Wilson, 2009). When considering the cost of rehabilitation programmes, it is useful to distinguish between direct and indirect costs (Wood *et al*, 1999). Direct costs refer to the cost of providing treatment and indirect costs refer to more social burdens such as time off work to attend programmes and the costs of benefits. It has been shown that rehabilitation undertaken within two years of injury results in improved outcomes and savings in care support (Wood *et al*, 1999). This, together with the benefits for the individuals with brain injury and their families, makes rehabilitation essential and not a luxury.

Different kinds of therapy/intervention

Cognitive remediation therapy (CRT) is an umbrella term that includes many approaches. These are mainly defined by their surface characteristics, for example, use of a therapist or computer, or types of tasks. The primary function of CRT is to improve thinking processes rather than thinking

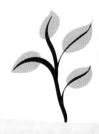

content by using cognitive exercises to improve thinking skills. CRT can be administered in individual or group settings (see chapter 10 for description of group programmes). It can be computerised, non-computerised, or a combination of both and can also be manualised.

Cicerone *et al* (2005) in a review of 87 studies found substantial evidence to support CRT for people with a traumatic brain injury (TBI). The aforementioned reviews have generally found some evidence to support the effectiveness of CRT after TBI. They also found the need to better describe and measure how the treatment is effective (SMART goals) and recognised the need to improve research methodology.

Restitution and compensation of memory impairments

Any illness or injury to the brain has a high degree of potential to affect memory. This, in part, is due to memory relying on many different systems, including the attentional system. Any factor that affects our ability to attend to information, such as anxiety, depression or pain, affects our ability to remember. Despite being among the most common of the deficits, the evidence base exploring the effectiveness of cognitive rehabilitation is small. Memories are organised and processed and are either used immediately or stored for long-term use. We have verbal, visual and motor memory channels. Deficits in memory are one of the most common cognitive impairments following brain injury (executive functioning including attentional impairments is the other common deficit). Difficulties in this area are also extremely upsetting and disabling for any person affected.

Strategies to help with memory impairments can be divided into: external memory strategies, environmental cues, strategies to help improve encoding and consolidation, strategies to help with retrieval, and strategies for those with strengths in verbal memory. External memory strategies include the use of notebooks, diaries, electronic organisers, alarms set on mobile phones as a reminder to take medication or attend appointments. Other external memory strategies include labelling cupboards or writing notes.

Strategies to help with encoding and consolidation include repeating information after it is presented, and allowing time for these processes to occur before new information is presented, asking questions to deepen encoding and learning to chunk information together (for example, the

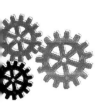

first three words in a list or putting things in categories). Strategies for those with strengths in verbal memory include taking notes of important conversations and tape recording meetings, for example, taking notes during a meeting with a GP. Strategies for those with strengths in visual memory include learning to use visualisation skills (for example, trying to remember that a man you have just met is called Mark, then imagining a dark mark across his eyebrows) and the use of pictures and flashcards.

Restoration of memory functioning involves attempting to restore lost functioning while compensation involves modifying the environment to aid recall and help a person with a neurological difficulty learn in a more effective way (Wilson, 2002). Several factors predict good use of compensation strategies for memory impairment (Evans *et al*, 2003), including a young age at the time of brain injury, less severe impairments, specific rather than global deficits and the previous use of coping strategies (eg. using a diary as a memory aid).

A study undertaken by Evans and Wilson (1992) found no evidence of memory improvement for members of a group programme in memory rehabilitation. Participants did, however, demonstrate improvements in the use of compensatory memory strategies and a lowering of anxiety and depression. The lowering of anxiety was possibly due to the participants being able to do more for themselves by using strategies.

Ryan and Ruff (1988) found only those with a mild impairment benefited from memory rehabilitation training. A review of the literature by Nair *et al* 2007 concluded that there is no evidence for the effectiveness of memory rehabilitation following stroke (Cochrane review). One study did find that the person and their carer/family reported improvements in memory following a structured memory group programme. These improvements were maintained one month later (Thickpenny-Davis & Barker-Collo, 2007). Studies into the effectiveness of visualisation have shown that this can improve memory retrieval (Incagnoli & Newman, 1985) but the transferability into real life situations is questionable. External memory strategies have been found to be useful for a variety of people, including those with traumatic brain injury and Alzheimer's disease (Pliskin *et al*, 1996). Of course because we can only recall what we can attend to, it is vital that attention is also considered in work on memory deficits.

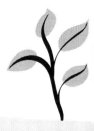

Case study 2

Terry is a 55-year-old man who suffered a right brain stroke while on holiday in Africa. He spent two weeks in an African intensive care unit and was then transferred to England to his local inpatient neuro-rehabilitation unit. He progressed very well in physiotherapy and presented himself well. However, one difficulty he did have was an impairment of impulse control, which was observed by all members of the MDT and family members and confirmed by neuropsychological assessment.

The results of the neuropsychological assessment and formulation were used to help Terry develop insight into this difficulty and he was then taught to break down what he was doing and use self-instruction. This work included eliciting the support of his wife.

Terry made significant improvements in his impulse control and only occasionally interrupted others. He also gained more control over his general impulse control as observed by family members and members of the MDT. More importantly, Terry recognised and valued his improvements.

Further evidence supporting the use of problem-solving retraining comes from Rath *et al* (2003) who compared a group of people receiving problem-solving training to a group of people receiving general CRT and social skills training. This study used neuropsychological tests, questionnaires and role play of problem-solving to assess outcome. The study found that those in the problem-solving retraining group showed improvements in their problem-solving ability and ability to manage emotions. These improvements were maintained six months later during the follow up.

von Cramon and Matthes-von Cramon (1992) conducted a single case study on a male with problems with planning and decision-making. They identified that many of the patient's difficulties were due to him jumping to decisions and not following any plan. The patient was taught to internalise an external checklist which helped him make the correct decisions. He was however, unable to transfer this learning to novel situations.

Case study 3

Ian was a 32-year-old man who had worked for the same company for 12 years. He suffered an acquired brain injury following a road traffic accident and spent a few weeks in an inpatient rehabilitation unit and was then discharged. He returned to work

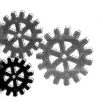

very quickly, although he had problems with problem-solving and decision-making but was not aware of these difficulties. Ian's job involved talking to customers on the phone and taking orders, tracking the orders and helping customers choose the right products. Following his injury Ian started to have problems at work and attended a vocational rehabilitation unit following a referral from his HR manager.

Ian received CRT to help with problem-solving and decision-making and was supported in his workplace with flow charts of potential issues at work. He was also given a clear worksheet detailing all his calls by his manager. He was able to remain in employment and began to appreciate some of the ways he would need to compensate in order to continue to achieve what he wanted.

Restitution and compensation of attention deficits

There are different types of attention. Focused attention refers to the ability to focus effects on one area, for example, reading a book or concentrating on one conversation while ignoring other irrelevant conversations. Divided attention is where we are able to focus on two forms of stimulation at any one time, for example, having a conversation while making a cup of tea. Sustained attention refers to our ability to focus on one activity for a reasonable period of time, for example to read this chapter. There is of course an overlap between these systems and it is not easy to separate them in everyday life (see chapter 3 for more information).

Attention is also required in order for us to perform other cognitive tasks, such as memorising and decision-making. Memory complaints that are frequently reported by suffers of multiple sclerosis (MS) may be attributable to difficulties with sustained attention and the time taken to process information (Lezak *et al*, 2004). One strategy for helping the individual manage this difficulty is for the family, friends or colleagues to limit the amount of information the person with MS is asked to process.

Some of the strategies to help with sustained attention include activity pacing and frequent breaks, helping the person with an activity log and increasing activities slowly while providing feedback, and scheduling activities when the person is at their most alert. A different set of strategies help with focused attention, for example, reducing distractions in the person's environment .This may involve the use of ear plugs or listening to music on headphones. Warning the person about possible distractions may

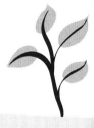

also be useful, as well as basic behavioural strategies such as rewarding focused attention. Strategies for helping with divided attention include structuring the person's environment so they are not put in situations where there are too many things to concentrate on and ensuring that multiple activities are not attempted. This will probably involve working with family members and colleagues. For an educational setting it may be helpful to give the person written handouts so they do not have to write, and listen. Checklists also help the client see what they have achieved.

Robertson (1999) reviewed a number of studies on the effectiveness of retraining programmes for attention. The majority of the studies reviewed used computerised presentation. The results of this review were mixed and some had methodological problems. Some of the studies did see positive changes over time, but it is difficult to conclude if these improvements were a direct result of the retraining programmes.

Cappa *et al* (2003) reviewed the literature and found evidence to support the use of attention and memory training for those with mild memory impairments. These results were found in the post-acute stage after traumatic brain injury (TBI) but not in the acute stage of recovery. Sohlberg *et al* (2003) reviewed the literature and found evidence for the effectiveness of direct attention training following TBI.

A further study by Ponsford and Kinsella (1988) found improvements in attention over time, however, the authors concluded that it was difficult to link these improvements directly to the computerised training. Sturm *et al* (1997) studied the effects of training-specific aspects of attention, for example, sustained or selective attention and found improvements in the type of attention targeted. Further research by Sturm *et al* (1997) found improvements in a range of neuropsychological tests for attention following CRT for attention disorders; this study used a matched control group. Sturm *et al* (1997) found some evidence to support the use of computerised cognitive training programmes for attention. Additional supporting evidence demonstrating the benefits of attention retraining comes from Gray and Robertson (1989) and Gray *et al* (1992).

Studies exploring the effectiveness of CRT for attention deficits show some improvements, but it is difficult to link this change directly to attention retraining. In addition, such change may not always generalise to everyday life. External compensatory strategies for attention do, however, appear to be useful and effective.

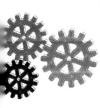

Case study 4

Jo is a 34-year-old woman who suffered a TBI following a car accident and returned to work quickly without any cognitive rehabilitation. Jo worked in a busy call centre with multiple distractions and experienced problems with sustained attention and divided attention at work. Jo found she was unable to concentrate and she began to feel distressed, which made the whole situation even worse. She was about to hand in her notice because she believed that she could no longer work.

Jo went to see a neuropsychologist who conducted a formulation and identified the problems Jo had with attention. The psychologist visited the work environment and gave Jo specific work-related advice on the importance of regular breaks and breaking her work into shorter periods of concentration, as she had previously been attempting to concentrate for up to four hours at any one time. She was also moved into a quiet office area where she was able to limit the amount of distracting information around her.

Jo reported that she was now able to achieve more in her working day as a result of increased concentration, and she recognised the importance of taking regular breaks and breaking tasks into shorter chunks of activity. She no longer wanted to leave her job and said she felt better about her abilities.

Restitution and compensation of visual-spatial difficulties

We rely on our visual-spatial abilities, for example when driving a car, using a computer, writing our name or even walking around in the supermarket buying food. There are now computerised rehabilitation packages for visual-spatial problems, however, their effectiveness has not been well documented. Repetition is the most widely used rehabilitation method; refractive lenses have been used as prescribed by an optometrist or ophthalmologist; magnifying sheets have also been used and computer monitors can enlarge information. Also providing a greater contrast between the background and any text needed to be read can also prove useful. There are numerous environmental strategies such as applying brightly coloured tape to the corners of rooms or furniture and adjusting any light in the environment. There are also many strategies to help improve spatial neglect, for example, helping the person appreciate the neglect and verbal cues, and in terms of restoration encouraging eye scanning movements.

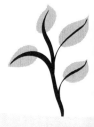

Research has found that rehabilitation results in increases in the efficiency, scope and accuracy of a visual search, however, the visual field deficit did not decrease (Pommerenke & Markowitsch, 1989). Bosley *et al* (1978) found that any improvements in visual fields following a stroke were limited to persons where the injury was outside the occipital lobes.

Take away message

Over the last 20 years researchers and clinicians have attempted to identify if neuropsychological rehabilitation is effective, and the general agreement is that it is (Cicerone, 1999). What is now being debated is whether is it better to focus on restoring lost functioning or teaching compensatory strategies. Prigatono (1999) argues that there is no evidence to suggest that neuropsychological rehabilitation can help with restoration of lost functioning for cognitive deficits. Thus we should focus our efforts on compensation not restoration and on helping people and their families adjust psychologically to the changes in their lives. Of course, in clinical practice these theoretical arguments are set aside and interventions such as restitutive and compensatory are offered.

There is increasing evidence that cognitive rehabilitation can be effective in improving cognitive functioning (Robertson, 1999). Of course we also need to consider the effect of mood on cognitive functioning, for example, if a person is depressed or anxious then this will have a significant effect on neuropsychological assessments and treatment. The evidence for the effectiveness of memory functioning following CRT is limited. What is evident is improvements in the use of strategies following such rehabilitation, and some improvements in mood. The evidence that executive functioning impairments can be restored is not convincing but using assessments to aid self-awareness does appear to be effective.

The CRT programmes with the strongest evidence are those that combine early intervention, teaching the benefits of compensatory strategies and supported employment (Carney *et al*, 1999). The evidence for CRT-based attention training is mixed but yields some positive findings. However, the most salient question is how to pragmatically transfer training to everyday life issues.

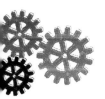

Perhaps the most useful forms may be those combining attention training with a solid transferability to everyday life, and the use of compensatory strategies.

Neuropsychological rehabilitation should hopefully continue to evolve despite the current demands to cut services. It is important to offer a quality rehabilitative service, and more robust research is required as many of the current studies consist of small numbers of participants and often have design flaws. This is a challenge for all those involved in neuro-rehabilitation, which is still a young and growing field of speciality.

Quiz

1. Define 'multidisciplinary neurorehabilitation'.

2. What is the 'gold standard' in terms of research design?

3. What does the term 'neuro-plasticity' stand for?

4. List the different types of recovery.

5. What are the most common deficits following brain injury?

6. What does CRT stand for?

7. What factors predict good use of compensation strategies for memory impairment?

8. What does the evidence on the effectiveness of CRT for attention demonstrate?

9. What is the general agreement over the effectiveness of neuropsychological rehabilitation?

10. In clinical practice, is it best to offer restitutive or compensatory interventions?

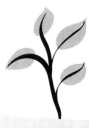

References

Almli C & Finger S (1988) Towards a definition of recovery of function. In: S Finger, TE LeVere, C Almli & DG Stein (Eds) (1988) *Brain Injury and Recovery: Theoretical and controversial issues.* New York: Plenum Press.

Ben-Yishay Y (1978) Reflections on the evolution of the therapeutic milieu concept. *Neuropsychological Rehabilitation* **6** (4) 327–343.

Bosley TM, Dann R, Silver FL, Alavi A, Kushner M, Chawluk JB (1978) Recovery of vision after ischemic changes: positron emission tomography. *Annals of Neurology* **21** 444–450.

Braun JJ (1978) Time and recovery from brain damage. In: S Finger (Ed) (1978) *Recovery from Brain Damage: Research and theory.* New York: Plenum Press.

Cappa SF, Benke T, Clarke S, Rossi B, Stemmer B and van Heugten CM (2003) Guidelines on cognitive rehabilitation: report of an EFNS task force. *European Journal of Neurology* **10** 11–23.

Caramazza A (1989) Cognitive neuropsychology and rehabilitation: an unfilled promise? In: X Seron & G Deloche (Eds) (1989) *Cognitive Approaches in Neuropsychological Rehabilitation.* Hillsdale: Lawrence Erlbaum Associates.

Carney N, Chesnut RM, Maynard H, Mann NC, Patterson P & Helfand M (1999) Effect of cognitive rehabilitation on outcomes for persons with traumatic brain injury: a systematic review. *Journal of Head Trauma Rehabilitation* **14** 277–307.

Chesnut RM, Carney N, Maynard H (1999) Summary report: evidence for the effectiveness of rehabilitation for persons with traumatic brain injury. *Journal of Head Trauma Rehabilitation* **14** (2) 176–188.

Cicerone KD (1999) Commentary: the validity of cognitive rehabilitation. *Journal of Head Trauma Rehabilitation* **77** 316–321.

Cicerone KD, Dahlberg MA, Malec JF, Langenbahn DN, Felicetti T, Kneipp S, Ellmo W, Kalmar K, Giacino JT, Harley P, Laatsch L, Morse PA & Catanese MA (2005) Evidence-based cognitive rehabilitation: updated review of the literature from 1998 through 2002. *Archives of Physical Medical Rehabilitation* **86** 1681–1682.

Coltheart M (1985) Cognitive neuropsychology and reading. In: MI Posner & OSM Marin (Eds) (1985) *Attention and Performance XI* 3–37.

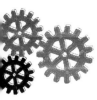

Evans JJ & Wilson BA (1992) A memory group for individuals with brain injury. *Clinical Rehabilitation* **6** (1) 75–81.

Evans JJ, Wilson BA, Needham PA & Brentnall S (2003) Who makes good use of memory aids? Results of a survey of people with acquired brain injury. *Journal of the International Neuropsychological Society* **9** 925–935.

Goldstein K (1942) *After Effects of Brain Injuries in War: Their evaluation and treatment.* New York: Grove and Stratton.

Gray J & Robertson IH (1989) Remediation of attentional difficulties following brain injury: three experimental case studies. *Brain Injury* **3** 163–170.

Gray J, Robertson IH, Pentland B & Anderson SI (1992) Microcomputer based cognitive rehabilitation for brain damage: a randomised group controlled trial. *Neuropsychological Rehabilitation* **2** 97–116.

Incagnoli T & Newman B (1985). Cognitive and behavioural rehabilitation interventions. *International Journal of Clinical Psychology* **4** 173–182.

Jennett B & Bond M (1975) Assessment of outcomes after severe brain damage. A practical scale. *Lancet* **i** 480–484.

Kolb B (1995) *Brain Plasticity and Behaviour.* New Jersey: Erlbaum.

Laurence S & Stein DG (1978) Recovery after brain damage and the concept of localisation of function. In: S Finger (Ed) (1999) *Recovery from Brain Damage.* New York: Plenum Press.

Leon-Carrion J, Doinguez-Morales MR, Barroso Y, Martin JM & Murga FM (2004) *Time and Course of Recovery of Post-TBI Cognitive Disorders After Neurorehabilitation* (2nd edition). Cambridge: Cambridge University Press.

LeVere TE (1980) Recovery of function after brain damage: a theory of the behavioural deficit. *Physiological Psychology* **8** 297–308.

Lezak MD (2004) *Neuropsychological Assessment* (4th edition). Oxford University Press: New York.

Nair RD, Lincoln N, Majid M & Weyman N (2007) *Cognitive Rehabilitation for Attention Deficits Following Stroke.* Cochrane Database of Systematic Reviews 3.

Plaut D (1996) Relearning after damage in connectionist networks: towards a theory of rehabilitation. *Brain Language* **52** 25–82.

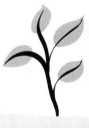

Pliskin NH, Cunningham JM, Wall JR & Cassissi JE (1996) Cognitive rehabilitation for cerebrovascular accidents and alzheimer's disease. In: P Corrigan & S Yodofsky (Eds) (1996) *Cognitive Rehabilitation for Neuropsychiatric Disorders* 193–222. Washington: American Psychiatric Press.

Pommerenke F & Markowitsch HJ (1989) Rehabilitation training of homonymous visual defects in patients with postgeniculate damage of the visual system. *Restorative Neurology and Neuroscience* **1** 47–63.

Ponsford J & Kinsella G (1988) Evaluation of a remedial programme for attentional deficits following closed head injury. *Journal of Clinical and Experimental Neuropsychology* **10** 693–708.

Prigatano GP (1999) Commentary: beyond statistics and research design. *Journal of Head Trauma Rehabilitation* **14** 308–311.

Rath JF, Simon D, Langenbahn DM, Sherr L & Diller L (2003) Group treatment of problem solving deficits in outpatients with traumatic brain injury: a randomised outcome study. *Neuropsychological Rehabilitation* **13** 461–488.

Robertson IH (1999) *Theory-driven Neuropsychological Rehabilitation: The role of attention and competition in recovery of function after brain damage.* In: D Gopher & A Koriat (Eds) (1999) *Attention and Performance XVII: Cognitive Regulation of Performance: Interaction of theory and application.* Massachusetts: MIT Press.

Ryan TV & Ruff RM (1988) The efficacy of structured memory retraining in a group comparison of head trauma patients. *Archives of Clinical Neuropsychology* **3** (2) 165–179.

Sohlberg MM, Avery J & Kennedy M (2003) Practice guidelines for direct attention training. *Journal of Medical Speech Language Pathology* **11** 19–39.

Sturm W, Willmes K, Orgass B & Hartje W (1997) Do specific attention deficits need specific training? *Neuropsychological Rehabilitation* **7** 81–103.

Thickpenny-Davis K L & Barker-Collo SL (2007) Evaluation of a structured group format memory rehabilitation program for adults following brain injury. *Journal of Head Trauma Rehabilitation* **22** (5) 303–313.

von Cramon D & Matthes-von Cramon G (1992) Reflections on the treatment of brain injured patients suffering from problem-solving disorders. *Neuropsychological Rehabilitation* **2** 207–230.

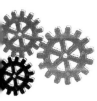

Walsh K (1987) *Neuropsychology: A clinical approach.* Edinburgh: Churchill Livingston.

Wilson BA (2002) Towards a comprehensive model of cognitive rehabilitation. *Neuropsychological Rehabilitation* **12** (2) 97–110.

Wilson BA (2009) In: BA Wilson, F Gracey, JJ Evans & A Bateman (2009) *Neuropsychological Rehabilitation: Theory, models, therapy and outcome.* Cambridge: Cambridge University Press.

Wood RLI, McCrea JD, Wood LM & Merriman RN (1999) Clinical and cost effectiveness of post-acute neurobehavioral rehabilitation. *Brain Injury* **13** 69–88.

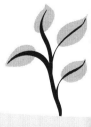

Chapter 10

What can be done II: approaches to rehabilitation

Roshan das Nair and Shirley Thomas

Aims of the chapter

This chapter aims to:

▶ outline the process of cognitive rehabilitation: when to begin it, where to offer it, and how to deliver it

▶ describe the various types of cognitive rehabilitation used in brain injury rehabilitation

▶ demonstrate how the biopsychosocial model maps onto cognitive rehabilitation

▶ identify rehabilitation approaches for mood problems

▶ evaluate and monitor process and outcome in cognitive rehabilitation.

Introduction

Overall perspectives and approaches to rehabilitation

The term rehabilitation means different things to different people and professions. The word comes from the Latin for '*to make fit again*' and this occupation with making fit again takes on a variety of forms even within healthcare, with professionals approaching rehabilitation from illness/disease-specific perspectives (such as cardiac rehabilitation, stroke rehabilitation, etc.) to highly specialised systemic forms of rehabilitation (such as neurorehabilitation). The aims and processes of rehabilitation vary. For instance, vocational rehabilitation focuses on finding, staying

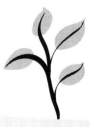

on or returning to work, while cognitive rehabilitation attempts to restore lost cognitive functions or circumvent problems caused by acquired cognitive deficits.

Rehabilitation professionals not only work with patients directly, but also work with carers, multidisciplinary teams, and can be consultants for environmental design or ergonomic rehabilitation. Rehabilitation itself is a multidisciplinary enterprise, with professionals from fields such as occupational therapy, clinical psychology, physiotherapy, rehabilitation medicine etc. focusing on different aspects – all with one common goal: to make people fit again.

With improvements in technology and healthcare provision, people are living longer even after severe injuries and insults to the brain. This raises a primary moral imperative within healthcare, which aims not only to increase the quantity of life, but also the quality of this life. This means that modern day healthcare, particularly rehabilitation, strives to help people get back to their premorbid levels of functioning, thereby making them less vulnerable citizens capable of independent living and achieving their potentialities. Furthermore, rehabilitation is also guided by socio-economic drivers, such as getting people back into the workforce, whether at home or outside, or reducing their care requirements.

Both these aspects of rehabilitation are particularly pertinent for those who experience cognitive deficits as a result of brain-related disorders or injuries. Cognitive rehabilitation is a specialised type of rehabilitation, defined by Cicerone *et al* (2000) as '*a systematic, functionally oriented service of therapeutic activities that is based on assessment and understanding of the patient's brain-behavioral deficits*'. Like other forms of rehabilitation, cognitive rehabilitation is provided at different levels and in different forms at different times by various professionals, sometimes in diverse settings. This complexity of delivery of cognitive rehabilitation is also reflected in a theoretical model proposed by Wilson (2002) in which she attempts to synthesise models of cognition, assessment, recovery, behaviour, emotion, compensation, and learning, in an attempt to provide a comprehensive framework for understanding the process of cognitive rehabilitation. This, therefore, makes cognitive rehabilitation a multi-modal, multidisciplinary, multidimensional activity.

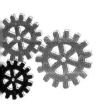

A biopsychosocial perspective

As cognitive rehabilitation is a complex endeavour that requires a theoretically broad-based approach and practically a multidimensional framework, it appears intuitive to consider it within a biopsychosocial model (Engel, 1977) (see chapter 1 for more details). Cognitive rehabilitation is one therapeutic approach that sits comfortably within the framework of this model because it relies on each of these components to succeed. Interestingly, the goal of rehabilitation to some extent also connects with the biological, psychological and social spheres.

Injury or illness is never only felt by the body, but by an individual, and the spaces he/she inhabits. The biopsychosocial model maps onto the World Health Organization's (WHO) classification of health and health-related domains, classified from body, individual and societal perspectives. This conceptualisation is enshrined within the International Classification of Functioning, Disability and Health (ICF) (WHO, 2001) (see chapter 1 for more information). What the ICF does is to normalise and mainstream the notion of illness and disability, creating space for the inclusion of society within the individual's experience of ill-health and disability. This shifts the onus of integration back into society not only from that of the individual but also from their surroundings. The ICF delineates (i) impairments of bodily functions, for example, mental, sensory, voice and speech functions etc.; and structures such as the nervous system, cardiovascular, respiratory etc. (ii) activity limitations and participation restrictions, for example, communication, mobility, self-care etc. (iii) and environmental factors such as the physical, social and attitudinal environment that facilitate or impede integration, for example, support and relationships; services, systems and policies; products and technology etc. For successful cognitive rehabilitation, the spirit of the ICF needs to permeate every aspect of rehabilitation, from planning, implementing, and assessing its effectiveness (Thomas & das Nair, 2010).

The importance of assessments in cognitive rehabilitation

If we are to liken cognitive rehabilitation to a process, there are three interconnected aspects that need to be considered. A good place to start this process would be with an assessment of the individual's cognitive functions. The aims of this assessment should be to answer the following questions.

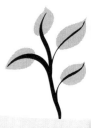

► Why is this person here at this time?

► What are the presenting complaints?

► What is the profile of his/her strengths and weaknesses? (See also chapter 7)

In order to answer these questions appropriate assessment tools need to be considered. The following questions may guide the choice of such tools.

► What tools will best describe the cognitive deficits in a systematic manner?

► What tools can be adequately used more than once?

► Will the tools help in developing a specific treatment plan for this individual?

► Are the tools appropriate for this individual (considering the standardisation of the tools, the normative data available, and the individual's specific limitations)?

The rationale for the assessment, and where appropriate, the rationale for specific tools need to be communicated to the person and their carers. This will ensure that they feel involved right from the beginning, thereby improving their motivation to take the assessments and making them feel less threatened by the whole experience. Feeding back the results of the study is a crucial stage in the cognitive rehabilitation process as it will set the stage for rehabilitation. When feeding back results, both strengths and limitations need to be addressed, so that a person can appreciate that they can capitalise on their strengths to circumvent or adapt to some of their weaknesses. In order to obtain such a detailed profile it is best to consider using multiple methods of collecting data, which can include standardised psychometric measures, questionnaires, structured interviews, observations, information from carers/others, across a variety of settings (Malia *et al*, 2004). Triangulating information from multiple sources will also offer information on similarities and differences between subjective reports of cognitive successes or failures versus others' reports.

The information gleaned though interviews with individuals and their carers, and others along with the assessment data would inform the formulation that will guide the intervention (see chapter 8 for more details). Formulations for interventions need to be planned in conjunction with the person and their carers, along with staff.

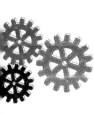

Goal planning

'A goal refers to the intended consequences of actions undertaken by the rehabilitation team' (Wade, 2009).

The importance of goal setting and involving the person in this process should not be underestimated. Goals are central to rehabilitation and changes or control of behaviour are likely to be easiest to accomplish if the individual wants to achieve the goal set (Wade, 1998). A common goal helps staff to co-ordinate their therapeutic approaches and keep the person motivated. In addition to the person and staff, it can sometimes be appropriate to include family members when agreeing goals. Having a realistic person-centred goal does not only give the person something specific to work towards but also allows staff to monitor progress. Therapists should identify with the person which goals or outcomes are important to them and this may also take into account carers' wishes which would be needed to accomplish each goal and the likelihood of the change (Wade, 2009). The agreed goals should be documented and made available to staff and patients. Goals can be short-term, medium-term or long-term and may relate to impairments, activities or social participation in the ICF framework. It is more effective to set both short-term and long-term goals rather than only long-term goals, as achieving short-term goals can motivate patients to strive to attain their long-term goals.

It is usually recommended that goals should be SMART: Specific, Measurable, Achievable, Realistic/Relevant and Time-bound (see also chapter 9). One approach for developing a goal is to specify the target activity (behaviour), the support needed (physical assistance, emotional support, prompting); quantify the performance (time, quantity, frequency) and specify the time period for achieving the goal (Bovend'Eerdt *et al*, 2009). This means that a goal should be well-defined but also that the rehabilitation plan for achieving the goal is outlined.

Examples of goals

▶ To be able to remember the names of work colleagues in the office using a mnemonic within six weeks.

▶ To be able to dress the upper body without verbal or physical prompts within eight weeks.

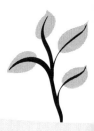

> ▶ To prepare a sandwich for lunch without verbal or physical assistance within four weeks.
>
> ▶ To complete a 100 piece jigsaw independently within two weeks.

Once the initial assessment has been completed the implementation of rehabilitation strategies can start. However, while teaching people these strategies, their uptake and effectiveness need to be constantly monitored, ideally both formally and informally. It is good practice to plan, right at the beginning when an appropriate time would be to conduct formal assessments. Such assessments should give a good indication whether or not an intervention is working as planned, and if not, what changes need to be introduced.

It is prudent to have a follow up assessment after some time has elapsed since the person was discharged from the rehabilitation programme. Such long-term follow ups have the potential to inform whether or not the person has continued to successfully employ the rehabilitation strategies that they were taught, and whether they have adapted these to suit their own environments, that is, generalisation and sustainability of the treatment gains.

When to begin cognitive rehabilitation

Immediately post-injury, there is evidence to suggest that some amount of spontaneous recovery takes place, and is achieved by reduction in oedema to the brain, neuroplasticity, recovery from trauma etc., which can extend to several months. However, following this period, it is generally accepted that plastic changes are minimal and therefore need to be augmented with intensive, focused rehabilitation (Cramer, 2008).

Some researchers have investigated the application of cognitive rehabilitation to people with reduced awareness such as those in comas, vegetative or minimally conscious states. Such rehabilitation has mostly been within sensory stimulation modalities and Wilson and McMillan (1993) conclude from their review of studies that such interventions not only have the potential to reduce the duration of coma, but can also alter the behaviour of the patient while in a coma. The Bekinschtein *et al* (2005) case report of a 20-year-old woman who sustained brain injuries following a road traffic accident summarises some of the challenges in conducting cognitive assessments and rehabilitation with a minimally conscious patient (for other case studies see Shiel, 2003). However, with a concerted effort from a multidisciplinary team of rehabilitation professionals employing several brain stimulation strategies, the person was able to make significant gains in her cognitive abilities. The researchers did, however, find persisting social skills deficits in this patient, which could not be tapped by the cognitive assessments they employed, and it was not certain whether remediation of such skills were attempted at the time. This suggests that cognitive rehabilitation should not be limited to inpatient settings, but should spill into community care as well. In fact, oftentimes, it is only when people return to their home and work settings that the cognitive deficits become apparent. It must also be acknowledged that the period of transition from hospital to home can be challenging and distressing, and therefore the person could benefit from extra support, perhaps in the form of an intervention to help them through this stage.

Rehabilitation has been found to be successful not only when provided during the period immediately following brain injuries, but even years later (Sbordone *et al*, 1995). This later onset rehabilitation has found its theoretical basis in research studies, which have found post-acute brain plasticity and cerebral functions not only solely localised to specialised regions of the brain, but to also being distributed (Kolb & Gibb, 2008). Plasticity and distributed function imply that even if one part of the brain is damaged, there is a possibility of another part of the brain (which is already involved in the function) to reorganise and provide some facility for the (impaired) function to be carried out. However, it must be added that plasticity is not a homogeneous process across people, in that plasticity has been found to be dependent on various factors, including age, IQ, education, awareness of deficits, aetiology, lesion (type, size and location) etc. (Robertson & Murre, 1999; Kolb & Gibb, 2008). Therefore, there is no time limit to when rehabilitation can be offered, but the type of rehabilitation may be guided by the time passed post-injury, and the outcomes are likely to be variable given that there are several factors that may account for success or failure of rehabilitation.

Where to offer cognitive rehabilitation

The decision of where to offer rehabilitation will be governed by several factors, not least of which includes the condition of the person when rehabilitation is attempted. However, as previously mentioned, cognitive deficits are often observed or are pronounced only when the individual is

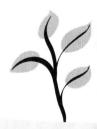

beginning to readjust to life outside of the hospital. This means that cognitive rehabilitation only becomes meaningful to the individual after they have been discharged and therefore, such rehabilitation will need to be offered on an outpatient basis. This is suitable for most people as it affords them an opportunity to put to test the skills they are taught during rehabilitation programmes in the environment in which they need to be used. Furthermore, because of the labour intensive nature of cognitive rehabilitation required to produce meaningful results (León-Carrión *et al*, 2004), with some researchers suggesting at least 100 hours (Prigatano, 1999) to over 400 hours of rehabilitation distributed over six months; this degree of intensive work cannot always be provided within inpatient settings.

Providing cognitive rehabilitation in the community has further advantages in terms of increasing patient choice. Some patients do not want to be seen in hospitals after they have been discharged, as hospitals may be linked with the traumatic events that brought them there in the first place. Alternative service provision is sometimes offered in stroke clubs and charities that deal specifically with an illness or injury. Specialist rehabilitation centres such as the Oliver Zangwill Centre can also offer more intensive and holistic rehabilitation programmes for people with acquired brain injuries of differing aetiologies. These can be residential centres or day centres and these kinds of centres provide opportunities for staff and patients to establish strong working alliances which also influence uptake of such services and eventual outcome. The significance of good working alliances, Prigatano (2000) asserts is one of the hallmarks of cognitive rehabilitation provided under the milieu-oriented approach to rehabilitation.

Ben-Yishay, a leading figure in neuropsychological rehabilitation, has advocated the 'therapeutic community' (Ben-Yishay *et al*, 1978) or 'therapeutic milieu' (1996). He draws on Goldstein's (1959) ideas about holistic neuropsychological rehabilitation, regarding the use of modified environments to help the patient cope with situations.

'*Within this framework, an individual's neurobehavioural and cognitive deficits, his or her intrapersonal and social-interactive difficulties, and problems resulting from the drastic alterations in the individual's status and role within the "significant others" network would be remedially tackled in an integrated and holistic fashion*' (Ben-Yishay, 1996).

His therapeutic model consisted of a very intensive programme, an almost one-to-one staff-patient ratio working in programmes that lasted seven hours daily, six days a week for one year, which integrated vocational placements within rehabilitation. While the utility of this kind of rehabilitation is noteworthy, in our current economic climate and working within the structure of the NHS, such communities may not always be feasible. However, the spirit with which these communities were set up and run and the ethos that they propagated could still guide us in providing comprehensive rehabilitation programmes.

Types of approaches used in cognitive rehabilitation

There are several types of rehabilitation approaches that are used, and the factors that influence the form and type of rehabilitation are equally myriad. Factors such as the possibility of plasticity (see above), lesion specifications, the patient's premorbid level of functioning, current lifestyle and attitude towards rehabilitation, external support systems etc., all have a valid place in decision-making. The final decision about the types of cognitive rehabilitation to be used, however, should be one that is made in consultation with the patient, carers, and other treating staff.

Compensation or restitution

From a theoretical perspective, clinicians may consider using strategies that promote compensation (sometimes referred to as substitution) or restitution (also referred to as restoration) of function (see Chapter 9 for a review of these theoretical positions). Compensatory strategies help individuals to circumvent their cognitive deficit by engaging in other learned behaviours. For example, people with memory deficits can be taught to effectively use a diary or mobile phone to remember to do things at a particular time. Restitutive strategies typically involve attempting to break down a cognitive function into its constituent parts and retraining each of these with drill and practice training. Such retraining for memory deficits would take the form of breaking down memory into attention, encoding, storage and retrieval. Each of these components is then targeted with specific exercises, for example cancellation tasks for attentional retraining, considering different ways to encode information etc. While the utility of restitutive approaches has been documented in some cognitive domains such as visual neglect (Mueller *et al*, 2008), in other areas such as memory rehabilitation, debate still ensues (Evans, 2006). In practice, however, despite these theoretical debates, clinicians sometimes offer interventions that consist of both restitutive and compensatory strategies.

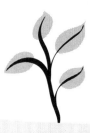

Single domain or holistic interventions

Cognitive rehabilitation can also be geared to address a specific deficit in isolation, for instance, training can be offered for dealing specifically with visual neglect or executive functions (see chapter 4). While these domain-specific approaches are common in research-related interventions, oftentimes in clinical practice it is simply not possible to only address one specific domain to the exclusion of others, due to the interactive nature of the various cognitive domains and other psychological factors such as affect, adjustment, motivation etc. Therefore, a more holistic approach is often attempted, of course, within the limits of what can be offered.

The seminal work by Prigatano *et al* (1994) on holistic, milieu-oriented rehabilitation programmes has demonstrated the utility of creating an ecologically valid training environment for patients to optimise generalisation of skills learned in training to their daily usual life, thereby improving functional outcomes. Such training typically involved an individual tailor-made programme to suit the individual's needs, provided by a multidisciplinary team in individual and group session formats. Therapeutic activities were also embedded in the programmes which simulate day-to-day experiences. The effectiveness of such a format of intervention has been established by Pepping and Prigatano (2003), Malec and Basford (1996) amongst others.

Individual or group formats

Cognitive rehabilitation can be offered in individual, group or combined formats. Both individual and group formats have their own advantages and disadvantages, so we advocate the combined format. In combined cognitive rehabilitation programmes, the patient is first assessed to obtain a profile of their cognitive abilities and deficits. A few individual sessions following this would help in identifying how these deficits affect the individual's activities of daily living (ADL) and to formulate the treatment goals. These sessions personalise the intervention, and after this, individuals can be seen together in a group setting. During these sessions, a good facilitator would ensure that all the material taught to the group is connected to the individual goals to make the information meaningful to each person attending the group programme.

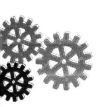

Group interventions

Any kind of a group intervention requires a significant amount of planning if it is to achieve its goals. It is therefore important to consider the aims of the group, who should be invited (the composition of the group), how many therapists/leaders will facilitate it, when and where it will take place, what resources will be required, how long each session will last, whether there will be a break during the session, how long the group will run for, and whether there will be booster or follow up sessions. It is advisable to clearly state the aims of the group and get the group to come up with some ground rules to achieve these aims. These can be simple and straightforward, such as giving everyone a chance to speak, not being judgemental or critical of others' views or lifestyles, sharing information only when people are comfortable in doing so, respecting privacy, confidentiality, etc.

Given that cognitive rehabilitation needs to be intensive in order for it to be useful, setting homework assignments is useful. This will not only give group members a chance to remind themselves of what they learnt during the session, but it will also enable them to try out some of these strategies at their own homes or work, thereby personalising use. If homework assignments are set, then opportunities to feed back people's experiences should also be provided.

To facilitate recall of ground rules and structure homework tasks, it is best advised that a manual or handbook is prepared for the entire rehabilitation programme. This way, group members can also see what they have covered and what they will cover in future sessions. They can also show others at home what was covered in each session. Such manuals are also useful in research settings to maintain consistency of delivery of cognitive rehabilitation where multiple groups may be run at various sites.

It is also important to consider what happens when the group ends. Ending a group should be a planned activity and group members need to be prepared for it. Some people keep in touch with others informally after the group has come to an end. Such informal meetings should be encouraged if they have the potential to create another source of support, in this case peer support, for members.

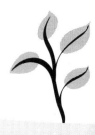

Advantages of groups

▶ Social support which may continue after the formal group ends

▶ People can learn practical tips from other group members

▶ Group members feel they are not the only one with their difficulties

▶ Some people feel better when they are helping others

▶ Sharing experiences and challenges

Disadvantages of groups

▶ Practical difficulties in identifying a time and venue suitable for all members

▶ Need to be well managed by group leaders, particularly if one person dominates the group

▶ May not be suitable for all people

▶ May have varying attendance from different group members (for example, some people with memory problems forget to come)

▶ The problems faced by those with more severe disabilities may frighten those with less severe disabilities (especially in progressive conditions such as dementia)

Example of a group-based memory rehabilitation programme

The Rehabilitation of Memory in Neurological Disabilities (ReMIND) study (Nair, 2007) employed a group format to deliver a memory rehabilitation programme to those who had sustained head injuries, or had strokes or multiple sclerosis. People were initially met for individual sessions to conduct assessments and formulate treatment goals before they went into a group. Each group consisted of four individuals with different aetiologies, but all experiencing memory problems. The aims of the groups were to (i) improve knowledge regarding brain damage and memory functioning, (ii) encourage the use of memory aids (iii) develop skills in coping with memory problems and their illness or condition, and (iv) provide peer support though the group sessions. As the groups were run according to a manual, all the groups were conducted in a consistent manner. Session one was mostly didactic and educational in nature, and consisted of introductions, setting of group rules, and explaining the entire programme in detail. Topics related to memory structure and brain damage were explored and homework assignments consisted of revision of the content covered in the session and permitted participants to apply what was learnt within their chosen environments.

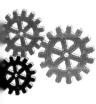

The structure for all other sessions consisted of a discussion of the week's activities for each participant, feedback regarding homework, a review of the previous week's session, a preview of the current session, the planned activity for the session, setting homework for the week, a review of the session, and a preview of the next session. During the remainder of the eight sessions, people were taught the use of memory aids and remembering strategies. Each session was planned to last about 1.5 hours, with a break of 10 minutes. The last session provided a review of the entire programme, and offered people an opportunity to share their views on attending the groups. Formal follow up assessments were conducted immediately after the end of the last session, and seven months thereafter. The last assessment was conducted to examine whether people were still using the strategies they were taught effectively in helping them deal with their memory problems.

In addition to the effects of a neurological condition or brain injury on cognitive functions, it is also relevant to consider the impact of such conditions on someone's mood. The next section summarises some of the approaches used as part of psychological treatments of mood problems.

Rehabilitation approaches and mood problems

Mood problems such as depression and anxiety can be common in people following a brain injury or neurological problems. Depression, combined with physical or cognitive difficulties, can present a more complex picture for rehabilitation (see also chapter 4). For example, a patient who is depressed may be less motivated to engage in rehabilitation activities, thus impacting on their recovery. It can be helpful to find out what the person's premorbid personality was like (ie. what they were like before their stroke or head injury) such as their behaviour patterns, what they used to enjoy doing, how they spent their time etc.

Cognitive behaviour therapy (CBT) is a psychological approach widely used to treat depression in people who are physically healthy and has also been applied to people with a physical or neurological condition. CBT is based on the cognitive model of depression and learning/behaviour theory. According to the cognitive model, people who are depressed have 'dysfunctional assumptions' where core beliefs that they have are unhelpful and can result in 'negative automatic thoughts' (negative self-talk) and negative views of the self, the world and the future. Behavioural theory suggests

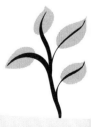

that depression can develop as a result of reduced positive reinforcement/reward (for example, due to low activity levels or being in an environment not conducive to activities). As mood lowers further, this leads to reduced motivation and engagement in activities and can perpetuate a vicious cycle. This can be applied to people with cognitive difficulties or physical disabilities, which can lead to changes in everyday functions, social roles and hobbies. CBT aims to bring about change in maladaptive thinking, behaviour and mood, thoughts and practising new behaviours, analysing faulty thinking patterns and learning more rational self-talk skills (Khan-Bourne & Brown, 2003). Therapeutic techniques include setting therapy goals, gradually increasing activity level, and identifying and reducing negative thinking about physical or cognitive losses and life changes.

Behaviour therapy or behavioural approaches are used as part of CBT. Behavioural approaches aim to increase 'pleasant events', such as the amount of time people spend doing things they enjoy. The theory is that if people are more often engaged in enjoyable activities, then this will be rewarding and improve their mood. As behavioural approaches are concrete and practical they may be suitable for people who have severe cognitive or communication difficulties. Components of behavioural approaches include the following.

Activity monitoring

Activity monitoring involves identifying how someone currently spends their time. As a 'homework' task between therapy sessions, the person can be asked to complete an activity diary. The diary allows the therapist and person to see changes in activity level currently and over time, and also periods of time where the person is doing very little. The level of detail for the diary can be varied according to the person's abilities – for example, the diary could show each hour of the day and the person writes in the space what they have done, or for people with severe communication or cognitive problems the diary can be divided into morning/afternoon/evening with velcro picture or word cards to stick onto the diary. In addition to recording activities it is informative to ask the person to rate their mood for each activity or period of the day. This can be done using simple rating scales (for example 0–10) or mood faces such as ☺/☹. This allows the therapist to explore how much enjoyment the person gets from particular activities.

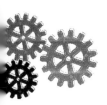

Table 1: An example of an activity diary

	Monday	Tuesday	Wednesday	Thursday	Friday	Saturday	Sunday
8am – 10am							
10am – 12noon							
12noon – 2pm							
2pm – 4pm							
4pm –6pm							
6pm –8pm							
8pm –10pm							

Table 2: Another example of an activity diary

	Monday
Morning	
Afternoon	
Evening	

Activity scheduling

Pleasant events and activities are planned in advance for each day. This gives a structure to the person's time and removes 'on the spot' decisions, which means they are more likely to do the activity. 'Pleasant events' will be agreed with the person and need to be realistic and should be activities that can be increased and done more often (Laidlaw *et al*, 2003). The activity diary can be used as a template for recording the activity schedule and again the format will be adapted to accommodate the person's abilities. Mood monitoring should continue so that the therapist and person can see whether a change in activity level corresponds to a change in mood.

Graded tasks

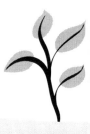

This is the process of breaking down an overall or complex activity into smaller more manageable steps and sub goals. As each step is more likely to be achieved this improves self-reward and increases the likelihood of succeeding at the overall goal.

Khan-Bourne and Brown (2003) and Grober *et al* (1993) have suggested some ways in which CBT approaches can be adapted when working with people who have cognitive difficulties. These include:

▶ using memory aids – written summary, cue cards, audio recordings

▶ simplifying techniques and homework according to the patient's abilities

▶ having shorter but more frequent therapy sessions

▶ regularly summarising and checking understanding

▶ involving a carer or friend to help remind the person or help with homework tasks where appropriate

▶ using supported communication for people with reception or expressive aphasia.

Case study

'Linda' is a 46-year-old woman who had a stroke eight months ago. Since the stroke she has a mild weakness down the right hand side of her body and walks with a stick. She sometimes has difficulty in finding the right words when she is speaking and may say the wrong word, and she also finds it difficult to follow a conversation when lots of people are talking. Currently she doesn't go out of the house on her own as she is not very confident.

A graded task was agreed with Linda with the final goal being for her to go into the local town centre and back on her own using the bus. The goal was broken down into smaller steps as follows.

1. To get the bus into the town centre and back with her daughter for a short visit (about 30 minutes).

2. To get the bus into the town centre and back with her daughter for a longer visit (about one and a half hours).

3. To get the bus into the town centre alone and for her daughter to meet her at the bus stop in town.

4. To get the bus into the town centre and back on her own.

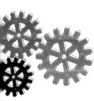

Supported communication for people with

aphasia or dysphasia

When having a conversation or therapy session with someone who has communication problems (for example aphasia or dysphasia) it helps to find a quiet environment, make sure the therapist has the person's attention before starting to speak and speak face-to-face. The therapist, relative or carer should encourage the person's residual communication abilities and be flexible in their approach during the conversation. It is helpful to summarise and check understanding frequently in case there is the need to recap or rephrase anything. Tiredness and stress can exacerbate someone's communication difficulties so regular breaks can be helpful. Also, it is important to remember that communication includes non-verbal elements, for example, body language, facial expression, gesture and voice tone. There is a wide range of communication resources that can be used to support communication, including (but not limited to) pen and paper and message board, picture cards, photographs, drawing, maps, diary or calendar, personal communication book, word lists and objects. Speech and language therapists may have additional resources to use. There is variation in patients' personal preferences for different resources, for example some patients like using 'clipart' or cartoon pictures while others have reported finding them childish and preferring photographs or other tools. When teaching someone methods of supporting communication, for example, using picture cards or a communication book, the therapist or carer should show the person how to use the communication 'ramps' rather than just telling them to use these tools. It is not necessarily helpful to use all of the techniques at once and the therapist or carer and person should try some out to see what works best for each individual. Finally, the importance of accessible written information should not be overlooked. Written documents for someone who has reading difficulties due to aphasia or dysphasia should have short phrases, one idea per sentence, bullet points rather than long paragraphs, and include familiar words (key words highlighted or in bold) and selected pictures may aid understanding.

The following **figure 1** and **figure 2** summarise advice on how to get your message in (ensuring that your message is clear to help the person with aphasia or dysphasia to understand) and how to help the person to get their message out (giving the person with communication difficulties the opportunity to express their message) (Kagan, 1998).

Figure 1: Getting your message in

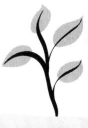

Getting your message IN (facilitating comprehension)

▶ Present one idea at a time in short chunks of information

▶ Make it clear when the topic of conversation is changing

▶ Use simple and familiar words

▶ Repeat or rephrase information if it has not been understood

▶ Write down key words

▶ Use visual cues

Figure 2: Getting their message out

Getting their message OUT (facilitating expression)

▶ Encourage any form of communication response, including non-verbal communication such as pointing and making other gestures

▶ Allow someone plenty of time to respond

▶ Encourage drawing and writing (always have pen and paper to hand)

▶ Use pictures or written choices

▶ Don't interrupt when someone is trying to find a word

▶ Clarify what you think the person means

A common concern from staff is how to be certain that they have correctly understood the person and whether the person's response was reliable. First, staff can check the consistency of the response by asking the patient the same question at different points during the session. Second, they can assess whether the patient's verbal response corresponds with an alternative response such as pointing to a picture, and third ask questions to clarify and find out whether the response is consistent with other sources (for example, medical notes, other staff, or carers). Sometimes a conversation may get 'stuck' where the person with communication problems finds it difficult to express what they want to say or the speaker without communication problems is having trouble understanding or explaining their point. When this happens it is acceptable to acknowledge that there is a difficulty and agree whether to come back to the point later. The following box gives 'top tips' on what not to do when working with

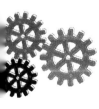

someone who has impaired communication.

What not to do

Do not:

▶ talk too fast

▶ use medical jargon

▶ pretend to have understood when you have not

▶ interrupt or talk over someone

▶ finish someone's sentences or find the words for them (unless already agreed)

▶ dismiss what someone says if you can't understand them

Who attends cognitive rehabilitation programmes?

Ideally, a comprehensive cognitive rehabilitation programme should include all those affected by the brain injury and this therefore would normally include the person, their carers or significant others. Rehabilitation programmes vary in terms of how information is imparted; some programmes include both patient and carer in each group session, while others have special sessions for carers that patients do not attend, and some others only invite carers to a few sessions along with the patients. In some instances, getting the support of carers is vital for the success of the rehabilitation programme, and therefore including them helps enlist this support. However, it is not always possible to involve carers for various reasons. In fact, sometimes, people prefer that carers are not involved in their rehabilitation process. In such instances, it may be useful to offer patients a written summary of the programme (or session) to take back with them.

Monitoring progress and evaluation

In relation to the ICF framework, outcomes following cognitive rehabilitation can be assessed at the level of impairment, activity or participation. Lincoln and das Nair (2008) suggest that for cognitive rehabilitation activity measures are the most important outcomes. Few measures exist that assess the impact of cognitive rehabilitation on social

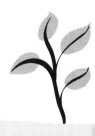

activities and participation. Outcomes should be relevant to the patient and considered in the context of the goals that were agreed. The decision about when to assess outcome – during treatment, at the end of treatment, or at a follow up point after treatment, has stopped and will also depend on the goals set. In addition to objective measures such as standardised assessments and direct observations of behaviour, interviews with the patient (and sometimes a relative or carer) provide useful qualitative details. Information from multiple sources can be helpful where patients have difficulty giving accurate accounts because of severe cognitive or communication difficulties or low mood.

One common method of assessing outcome is using a standardised assessment (see Chapter 7). When choosing an outcome assessment the psychometric properties should be reviewed to inform the decision of which tool to use. For example, an assessment that is used to screen patients to identify those who may have an impairment may not be suitable for evaluating outcomes following an intervention. Outcome measures should have the following properties reliability, validity, sensitivity and practicality (Lincoln & das Nair, 2008).

Reliability

A reliable measure is one which provides consistent results if completed by different assessors (inter-rater reliability), the same assessor on different occasions (intra-rater reliability) and the same patient on different occasions during which a change is not expected (test-retest reliability).

Validity

A valid measure is one which measures what it intends to measure. The scale items should reflect the construct being assessed (for example, does it cover all symptoms of depression?), should correlate with other measures of the same construct, and the results of a measure should follow the theory upon which the measure is based.

The ecological validity of a test refers to *the degree to which test performance corresponds to real-world performance* (Chaytor & Schmitter-Edgecombe, 2003). For a test to have ecological validity the task needs to be similar to the cognitive skills needed for an everyday task or the performance on a test needs to be looked at to see if it corresponds to everyday functioning. However, a word of caution is necessary here: the

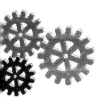

goal of rehabilitation is not to improve a test score but the performance in everyday life that is relevant to the individual.

For instance, outcomes for memory rehabilitation can be an improvement in list recall, an increased score on a test like the RBMT-E (Wilson *et al*, 1999 (see chapter 7); or updated versions of such tests), or forgetting less often the names of one's grandchildren. We advocate that cognitive rehabilitation should focus on the latter, if for a person that is the most significant goal. This relates to an alternative method for evaluating outcomes, which is using a technique called 'goal attainment scaling' (GAS), which quantifies the extent to which a goal is achieved (Turner-Stokes, 2009). This allows the therapist to personalise the outcome measure for a particular patient and can relate to any of the ICF levels. Instead of simply recording that someone has or has not met their goal, GAS records the level of success: goal achieved – expected level (0), better than expected (+1), much better than expected (+2), less than expected level (-1) and much less than expected level (-2) (Turner-Stokes, 2009; Bovend'Eerdt *et al*, 2009). Goals can also be weighted according to their importance and difficulty.

Sensitivity
An outcome measure should be sensitive to (ie. able to detect) change that has occurred, for example, a change in mood.

Practicality
It is important that the measure is short and straightforward to complete. Staff should also consider whether they need to be trained to use and score a measure, and how easily the results can be communicated to other people. Tests should also be suitable for repeated administration; otherwise someone's performance may improve as a result of practice.

Assessing mood as an outcome
A common way of assessing mood (depression and anxiety) is using questionnaires with multiple choice response options. There are several self-report questionnaires for assessing mood. A limitation of these questionnaires is that most were not designed specifically for people who have experienced a brain injury or cognitive problems. This means that some of the questionnaire items may be affected by someone's physical disability and so may not be accurate at detecting changes in mood.

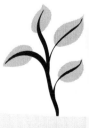

Examples of mood questionnaires that are used with neurological patients include:

▶ Hospital Anxiety and Depression Scale (HADS) (Zigmond & Snaith, 1983) – this is a 14-item scale which gives separate scores for the severity of depression and anxiety. It was designed to exclude physical indicators of distress although some items could still be affected by physical disability. It may be more appropriate as a screening measure rather than outcome assessment (Lincoln & das Nair, 2008).

▶ General Health Questionnaire (GHQ) (Goldberg & Williams, 1988) – is a widely used questionnaire to assess general psychological distress, which has been found to be sensitive to change following interventions. There are 30, 28 and 12 item versions.

▶ Beck Depression Inventory II (BDI-II) (Beck *et al*, 1996) – this is a commonly used 21-item questionnaire designed to assess the severity of depression, which has been used with neurological patients. A limitation of this questionnaire is that some patients find it lengthy to complete and it includes some somatic (physical) items such as changes in sleep and appetite and loss of libido, which are not always appropriate, particularly in an inpatient setting.

People with communication difficulties (such as aphasia or dysphasia) often find it difficult to reliably complete self-report questionnaires. For example, a person may have difficulty reading, understanding verbal instructions, or giving their response to a question. However, it is important not to exclude people with communication difficulties when assessing mood outcomes. An alternative to a written or verbal questionnaire is a picture-based (visual analogue) tool. The Visual Analog Mood Scales (VAMS) (Stern, 1997) was developed for people with neurological problems and assesses eight mood items, which are each presented as a 'neutral' cartoon face at the top of a vertical line and the 'mood' face and label (for example, 'happy' or 'sad') at the bottom of the line. The patient marks on the connecting line how they are currently feeling. In addition to self-report tools it can also be informative to gather impressions about someone's mood from nursing staff or relatives. The Stroke Aphasic Depression Questionnaire (SADQ) (Lincoln & Sutcliffe *et al*, 2000; Sutcliffe & Lincoln, 1998) was developed to assess mood in people with aphasia by asking nursing staff or relatives to answer questions about the frequency of behaviours associated with depression (for example, weeping spells, initiating activities, taking an interest in events around them). Both the VAMS and SADQ are appropriate for people

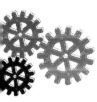

with communication difficulties although their sensitivity to detect change following intervention needs to be evaluated.

Does cognitive rehabilitation work?

This is the wrong question! A more appropriate question would be 'When and in what ways does cognitive rehabilitation work best for this individual, given his/her circumstances at the present time?'

When the effectiveness of each cognitive domain is considered separately, there is considerable heterogeneity of findings. For instance, Cochrane reviews by Bowen *et al* (2007) found no evidence of effectiveness of memory rehabilitation following stroke; Bowen *et al* (2007) found some evidence for the effectiveness of rehabilitation for spatial neglect, but only on impairment measures and not functional measures; and Lincoln *et al* (2000) concluded that there was no evidence to support or refute the use of cognitive rehabilitation for attention deficits to improve functional independence following stroke. The reasons for these differences in conclusions have most often been attributed to a range of people, conditions, interventions and outcomes studied, small sample sizes in the research trials, and limited number of good quality studies. However, there have been several attempts to synthesise research findings to evaluate the effectiveness of cognitive rehabilitation as a whole (Cicerone *et al*, 2000; Cicerone *et al*, 2005; Carney *et al*, 1999; Chestnut *et al*, 1999; Cappa *et al*, 2003; Cappa *et al*, 2005). Most of these reviews have concluded substantial effectiveness of cognitive rehabilitation in reducing cognitive dysfunctions, or the deleterious effects of these deficits.

Take away message

Cognitive rehabilitation is diverse in its approaches, which are embedded within a biopsychosocial model. Therefore, holistic approaches to cognitive rehabilitation should be considered, which view the person as greater than the sum of their cognitive functions. Other factors, such as mood problems can affect cognitive rehabilitation, and therefore, need to be monitored and treated alongside the cognitive deficits. For it to be meaningful to the patient, it should tap into the various domains of the ICF, particularly targeting activity limitations. It needs to be driven by findings from

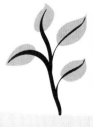

individual assessments, goals and formulations, and evaluated consistently during the intervention, and after.

Quiz

1. What are the three components of the ICF?

2. What are the three (interrelated) phases of cognitive rehabilitation?

3. What does SMART stand for in relation to goals?

4. In what kind of settings is cognitive rehabilitation offered?

5. What are the advantages of offering cognitive rehabilitation in groups?

6. Outline the three behavioural approaches to treat mood problems:

7. What resources may be used to support communication?

8. What are the four properties to look for when selecting outcome measures?

9. What are assessments used for in cognitive rehabilitation?

10. There are mixed conclusions about the effectiveness of rehabilitation for specific cognitive deficits as demonstrated in systematic reviews. What are the reasons for these differences?

References

Beck AT, Steer RA & Brown GK (1996) *Beck Depression Inventory Manual* (2nd edition). San Antonio: The Psychological Corporation.

Bekinschtein T, Tiberti C, Niklison J, Tamashiro M, Ron M, Carpintiero S, Villarreal M, Forcato C, Leiguarda M & Manes FF (2005) Assessing level of consciousness and cognitive changes from vegetative state to full recovery. *Neuropsychological Rehabilitation* **15** 307–322.

Ben-Yishay Y (1996) Reflections on the Evolution of the Therapeutic Milieu Concept. *Neuropsychological Rehabilitation* **6** (4) 327–343.

Ben-Yishay Y, Ben-Nachum Z, Cohen A, Gross Y, Hoffien D, Rattock J & Diller L (1978) Digest of a two-year comprehensive clinical research program for outpatient head injured Israeli veterans. In: Y Ben-Yishay (Ed) (1978) *Working Approaches to Remediation of Cognitive Deficits in Brain Damaged Persons (Rehabilitation Monographs No. 59)*. New York:

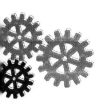

New York University Medical Center.

Bovend'Eerdt, TJH Botell, RE & Wade DT (2009) Writing SMART rehabilitation goals and achieving goal attainment scaling: a practical guide. *Clinical Rehabilitation* **23** 352–361.

Bowen A, Lincoln NB & Dewey M (2007) Cognitive rehabilitation for spatial neglect following stroke. *Cochrane Database of Systematic Reviews* **2**.

Cappa S, Benke T, Clarke S, Rossi B, Stemmer B & van Heugten C (2003) EFNS guidelines on cognitive rehabilitation: report of an EFNS task force. *European Journal of Neurology* **10** 11–23.

Cappa SF, Benke T, Clarke S, Rossi B, Stemmer B & Van Heugten CM (2005) EFNS guidelines on cognitive rehabilitation: report on an EFNS task force. *European Journal of Neurology* **12** 665–680.

Carney N, Chesnut R, Maynard H, Mann NC, Patterson P & Helfland M (1999) Effect of cognitive rehabilitation on outcomes for persons with traumatic brain injury: a systematic review. *Journal of Head Trauma Rehabilitation* **14** 277–307.

Chaytor N & Schmitter-Edgecombe M (2003) The ecological validity of neuropsychological tests: a review of the literature on everyday cognitive skills. *Neuropsychology Review* **13** 181–197.

Chestnut RM, Carney N, Maynard H, Patterson P, Mann NC & Helfand M (1999) *Rehabilitation for Traumatic Brain Injury: Evidence report/ technology assessment No* **2**. Rockville: Agency for Health Care Research and Quality Publication.

Cicerone KD, Dahlberg C, Kalmar K, Langenbahn DM, Malec JF, Bergquist TF, Felicetti T, Giacino JT, Harley JP, Harrington DE, Herzog J, Kneipp S, Laatsch L & Morse PA (2000) Evidence-based cognitive rehabilitation: recommendations for clinical practice. *Archives of Physical & Medical Rehabilitation* **81** 1596–1615.

Cicerone K, Dahlberg C, Malec JF, Langenbahn D, Felicetti T, Kneipp S, Ellmo W, Kalmar K, Giacino JT, Harley JP, Laatsch L, Morse P & Catanese J (2005) Evidence-based cognitive rehabilitation: updated review of the literature from 1998 through 2002. *Archives of Physical Medicine & Rehabilitation* **86** 1681–1692.

Cramer SC (2008) Repairing the human brain after stroke: I. Mechanisms of spontaneous recovery. *Annals of Neurology* **63** (3) 272–287.

Engel G (1977) The need for a new medical model: a challenge for biomedicine. *Science* **196** 129–136.

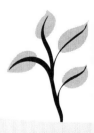

Evans JJ (2006) Memory rehabilitation: should we be aiming for restoration or compensation? Commentary on Hildebrandt H, Bussmann-Monk B & Schwendemann G. In: Group therapy for memory impaired patients: a partial remediation is possible. *Journal of Neurology* **253** 520–521.

Goldberg D & Williams P (1988) *A User's Guide to the General Health Questionnaire.* Windsor: NFER-Nelson.

Goldstein K (1959) Concerning the concreteness in schizophrenia. *The Journal of Abnormal and Social Pychology* **59** (1) 146–148.

Grober S, Hibbard MR, Gordon WA, Stein PN & Freeman A (1993) The psychotherapeutic treatment of post-stroke depression with cognitive-behavioral therapy. In: WG Gordon (Ed) (1993) *Advances in Stroke Rehabilitation.* Andover: Andover Medical Publishers.

Kagan A (1998) Supported conversation for adults with aphasia: methods and resources for training conversation partners. *Aphasiology* **12** 816–830.

Khan-Bourne N & Brown RG (2003) Cognitive behaviour therapy for the treatment of depression in individuals with brain injury. *Neuropsychological Rehabilitation* **13** 89–107.

Kolb B & Gibb R (2008) Principles of neuroplasticity and behaviour. In: DT Stuss, G Wincour & IH Robertson (Eds) (2008) *Cognitive Neurorehabilitation* (2nd edition). Cambridge: Cambridge University Press.

Laidlaw K, Thompson LW, Dick-Siskin L & Gallagher-Thompson D (2003) *Cognitive Behaviour Therapy with Older People.* Chichester: John Wiley & Sons.

León-Carrión J, Dominguez-Morales MR, Barroso y Martin JM & Murga FM (2004) Time and course of recovery of post-TBI cognitive disorders after neurorehabilitation. *Revista Española de Neuropsicologia* **6** (3–4) 187–200.

Lincoln NB & das Nair R (2008) Outcome measurement in cognitive rehabilitation. In: DT Stuss, G Wincour & IH Robertson (Eds) (2008) *Cognitive Neurorehabilitation* (2nd edition). Cambridge: Cambridge University Press.

Lincoln NB, Majid MJ & Weyman N (2000) Cognitive rehabilitation for attention deficits following stroke. *Cochrane Database System Review* **4**.

Lincoln NB, Sutcliffe LM & Unsworth G (2000) Validation of the Stroke Aphasic Depression Questionnaire (SADQ) for use with patients in hospital. *Clinical Neuropsychological Assessment* **1** 88–96.

Malec JF & Basford JS (1996) Postacute brain injury rehabilitation. *Archives of Physical Medicine and Rehabilitation* **77** 198–207.

Malia K, Law P, Sidebottom L, Bewick K, Danziger S, Schold-Davies E, Martin-Scull R, Murphy K & Vaidya A (2004) Recommendations for Best Practice in Cognitive Rehabilitation Therapy: Acquired brain injury [online]. Available at: www.resursteamet.se/det_har_ar_resursteamet/kognitiv%20rehab.pdf (accessed December 2010).

Mueller I, Gall C, Kasten E & Sabel BA (2008) Long-term learning of visual functions in patients after brain damage. *Behavioural Brain Research* **191** (1) 32–42.

Nair R (2007) *Effectiveness of Memory Rehabilitation Following Brain Damage*. Unpublished PhD Thesis. Nottingham: University of Nottingham.

Pepping M & Prigatano G (2003) *Psychotherapy After Brain Injury: Costs and benefits*. In: GP Prigatano & NH Pliskin (Eds) (2003) *Clinical Neuropsychology and Cost Outcome Research: A beginning*. New York: Psychology Press.

Prigatano GP (1999) Commentary: beyond statistics and research design. *Journal of Head Trauma Rehabilitation* **14** (3) 308–311.

Prigatano GP (2000) Rehabilitation for traumatic brain injury. *Journal of the American Medical Association* **284** 1783–1784.

Prigatano GP, Klonoff PS, O'Brien KP, Altman IM, Amin K, Chiapello D, Shepard J, Cunningham M & Mora M (1994) Productivity after neuropsychologically oriented milieu rehabilitation. *Journal of Head Trauma Rehabilitation* **9** 91–102.

Robertson IH & Murre JMJ (1999) Rehabilitation of brain damage: Brain plasticity and principles of guided recovery. *Psychological Bulletin* **125** 544–575.

Sbordone RJ, Liter JC & Pettler-Jennings P (1995) Recovery of function following severe traumatic brain injury: A retrospective 10-year follow-up. *Brain Injury* **9** (3) 285–299.

Shiel A (2003) Rehabilitation of people in states of reduced awareness. In: B Wilson (2003) *Neuropsychological Rehabilitation: Theory and practice*. Lisse: Psychology Press.

Stern RA (1997) *Visual Analog Mood Scales Professional Manual*. Odessa: Psychological Assessment Resources.

Sutcliffe LM & Lincoln NB (1998) The assessment of depression in aphasic stroke patients: the development of the Stroke Aphasic Depression Questionnaire. *Clinical Rehabilitation* **12** 506–513.

Thomas SA & das Nair R (2010) Psychological outcome measures to evaluate exercise interventions. In: H Blake (Ed) (2010) *Physical Activity in*

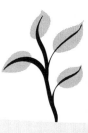

Rehabilitation and Recovery. New York: Nova Science Publishers.

Turner-Stokes L (2009) Goal attainment scaling (GAS) in rehabilitation: a practical guide. *Clinical Rehabilitation* **23** 362–370.

Wade DT (1998) Evidence relating to goal planning in rehabilitation. *Clinical Rehabilitation* **12** 273–275.

Wade DT (2009) Goal setting in rehabilitation: an overview of what, why and how. *Clinical Rehabilitation* **23** 290–295.

World Health Organization (2001) *International Classification of Functioning, Disability and Health*. Geneva: World Health Organization.

Wilson BA (2002) Towards a comprehensive model of cognitive rehabilitation. *Neuropsychological Rehabilitation* **12** 97–110.

Wilson BA, Clare L, Baddeley AD, Cockburn J, Watson P & Tate R (1999) *The Rivermead Behaviour Memory Test – Extended Version*. Bury St. Edmunds: Thames Valley Test Company.

Wilson SL & McMillan TM (1993) A review of the evidence for the effectiveness of sensory stimulation treatment for vegetative states. *Neuropsychological Rehabilitation* **3** 149–160.

Zigmond & Snaith (1983) The Hospital Anxiety and Depression Scale. *Acta Psychiatrica Scandinavia* **67** 361–370.

Useful contacts and organisations

Headway – the brain injury association [online]. Available at: www.headway.org.uk (accessed December 2010).

The Stroke Association [online]. Available at: www.stroke.org.uk (accessed December 2010).

Epilepsy Action [online]. Available at: www.epilepsy.org.uk (accessed December 2010).

Multiple Sclerosis (MS) Society [online]. Available at: www.mssociety.org.uk (accessed December 2010).

Speakability [online]. Available at: www.speakability.org.uk (accessed December 2010).

Connect [online]. Available at: www.ukconnect.org (accessed December 2010).

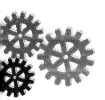

Chapter 11

Treatment, the recovery process and wider considerations following brain injury

Claire Pavlou and Robert Poppleton

Aims of the chapter

This chapter aims to:

▶ understand the treatment process of brain injuries

▶ understand different levels of brain injury severity

▶ understand the wider consequences that can affect family, work and finance.

Introduction

'No injury is too serious to despair of, nor too trivial to ignore.'
(Hippocrates, 400BC)

A brain injury will affect the whole family, but in different ways. Both the person with the brain injury and their family will have to try to come to terms with the consequences of the injury, and it may not be an easy adjustment to make. A brain injury can cause subtle changes, for example, a person may be more forgetful than before or there may be more moderate and severe changes, such as changes in personality and behaviour that can lead to frustration or verbal and physical aggression.

These changes can cause significant distress to families and people who have had a brain injury when they try to resume their previous activities

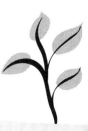

and roles ie. try to resume what was their 'normal family life'. Research shows that there are significantly higher rates of divorce in younger couples when one of them has suffered a brain injury. People may also find it difficult to return to work and there may be financial implications if the household income is reduced, which can put further pressure on relationships and the family as a whole.

This chapter will focus on the wider implications of brain injury. It will describe a patient's journey from the acute phase and what is typical of a hospital process, through to considering the range and effects of different levels of severe brain injury. It will go on to describe the emotional consequences of brain injury, particularly frustration, anger and depression (see also chapter 4), and the implications for family and work life.

The patient journey

Initial injury

A brain injury of any sort is usually unexpected and very distressing not only to the patient but also to the people around them, especially during the early stages when the injury may be life threatening.

A brain injury can be classed as non-traumatic or traumatic depending on the cause of the injury. **Non-traumatic** brain injuries are those which occur as a result of an internal problem in the body or brain, such as a stroke, or metabolic problems, for example, diabetes or tumour. **Traumatic** brain injuries are those that occur because of an outside force, for example, a bang on the head from an assault, or a fall down stairs. Traumatic injuries can be further sub-divided into two categories of 'open' or 'closed'. **Open (or penetrating)** brain injuries occur when an object, such as a bullet, fractures the skull and enters the brain, tearing the soft tissue. **Closed** brain injuries are more common and can result from an extreme movement of the brain, such as acceleration, deceleration or rotation of the brain. For example, in a car crash when the brain keeps moving in the instant after the head has stopped moving after the initial impact. Nerve fibres can be damaged and then the chemical processes can be disrupted. The brain can also be damaged from the inside by bony ridges in the front of the skull when the brain moves as a result of a force.

Emergency and paramedics

At this initial stage, the focus is on saving the person's life. Paramedics use a standard process known as ABC: airways, breathing and circulation. This period is also known as the 'golden hour' as it is a crucial time that can have significant implications for the person's recovery. During this time it is vital that the blood supply is not disrupted otherwise brain cells get starved of food and oxygen and will die. The oxygen supply can be interrupted in the event of extreme blood loss, chest injuries or a blocked windpipe. Sometimes an emergency blood transfusion may be necessary. A tube called a tracheotomy may be inserted into a person's windpipe to help them breathe more easily.

Accident and emergency at hospital

The accident and emergency (A&E) stage consists of interventions to try and prevent death and stabilise the person's condition. It is also the stage where the extent of damage to the body and brain will be investigated and clarified as far as possible. A main concern for the brain at this stage is monitoring the pressure inside the skull and the brain (intracranial pressure). The tearing and bleeding of blood vessels and leakage of other bodily fluids can cause the brain to swell and pressure to build up. The brain may then press against the skull, which could cause further damage and swelling of the brain also pushes on arteries, which can reduce blood circulation. To try to prevent the brain from swelling, it is important to keep oxygen levels and blood pressure high. Sometimes, if a blood clot forms in the brain, this can increase the pressure and surgery may be needed to remove it. If pressure within the skull increases, part of the skull may be removed (craniotomy), which can later be put back in place.

Acute hospital treatment

This stage occurs when a person is medically stable and at a point when they do not need emergency care, however, further medical intervention and close monitoring of the person's condition is needed. The main aim during this stage is to reduce complications and restrict the degree of the damage from the injuries. Attempts are made to aid the natural healing process, for example, by trying to provide oxygen to the brain and a good nutrient source via the blood. Initial rehabilitation may be started in this early stage, particularly physiotherapy to help with simple movements and minimise muscle weakness.

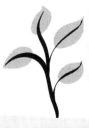

Inpatient neuro-rehabilitation

A person may be admitted to a specialist ward, such as a stroke ward, or a specialist hospital such as a rehabilitation centre. A large team of professionals, such as the following, is usually involved at this stage.

Physiotherapists aid the physical recovery of patients in areas such as the use of muscle and joints for movement, balance, co-ordination and strength.

Speech and language therapists are involved in maximising a person's communication skills, for example, voice and language skills, and assessing and minimising any swallowing problems. They can also advise on how best to communicate with a patient if they find understanding others difficult, or if people have difficulty being understood.

Occupational therapists help people get back to doing everyday tasks. This may involve helping a person relearn how to feed and wash themselves, or how to plan and organise when and how to do household tasks such as cleaning, washing and making meals. An occupational therapist may work with a patient on their hand function and may make splints to help keep their hands straight and in a good position.

Neuropsychologists assess behavioural, emotional and cognitive changes that a person may experience as a result of their brain injury. They may work with a patient to help them understand their difficulties and find strategies or things to practise to help a person compensate for difficulties that they may be experiencing. It may be that a person requires a talking therapy to help them understand and come to terms with what has happened and understand the new challenges that they face.

Community neuro-rehabilitation

In some areas, where community neuro-rehabilitation is available, the patient may receive input from a community physiotherapist, occupational therapist, speech and language therapist, psychologist or rehabilitation assistant. Community rehabilitation may take place in a specifically designed community home or in the person's own home. It is likely that assessments will take place to see how the person manages in their home environment, and strategies, equipment or assistance will be recommended.

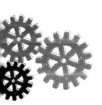

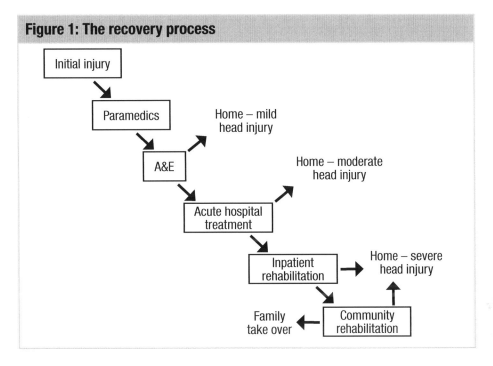

Figure 1: The recovery process

(Adapted from Powell, 2004)

Severity and recovery

Post-traumatic amnesia

Initially, after people regain consciousness they experience a period of post-traumatic amnesia (PTA), which refers to a period of confusion following a head injury when there is disorientation and loss of memory for events after the injury. The length of PTA can be used as a guide to the severity of the brain injury ie. the longer the length of PTA, the more severe the brain injury.

Mild brain injury

It is difficult to determine how many people experience a mild brain injury because it is likely that a lot of injuries are unreported as people do not go to hospital. However, it is thought that the majority of head injuries are mild, which could be as much as 75–80% (Headway, the Brain Injury Association). The medical definition of a mild head injury is a period of unconsciousness experienced for 0–30 minutes and a period of PTA for one day or less. It is likely that people with mild brain injury may develop 'post-concussion

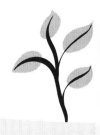

syndrome', where symptoms include nausea, headaches, dizziness, usually followed by cognitive changes (for example, memory loss or physical problems such as reduced co-ordination) and emotional and personality changes such as low mood and feeling depressed.

While often considered to be the least detrimental, mild head injuries may cause considerable distress. For most people, the symptoms clear within a few days or weeks, but it is also possible for them to last many months. Treatment is often not prescribed as recovery often takes place by itself.

Due to the 'minor' classification, healthcare professionals may give people a lower priority and may, therefore, not provide patients with detailed information about how the injury is likely to affect them. When people return home and try to resume their daily life, the difficulties experienced may not always be expected and this can lead to patients becoming frustrated and blaming themselves for their difficulties and altered functioning.

Cognitive changes

One of the most common cognitive symptoms experienced is attention difficulties. People become 'overloaded' and are unable to take in as much information as quickly as they did before, which can then affect their memory.

Memory problems resulting from a mild head injury are likely to be subtle. They are inconvenient and may cause slight irritation and frustration, but may not cause a major problem. People who report short-term memory problems may have difficulty remembering names, appointments and what they have to do. They may forget to pay a bill, but then once they have received a reminder will remember that they have not paid it, and will do so. This is understandably very frustrating.

There are, however, some ways these problems can be helped, for example, by using short-term memory aids and simple strategies such as calendars, diaries, lists, notebooks and phone alarms.

Fatigue

Another commonly experienced symptom following brain injury is fatigue (see chapter 6). This can cause frustration in all aspects of daily life. It is important that people recognise and accept that they can become excessively tired very quickly and to learn that they should not continue to push themselves to the point of exhaustion as this will intensify other symptoms. People should try to pace themselves, structuring activities

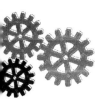

within set time limits and taking more breaks than they normally would do. They should try to ensure that people around them are aware of what fatigue means and how it affects them, so that they are not pushed into doing too much by people who do not recognise the signs.

Physical changes

Fine motor impairments may result from a mild brain injury and these are likely to be fairly minor. For example, a person may have some difficulty walking on an uneven surface, but with extra time and care they will manage it.

Emotional changes

As patients with mild head injuries look the same as they did before their injury, it is usually the case that they are expected to function in the same way too, and this can put added pressure on them. People who do not understand the unseen 'silent' and 'hidden' effects of mild head injuries may accuse people of making up their symptoms. This can be depressing for people and a demanding task if they need to try to convince others around them that they are experiencing serious difficulties.

As a person with a mild brain injury is likely to have more awareness (insight) into their difficulties and limitations (Sawchyn *et al*, 2005), and are aware of differences between how they are following the injury and how they were before, they may experience anger and depression. Increased irritability, lower tolerance and anger outbursts can be common. There is some evidence that suggests people who have had a mild traumatic brain injury are likely to experience anxiety, which can then affect a person's recovery (Moore *et al*, 2006). The person may need reassurance and understanding to help support them through difficult times.

Moderate brain injury

A head injury is classified as moderate if there is a loss of consciousness for between 30 minutes and a day. Post-traumatic amnesia can last from one to seven days. Patients may be observed in hospital and discharged relatively quickly if there are no obvious complications. Again, patients may not have any obvious outward signs of injury but may experience symptoms including fatigue, headaches and dizziness. It is also likely that more obvious cognitive problems will be evident than with that of a mild injury, for example, problems with attention, memory, planning and organisation. These, again, result in worry and anxiety, which can make symptoms

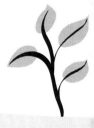

worse, causing an ongoing cycle from which it can be difficult to escape. A person's recovery from a moderate brain injury is likely to be longer than that from a mild injury, as symptoms have a greater impact on everyday functioning. It could take up to 12 months for the symptoms to improve and for people to adjust to the difficulties they have experienced.

Cognitive changes

There may be a greater range of cognitive problems affecting memory, concentration, planning, and problem-solving and attention to detail. More severe memory problems may be more frequent and cause bigger problems. As with mild injuries, a person may forget to a pay a bill for example, but may also lose track of their outgoings if they repeatedly forget to pay lots of bills.

Physical changes

Motor (movement) problems are likely to be a consequence of a moderate head injury and may cause gross motor problems in addition to fine motor problems. For example, a person may have difficulty walking and controlling or moving one of their hands or arms. They may need a wheelchair to help them get around, particularly if they need to walk long distances.

Emotional changes

Emotional and behavioural symptoms resulting from a moderate brain injury are likely to be more marked because of the extent of the difficulties people experience. These may pose big problems for the family. Anger may last for longer periods and tolerance may be even lower, for example, it may not be so easy to calm the person down. This can result in the person and their family feeling resentful and distressed. If cognitive problems are more severe, it may also be difficult for the person to work out why they are feeling so different and responding so differently compared to how they would usually react to difficult situations. They may also become frustrated with other people if they cannot see how their own behaviour has changed, that is, if they lack awareness (insight) into their difficulties.

Severe head injury

A severe head injury is defined by the person being in a coma for more than one day, and post-traumatic amnesia lasting for seven days or more. Patients who have experienced a severe head injury are extremely likely to be hospitalised and require rehabilitation. Patients who have experienced a longer period of a loss of consciousness and longer time in a coma state are at greater risk of having more serious physical disabilities.

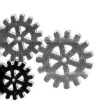

One of the greatest barriers to recovery from severe brain injury is the lower level of insight and self-awareness that people have. Over-estimation of abilities and under-estimation of limitations is a common problem among people with severe brain injuries. If deficits are not acknowledged, steps are not taken to compensate for these. This is linked with poor long-term adjustment, poor rehabilitation outcomes and relationship breakdown.

Cognitive changes
Again there is likely to be a greater range of cognitive difficulties. Following a severe head injury the memory problems experienced may present a major issue. These are likely to become very frustrating and have a much bigger impact on the life of the person. For example, bills may be forgotten about entirely and this could lead to financial difficulties, calls from debt collectors and legal processes.

Physical changes
Major motor problems may be acquired following a severe head injury. These are likely to have a large impact on the life of the person, for example, they may lose the ability to walk and become wheelchair bound.

Emotional changes
Following a severe head injury, emotional and behavioural issues are likely to be much more serious. It is likely that this will cause distress and disruption to the person and those around them, and can be very threatening and intimidating. The individual may anger extremely easily and this emotion may last for long periods of time – they may require specialist support to help them calm down.

Very severe head injury

A minority of head injuries are very severe and result in the person experiencing a prolonged state of coma or low awareness. If improvements do not occur a person can remain in a minimally conscious state or a permanent vegetative state (PVS).

Coma
Coma is diagnosed when a person is in a state of unconsciousness. Their eyes are usually closed and there is no evidence of sleep–wake cycles. Hopefully coma does not last for very long and people will regain consciousness and slowly 'wake up', however, when a brain injury is very severe a person may not recover quickly. They may go on to progress to a

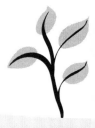

minimally conscious state and then improve further, but with significant cognitive problems. It is possible that they may only progress to a vegetative state which, if this continues for a long time, may become a permanent vegetative state.

Minimally conscious state
When a person shows 'minimal but definite evidence of awareness at times' (Royal College of Physicians, 2003) they may be diagnosed as being 'minimally conscious'. Other terms that are used to describe this are 'minimally responsive' or 'low awareness' state. People may have improved from a level of vegetative state and may go on to improve further, however, they may also stay at this level of recovery for the rest of their life. Prediction of the actual level of recovery that a person will experience is very difficult.

The lack of certainty as to whether or not a person will further improve can be very difficult for people to understand and accept. It is particularly difficult when a loved one is at a level of being 'minimally conscious' because there are times when the person seems to be awake and alert. They may for example be able to do a task, such as put a spoon in a cup or put a tissue to their mouth, but at other times not respond at all. This can give hope to the family that the consistency of a person's responses will improve and that they will get better, but, sadly, this may not be the case.

The vegetative state
This refers to when a person appears wakeful at times, although there may not be any detectable awareness. Physiological functions, such as breathing and sleep–wake cycles continue, but it is likely that all cognitive and emotional functioning ceases.

The Royal College of Physicians (2003) define this type of brain injury as:

'A patient in the vegetative state (VS) appears at times to be wakeful, with cycles of eye closure and eye opening resembling those of sleep and waking. However, close observation reveals no sign of awareness or of a 'functioning mind': specifically, there is no evidence that the patient can perceive the environment or his own body, communicate with others, or form intentions. As a rule, the patient can breathe spontaneously and has a stable circulation. The state may be a transient stage in the recovery from coma or it may persist until death. The vegetative state can follow a variety of severe insults to the brain, most commonly traumatic or hypoxic-ischemic brain injuries.'

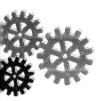

The chance of recovery from VS is dependent on the extent of the head injury. Generally, younger patients are more likely to recover. Unfortunately, if people are in a vegetative state following a non-traumatic event, then less than one-fifth of people recover awareness within a month.

After a year in persistent vegetative state (PVS), the likelihood of regaining consciousness is very low and the majority of patients who do emerge from this state endure significant disabilities. It is often the case that the greater the duration of VS, the greater the severity of the resulting disabilities. While rehabilitation may contribute to slight improvements, very few patients ever reach the point of recovery at which they are able to take care of themselves.

Patients in VS are unable to speak to their family or even acknowledge their presence, and show no understanding of their family's attempts at communication. They are likely to have their eyes open but will not respond to external stimuli. This is very distressing for families to witness particularly when first encountered, as family members are unlikely to know what to expect and may underestimate the severity of the condition. It is difficult for family members to know how to react but they should be encouraged to:

▶ talk to their relative (although it is not known what or how much information people can understand)

▶ speak calmly, slowly and clearly to the person

▶ explain who is with them and what they are doing (for example, say that you are going to hold their left hand and sit next to them)

▶ explain things that are happening around them.

Children may find it especially difficult to understand why their father, for example, is looking at them but will not listen to their stories or respond to their cuddles. However, children are often very resilient and still like to be involved in helping support their parent.

Persistent vegetative state/continuing vegetative state
When a person has been in a vegetative state for four weeks or more it is likely they will be given a diagnosis of being in a 'persistent vegetative state' and in previous guidance it has been called 'continuing vegetative state'. Persistent vegetative state can be easily confused with permanent vegetative state.

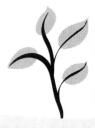

Permanent vegetative state

People will be considered to be in a 'permanent vegetative state' if their condition does not appear to change after six to 12 months.

'When the VS is deemed permanent, a prediction is being made that awareness will never recover. This prediction cannot be made with absolute certainty. However ... the chances of regaining awareness diminish considerably as the time spent in the VS increases.' (Royal College of Physicians, 2003)

'Locked in' state

In people who have had a brain injury following very severe physical symptoms and resulting in body paralysis, it is sometimes possible that their cognitive functioning remains intact. This is likely to occur if a person has had a brain injury that has affected the brain stem (see chapter 2). A person will definitely have observable sleep–wake cycles and may be able to communicate through movement of their eyes or by blinking. Sometimes a person may be able to communicate through movement of one small part of their body such as a thumb movement or slight turn of their head to one side. If it can be established that a person understands what is being said to them, for example by indicating 'yes' or 'no' correctly to questions and can make choices and decisions, then it is possible that their cognitive skills are relatively unaffected by their brain injury.

Table 1: Severity and symptoms			
Severity	**Cognitive**	**Physical**	**Emotional**
Mild	Occasionally forgetting people's names, to pay bills, where they have put things, etc.	Fine motor problems – difficulty walking on uneven surfaces	Occasional excess irritability and poor tolerance. Loss of temper is usually short lived and they calm down, for example, if reassurance is given
Moderate	Frequently forgetting important information such as appointments and bills	Gross motor problems – difficulty walking on flat surfaces	Poor tolerance and frequent strong anger in reaction to annoyances. Loss of temper is likely to last for considerable periods. More difficult to cope with

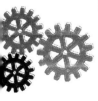

Severity	Cognitive	Physical	Emotional
Severe	Persistently forgetting important information	Inability to walk – wheelchair bound	Regular outbursts of anger and physical aggression with little warning, for example, it can be quite impulsive. Loss of temper may be prolonged. It can be difficult to cope with or manage these outbursts

Table 2: Very severe brain injury			
	Level of awareness	Physical skills	Prognosis
Coma	Absent	No purposeful movement	Recovery, vegetative state or death
Vegetative state	Absent	No purposeful movement	Variable: if permanent, continued vegetative state or death
Minimally conscious	Present (variable at times)	Some consistent or inconsistent verbal or motor behaviour	Variable
Locked in syndrome	Present	Vertical eye movements and eye blinking only	Depends on cause but full recovery is unlikely

(Adapted from Royal College of Physicians (2003) *The Differential Diagnosis of the Vegetative State)*

Emotional responses

Whatever the severity of brain injury experienced, emotional reactions are to be expected (see **figure 2**, patient bereavement reaction and see also chapter 8). People react in very different ways and there is no right or wrong way of reacting or coping. It has even been suggested that there are over 44 different identifiable ways of coping that people use following a brain injury (Kendall *et al*, 2009) and here are some common responses.

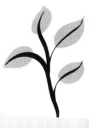

Frustration

Frustration is a very common emotional reaction that people experience, often when they realise that they are unable to do things as easily or as quickly as they did before, but still want to be able to do the task or activity. This frustration can then lead to anger and sometimes aggression that can be directed at the person themselves, or at other people around them. Combined with possible cognitive problems, for example, executive difficulties, that may cause a person to react more than they did before or in a more extreme way, frustration can become very difficult for people to manage and can lead to depression.

Anger

Anger is a very common reaction experienced after a brain injury. There can be many reasons why people feel angry but a common cause is that people are angry at having lost their previous 'life' and want to return to what they were used to. Sometimes the previous life becomes 'idealised' and people grieve for what they feel was perfect before.

If certain parts of the brain have been damaged, particularly the frontal lobe area, then anger may be expressed much more easily than before the injury as the brain's 'breaks' do not work so quickly. Other cognitive problems can cause people to see things differently and people may 'misjudge' situations. This may make them angry if they have misinterpreted what someone meant. Anger is common if people do not have awareness (insight) into their problems and so cannot see reasons why problems occur, or why they may need help to do things.

Depression

Depression is a common experience, if not one of the most common experiences following brain injury. Some executive problems look the same as symptoms of depression, for example, lack of motivation (withdrawal from activity) and lack of initiation, for example, not starting conversations or doing activities that a person would normally do. It is, therefore, important to determine the extent of cognitive problems and/or symptoms of depression so that the best help and treatment can be found.
It is thought that people who have coping styles that include worry, avoidance, wishful thinking, self-blame and using drugs and alcohol, have higher levels of anxiety and depression, as well as lower self-esteem (Anson & Ponsford, 2006).

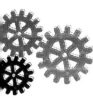

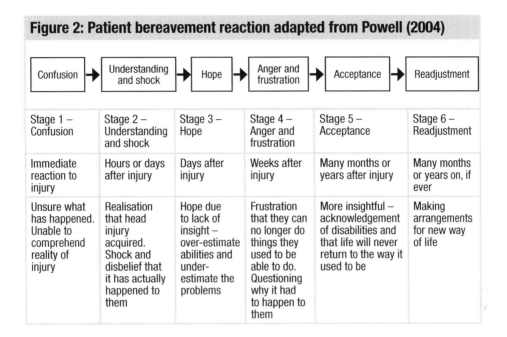

Figure 2: Patient bereavement reaction adapted from Powell (2004)

Stage 1 – Confusion	Stage 2 – Understanding and shock	Stage 3 – Hope	Stage 4 – Anger and frustration	Stage 5 – Acceptance	Stage 6 – Readjustment
Immediate reaction to injury	Hours or days after injury	Days after injury	Weeks after injury	Many months or years after injury	Many months or years on, if ever
Unsure what has happened. Unable to comprehend reality of injury	Realisation that head injury acquired. Shock and disbelief that it has actually happened to them	Hope due to lack of insight – over-estimate abilities and under-estimate the problems	Frustration that they can no longer do things they used to be able to do. Questioning why it had to happen to them	More insightful – acknowledgement of disabilities and that life will never return to the way it used to be	Making arrangements for new way of life

Wider consequences

Relationships

Relatives
There is a need for long-term support for both people who have had a brain injury and their relatives, for example, for at least two–five years from the time of injury (Ponsford & Schonberger, 2010).

Adapting to the changes caused by a brain injury can be difficult and sometimes confusing. Relatives often experience a mixture of emotions (see **figure 3**). It is not uncommon that people feel relief that their relative has survived, yet feel guilty when they experience negative emotions towards their relative if they realise that their relative's personality or behaviour has changed.

It can be a difficult time if a person has sustained a severe injury and may require care support to help them. Often relatives feel that it is their responsibility to do the washing and dressing that is needed, however, realistically they may not have the time to be a carer if they work or have children to look after.

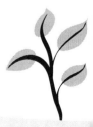

Sometimes relatives think that there are only two options: to be a full-time carer, or not. This should not be encouraged but instead, relatives should be supported to adjust to the new change in the relationship between them and their relative, and decide over a period of time how much support they feel they can give. It should not be assumed that husbands, wives or parents should automatically become the main carer.

Children

It can be hard to decide whether or not it is appropriate to take a child to visit a family member who has suffered a head injury, but it is generally thought that having family around can aid the recovery of patients. Children are likely to be worried about seeing someone they love looking very ill but it can often help them to see that the patient is alive and breathing. However, it is important to understand that children will need time to take in what is happening and to try and make sense of the situation. They must not be made to feel guilty if they do not feel ready to support their family member straightaway. It is a good idea to take some books and games to the hospital as if they do not feel up to seeing the patient, or get bored or upset, these can help to distract the child.

The person with the head injury may not want the child to be around them because they do not want them to see them struggling. This is also something that should be considered.

Children can become very impatient with their family member for not being able to do things that seem easy. It is also common for children to feel embarrassed about their family member's behaviour following a head injury. Their relative, for example, may wet themselves in public or shout at the child's friends – these changes will be hard for a child to understand. While it is important that children do not 'bottle up' their feelings, it may be helpful to encourage them not to express their frustration or embarrassment at the patient as it will make the person sad if they are unable to be who the child wants them to be. People may stare at the child and their brain injured relative when they are out and this is also likely to upset and embarrass the child. It may help to remind the child that it is natural for people to be curious and they are just trying to work out what has happened.

Children may try to think of reasons why someone they love has a brain injury and may start to blame themselves. The may feel sad and angry and can question why it happened to their family when none of their friends are affected. Children must be reassured that anyone can acquire a brain injury; there is no reason and there is no one to blame. They should be encouraged to talk about how they are feeling with their family, but also with people from outside their family. Many children find it useful to undergo counselling to discuss the complex feelings arising from having someone with a head injury in the family.

If it is the child's mother or father who suffers the head injury, the child is likely to experience greater emotional and behavioural problems and perform more poorly at school. As well as dealing with the changing and challenging behaviour of their brain injured parent, their other parent will spend vast amounts of time supporting their spouse and meeting their demanding needs. It may be helpful to seek support from the child's school as there may be access to pastoral care.

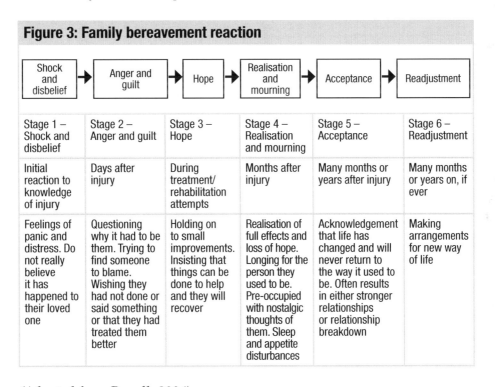

Figure 3: Family bereavement reaction

Shock and disbelief	Anger and guilt	Hope	Realisation and mourning	Acceptance	Readjustment
Stage 1 – Shock and disbelief	Stage 2 – Anger and guilt	Stage 3 – Hope	Stage 4 – Realisation and mourning	Stage 5 – Acceptance	Stage 6 – Readjustment
Initial reaction to knowledge of injury	Days after injury	During treatment/ rehabilitation attempts	Months after injury	Many months or years after injury	Many months or years on, if ever
Feelings of panic and distress. Do not really believe it has happened to their loved one	Questioning why it had to be them. Trying to find someone to blame. Wishing they had not done or said something or that they had treated them better	Holding on to small improvements. Insisting that things can be done to help and they will recover	Realisation of full effects and loss of hope. Longing for the person they used to be. Pre-occupied with nostalgic thoughts of them. Sleep and appetite disturbances	Acknowledgement that life has changed and will never return to the way it used to be. Often results in either stronger relationships or relationship breakdown	Making arrangements for new way of life

(Adapted from Powell, 2004)

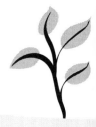

Return to work

There are several factors that can influence a person's return to work. These include environmental factors, such as having a supportive work environment; factors about the person, such as their age, type of job, level of self-awareness; and coping skills and cognitive problems. It has been shown that certain types of cognitive rehabilitation can help people in their return to work, specifically rehabilitation strategies that help with attention, memory and executive problems. However, social and emotional changes (for example, anxiety and depression) can impact on how people manage at work after a brain injury. Psychological interventions targeting this can be helpful (Mateer & Sira, 2006).

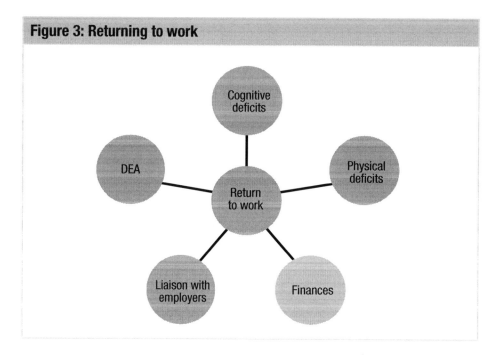

Figure 3: Returning to work

A key concern for many people who have suffered a brain injury is when they will be able to return to work. In reality, the percentage of people who have suffered a significant brain injury who have returned to full- or part-time work five years after their injury is approximately 19–29% (Powell, 2004). It is very important that brain injury sufferers do not attempt to return to work too soon. Government guidelines state that, following a severe head injury, the person should not return to work for at least a year. If a return to work is undertaken too soon, the person is more likely to experience difficulties and the return may fail. This is likely to seriously dent a person's confidence and could restrict them in getting another job.

Cognitive changes

Good physical recovery can make some people assume that cognitive recovery is also good. This can result in returning to work too early or resuming full duties too quickly. The person is then likely to find that they are unable to cope and experience fatigue, anxiety and depression, all of which exacerbate the extent of the difficulties. The common cognitive symptoms limiting work performance are poor memory, poor concentration, poor stamina and tiredness, slowed thinking, irritability and lowered tolerance. Executive difficulties, such as difficulties with planning and organising, judgement and problem-solving, analysing situations and using initiative, are also likely to limit the success of returning to work.

Physical changes

Physical changes after a head injury can also impact upon a person's ability to return to work. In some cases, services are available to make these less limiting, for example, work-related assessments may be carried out by employers in order to make the working environment as comfortable as possible for the person, such as a specialist chair to support the spine. People with speech problems can be supported by specialist computers, signers can be provided for the hearing-impaired, and a person with visual problems may be provided with a reader. Occupational therapists can also work with people and their employers to advise on any aids and adaptations that might be beneficial. This may only be possible in cases where funding is available, such as from the Access to Work programme.

Emotional changes

Emotional difficulties can impact on a person's return to work. Initially it can be anxiety provoking to return to work, for example, in knowing what to say when people ask about the brain injury. It can be helpful to practise what a person will say if they are asked what happened to them. It is common that people try to hide their difficulties as far as possible, however, although it may again be anxiety provoking at first, it is often useful to explain to employers and colleagues what potential problems might occur, and what they need to do in response, so that they do not panic or back off.

Sometimes people can get very tearful or anger more quickly than before and at times this can be embarrassing for the person with a brain injury. It can be useful to tell people that this might happen so that it is not such

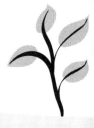

a big surprise. If people know what a problem is and why it is happening, then they are more likely to offer support rather than criticism.

Vocational rehabilitation

Vocational rehabilitation has been found to be particularly effective in improving work prospects. This involves interventions to promote the recovery of the cognitive skills necessary for work and learning coping strategies for dealing with work pressures and responsibilities. Tolerance on simulated work tasks is built up and retraining on tasks specific to the person's job are undertaken. Vocational rehabilitation courses are offered by some education establishments but availability is not universal due to limited funding.

Disability employment advisors

Disability employment advisors (DEA) are a source of support and guidance for those in the UK who are thinking about returning to work following a head injury. They offer specialist advice and can provide access to Jobcentre Plus services, which include Access to Work, Work Preparation and Workstep.

Access to Work
Access to Work provides practical support for disabled people and employers. This can include a grant towards extra costs resulting from a disability, such as communication support and adaptations to buildings. The value of the grant will take into consideration the length of employment, whether the person is an employee or self-employed, and what support is needed.

Work preparation
Work preparation is an individually tailored programme with specific support for people with head injuries who wish to return to work. The programme focuses on job finding behaviour, development needs, occupational decision-making and job keeping behaviour.

Workstep
Workstep provides supported job opportunities for people with disabilities. Providers offer workplace support, such as monitoring and coaching, and agree a plan for development with the person and their employer to ensure that they get the training and support needed to progress.

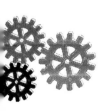

Government-funded programmes vary geographically and are subject to change, but the latest details of the programmes available can be found at www.uk-rehab.com and www.direct.gov.uk.

Liaison with employers

If a person is considered ready to return to work and is under the care of the NHS, a clinical neuropsychologist, consultant in rehabilitation medicine or occupational therapist may contact the employer to negotiate their return. They may also visit the workplace to give advice and support, but this will be time limited. If this is not the case, the person should liaise with the human resources department of their company or the occupational health worker, if one is in place. The length of their absence may have some bearing on whether or not they can return to work or to their former position, as someone else may be doing the job in their absence. The circumstances will be different for each person but it is important to make contact with employers.

Finances

Financial issues can often cause people who have experienced brain injury to return to work before they are ready as the worry of how they will continue to support their family can be great. It is important for people to check the terms and conditions of their employment contract as some employees may be entitled to pay despite their absence. However, this will be time limited and dependent upon many factors, including length of service and whether the individual held a permanent or a temporary position. There are many benefits available to individuals who are unable to work or limited in the work they can do due to disability. These are complex and ever changing but up-to-date information and advice can be found at www.direct.gov.uk and www.citizensadvice.org.uk. It is also worth considering meeting with an advisor such as those at the Citizens Advice Bureaux. Although difficult, the sooner that finances are looked at and realistic options considered and changes made, the easier it will be to cope in the longer term.

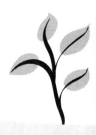

Quiz

1. Give an example of an 'open' traumatic injury.

2. The initial crucial period of time following a brain injury during which paramedics may be involved is called what?

3. What is a common way that people with 'locked-in' syndrome communicate?

4. What does PVS stand for?

5. What does DEA stand for?

References

Anson K & Ponsford J (2006) Coping and emotional adjustment following traumatic brain injury. *The Journal of Head Trauma Rehabilitation* **21** 3 248–259.

Headway [online]. Available at: www.headway.org (accessed January 2011).

Hippocrates 400BC quote [online]. Available at: www.titololawoffice.com/docs/DefiningMildTraumati%20BrainInjury.pdf (accessed January 2011).

Kendall E, Kendall M & Muenchberger H (2009) *Disabilities: Insight from across fields around the world Vol 1: The experience: definition, causes and consequences*. London: Greenwood Publishing Group.

Mateer C & Sira CS (2006) Cognitive and emotional consequences of TBI: intervention strategies for vocational rehabilitation. *Neurorehabilitation* **21** (4) 315–326.

Moore E, Terryberry-Spohr L & Hope D (2006) Mild traumatic brain injury and anxiety sequelae: a review of the literature. *Brain Injury* **20** (2) 117–132.

Ponsford J & Schonberger M (2010) Family functioning and emotional state two and five years after traumatic brain injury. *Journal of the International Neuropsychological Society* **16** (2) 306–317.

Powell T (2004) *Head Injury: A practical guide*. London: Speechmark Publishing.

Royal College of Physicians (2003) *The Vegetative State. Guidance on diagnosis and management. Report of a working party of the Royal College of Physicians*. London: Royal College of Physicians.

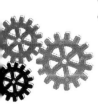

Sawchyn J, Mateer C & Suffield J (2005) Awareness, emotional adjustment and injury severity in postacute brain injury. *The Journal of Head Trauma Rehabilitation* **20** (4) 301–314.

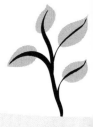

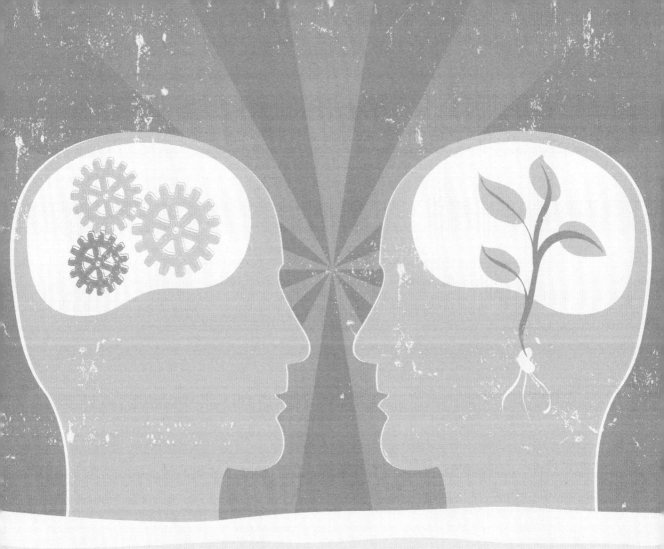

Part 3:
Two further applications

Chapter 12

Applying neuropsychological ideas to mental health problems: schizophrenia and disorders of anxiety

Louise Braham

Aims of the chapter

This chapter aims to:

▶ introduce mental health difficulties within a neuropsychological framework

▶ develop an understanding of the current neuropsychological thinking around schizophrenia

▶ develop an understanding of the current thinking around cognitive functioning and anxiety disorders

▶ understand the typical cognitive difficulties that people with schizophrenia experience

▶ gain a sense of what this 'looks like' in real people and how they present behaviourally

▶ consider changes in brain structure in people with mental health problems

▶ understand the types of cognitive or neuropsychological assessments that can be carried out

▶ consider what neuropsychological and cognitive models can add to your knowledge base and understanding of mental health problems.

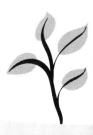

Introduction

This chapter considers the neuropsychological and cognitive aspects of mental health problems. The focus of the text is on schizophrenia with in-depth discussions around the presentation, cognitive deficit and neuropsychological functioning. The main cognitive difficulties in schizophrenia are discussed, but it is notable that they are common to many other areas of mental health problems. The areas considered include memory, executive functioning and attention; anxiety disorders including post traumatic stress disorder (PTSD) and obsessive compulsive disorder (OCD) are also considered although in less detail.

Mental health problems and the brain

Mental health problems are not unusual within our society with many people experiencing some form of difficulty. There are many different kinds of mental health problems, some of which can be debilitating and chronic. Such difficulties are considered to be a combination of a range of genetics and biology alongside experience and environment, as highlighted by the biopsychosocial functioning model in chapter 1.

Mental health problems can exhibit a range of presentations from mild depression or anxiety through to more debilitating difficulties such as obsessive compulsive disorder (OCD) or schizophrenia. Mental health problems often encompass social and emotional difficulties alongside behavioural and cognitive difficulties.

Cognitive functioning is that ability that humans have to function in a complex society. Such abilities allow us to make choices; weigh up risk; attend to things; communicate with each other (language); express ideas; execute decisions and remember things etc. – all those mental processes can be considered examples of cognition (Sharma & Antonova, 2003). When such functioning, much of which is taken for granted, is disrupted and the person is left with specific difficulties in some of those areas, then this is what we can term *cognitive deficit*.

All the functions discussed above fall broadly into four areas of cognitive functioning. The first is the receptive functions, this is the group of abilities that allow you to select and formulate or think about information received. It includes classifying information in a way that makes it understandable

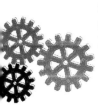

to the individual. The second group of abilities is expressive functions. These are the skills which allow a person to communicate with others behaviourally as well as verbally. Memory and learning functions are the third broad group, and these include the ability to store and retain information, and organise and retrieve it when necessary. The last group of functions is the executive and thinking functions. These abilities include being able to organise, manipulate and reformulate ideas and information, to reorganise it when needed. Each of these broad areas described actually comprises of many smaller functions such as being able to sustain attention, or memory to recall faces.

Neuropsychology is concerned with understanding the brain and behaviour relationship – it is essentially the behaviour resulting from the functioning of the brain. It is still not a well understood concept and a traditional approach has been to consider lesions relating focal brain damage and patterns of impaired functioning compared to preserved cognitive functioning. Within psychiatric conditions many types of brain abnormality are seen, but in the majority of psychiatric or mental health disorders a clear, focal brain lesion is not evident and the brain–cognition relationship no easy undertaking to understand.

Neuropsychological thinking can be applied to mental health difficulties, or aspects of them, such as mood disorders or schizophrenia. This will be considered in this chapter with a focus on schizophrenia. Psychological thinking has been applied to such difficulties for a number of years, and neuropsychology has more recently offered some very helpful ideas to understanding the difficulties further. Neuropsychology may be considered to more closely represent the medical model, which continues to largely dominate our health culture within mental health services. However, there are still a large percentage of people with such disorders considered to be 'treatment resistant' due to their lack of response to medication in relation to their mental health difficulty. Furthermore, there has been criticism offered toward the medical model and this is specifically in relation to the belief that medical or biological based diagnosis based on symptoms offers poor reliability and validity (Bentall *et al*, 2004). As stated in Chapter 1, using only the 'bio' or biology alone in the 'biopsychosocial model' can be limiting. In more recent times, however, schizophrenia has been broken down into subgroups minimising the heterogeneity within each group, and specifying more closely the diagnosis. However, this still does not remove the many difficulties in understanding, even these broken down aspects based on diagnosis alone.

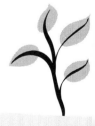

Understanding the functioning and changes of the brain in people with schizophrenia as well as the disease itself has managed to evade scientists, medics and psychologists for years. Even with all the technology available today, we still do not have the answers. Therefore, can neuropsychology offer something else by way of understanding these difficulties? In recent times advances in knowledge have allowed us to consider cognitive analysis at a more specific level. Development of neuropsychological assessment has allowed closer scrutiny of specific domains in different conditions and this can help target cognitive deficits in terms of rehabilitation as well as measuring outcome.

Assessing cognitive difficulties

When neuropsychologists assess aspects of functioning they do it two ways. First they take an account of or observe the difficulties where possible. This is to try and understand the functional or everyday behavioural aspects of a deficit. This information is then combined with test results of specific 'tools' designed to consider aspects of functioning in a discrete way. These are considered further below. Carrying out such assessments can aid diagnosis, providing specific information on deficits and helping differentiate between psychiatric and neurological problems. However, perhaps more importantly, neuropsychological assessment can now help patient care and treatment and help in understanding behaviour in relation to brain functioning. It can also help highlight those areas of strength.

Functional impairments are those impairments that make everyday life more difficult. Many people with such a disorder often need daily help and support in day-to-day activities. This may include being unable to sustain a job, or having difficulties in initiating and maintaining social relationships and many more are unable to live independently. Thus those cognitive difficulties highlighted in the next section are those which mainly impact upon daily functioning.

In relation to testing there are some basic ideas that we need to have in mind when considering tests. First, most tests come with 'norms', which are a range of scores gained by groups of people with and without various difficulties. This then allows comparison of any one individual's results on a test with a group of people in the same age group, of the same gender without known cognitive deficits or mental health problems. This allows the assessor to judge how far

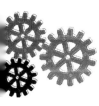

from the average the examinee is and thus what the main areas of deficit might be. Some tools do also provide information about scores gained by people with a history of such things as head injury or mental health problems, but this is not, however, the only way that tests can be used. Testing can also be used to see how an individual's functioning changes over time either to improve or decline, or to see specific weaknesses and strengths that can be built upon. Testing can help gauge how well a person might cope independently and can further aid diagnosis and rehabilitation and help target those areas most in need. This is the case used for all the tests used with the disorders discussed in this chapter.

Schizophrenia

What is schizophrenia?

The term schizophrenia often conjures up an image of crazy people acting in bizarre ways and doing unusual things, and the media does little to help this image. Only in more recent times have movies such as *A Beautiful Mind* offered a more compelling and realistic, although dramatised, view of the disorder. In fact, when translated, the word schizophrenia broadly means 'splitting of the mind'; it comes from the Greek language with Eugen Bleuler in the early 20th century first coining the term to account for the apparent separation in thinking, memory and perception. Indeed it is this translation which often leads to the misunderstanding that schizophrenia is an illness that leads to more than one personality or a split between personalities. The difficulties with definition perhaps reflect the difficulties in understanding this complex disorder.

Schizophrenia itself is really an umbrella term for a range of difficulties that may include, to a greater or lesser degree, a combination of the following symptoms: thought disorder; poor concept formation; delusions, often persecutory, paranoia; bizarre behaviour; social inappropriateness including sexualised or disinhibited behaviour, withdrawal; hallucinations, mostly auditory that is hearing voices; blunted affect that is, decreased expression of emotions; lack of relating to other people. Social functioning is impaired and a lack of motivation is common. It is often chronic, meaning long-term and persistent, and may be peppered with acute, short, sharp, perhaps extreme phases.

Many people at some point during their lifetime may experience a brief psychotic episode but a diagnosis of schizophrenia is only given to a long

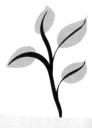

standing and often debilitating disturbance of thought, emotion and behaviour. The sorts of symptoms they might exhibit include those that are described as positive symptoms, which are experiences that most people do not have but that are present in those with schizophrenia, such as delusions or hallucinations. Negative symptoms on the other hand are those behaviours or experiences normally found in other people that are missing from the person with schizophrenia. These are things like a lack of motivation, blunted affect, inability to experience pleasure and poverty of speech. Clearly then you can see how such behaviours may influence a person's quality of life and ability to function in our society.

Case study 1

James was 26 years old when he was diagnosed with schizophrenia. At the time the development of the illness was most distressing to him and impacted upon his daily behaviours and thinking. He had recently taken a job as a newly qualified dentist and found he could not 'think straight' or remember which patient was coming in for which treatment without checking his notes two or three times. On occasion, he would forget the patient's name halfway through a 20-minute consultation or he found himself considering an intervention that was not useful to that patient. Further, he would describe ideas coming into his head that seemed sensible at the time, but as pointed out by his dental nurse, had no relevance to dentistry. He was finding it ever more difficult to communicate to people and he would describe feeling angry and irritated on one day and completely cut off and emotionless on another. He described what he would call 'whispering' in his ears when he was with patients – this voice would give him a running commentary on what he was doing or criticise him for treating a patient in a particular way.

James made an appointment with his GP following feedback from his dental nurse and wife that his behaviour was 'strange'. He attended the appointment with his wife who was able to describe her observations of him, and the GP referred James to the local community psychiatric team where he was diagnosed with schizophrenia. He is now well for the majority of the time following a range of medical and psychological treatment but describes his presentation when unwell as being 'bizarre'.

There are antipsychotic drugs available to help some of those with this disorder who can then go on to live a full life but there are also a great number of people who do not respond well to medication and for whom these symptoms become part of their everyday experience and life.

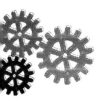

Onset and diagnosis of the disorder

Schizophrenia is usually seen to develop in the late teenage years, often before the age of 19. The initial phase of the illness is referred to as the 'prodrome' and this can be seen many months before the onset of the symptoms of schizophrenia. In this period, the person may begin to experience some of the symptoms which may include withdrawal from others, irritability or other non-specific symptoms. They may be transient or short-lived, but will affect the individual's day-to-day functioning.

One of the places where schizophrenia is defined is in the Diagnostic and Statistical Manual of the North American Psychiatric Association (DSM-IV, 2000), which defines schizophrenia as a disturbance that lasts for at least six months and includes at least one month of two or more active symptoms, that is delusions, hallucinations, disorganised speech, grossly disorganised or catatonic behaviour or negative symptoms that have been present for a significant period of time. Major areas of social or occupational functioning are also disturbed in one or more domains such as self-care, interpersonal relationships or work.

Schizophrenia it seems, therefore, is a complex and often debilitating condition which causes major stress and distress to the patient and family. However, as discussed earlier, the diagnosis of schizophrenia does not tell us very much about what we may see in an individual's behaviour. Certainly professional carers and families need to know more about the specific experience of each individual to allow for the appropriate support or help to be offered. Furthermore, as discussed earlier, there continues to be controversy surrounding the validity of the definition of schizophrenia (Boyle, 2002). With this in mind and the overlap in presentation with diagnoses such as major depression or bipolar disorder, measuring as well as understanding the disorder is always difficult.

The origins of schizophrenia

Genetics and hereditary

There have been many studies over the years trying to figure out the course, cause and development of schizophrenia and there is still no absolute conclusion and debate still abounds. The genetic hypothesis is one which has gained much support from twin and family studies from as early as the 1950s. It is thought that schizophrenia is a condition of complex inheritance, with many different potential genes each of small effect, with different

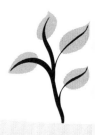

pathways for different individuals. Some have suggested that several genetic and other risk factors need to be present before a person becomes unwell but this is still uncertain (Owen *et al*, 2005). These ideas are still largely held to be true and this genetic link is often seen in clinical practice. Twin and adoption studies have indicated a high degree of heritability (O'Donovan *et al*, 2003). There are also now some hypotheses about particular chromosomal regions which may be affected in schizophrenia (Purcell *et al*, 2009) or particular proteins (O'Donovan *et al*, 2009) that may be exerting an effect on development of the disorder.

Environmental ideas

Having said that, there is evidence for genetic or hereditary factors, there is also thought to be a strong environmental link captured in the idea of the stress-vulnerability model. This model proposed that a person has an individual level of vulnerability to stressors according to their biology and life experience to date. When such stressors in the environment outweigh the ability to cope adequately with them, schizophrenia may develop as a response to the inability to cope with the given situation. Evidence suggests that genetic and environmental factors can act in combination to result in schizophrenia (Harrison & Owen, 2003). Thus, the diagnosis of schizophrenia must be considered to have a significant heritable component but that onset is significantly influenced by environmental factors or stressors. The idea of an inherent vulnerability or *diathesis* in some people is also known as the *stress-diathesis model* (Corcoran *et al*, 2003). An alternative model is that biological, psychological and social factors are all important and is known as the 'biopsychosocial' model. All of these ideas, stress-diathesis, stress-vulnerability and biopsychosocial models essentially agree that schizophrenia develops due to both genetic/biological, psychological and environmental, including social factors (see chapter 1 for further information on the biopsychosocial model).

Some studies have considered the impact of social or environmental experience on the development and course of schizophrenia. A number of areas are believed to be risk factors or things that contribute to make the development of the disorder more likely. These include being socially disadvantaged (Musser & McGurk, 2004) including poor housing or unemployment. Other experiences of social adversity such as racial discrimination or family discord are also thought to be risk factors. Unsurprisingly, given the discussion above around the idea of a genetic vulnerability plus stressors influencing the development of schizophrenia, a major stressor such as trauma is also considered to be a possible risk factor for development of the disorder. Such trauma may include sexual or psychical abuse (Schenkel *et al*, 2005). Given those risk factors we must still remember that one needs the vulnerability in the first place and that trauma or poor social experiences alone do not cause schizophrenia.

Whatever the cause of schizophrenia, the course and development of the disorder is individual in terms of experience, functioning and length of time over which it happens. The symptomology may often appear similar for example experiencing auditory hallucinations and social withdrawal, but the content, emotional response and ability to cope with it are unique to the individual and often have some sort of psychological link.

What is happening in the brain?

Areas of the brain

As early as the 1940s Bender (1942) believed schizophrenia to have developed from disordered neurological development or poorly developed CNS organisation alongside undisturbed development of the brain. Brain abnormalities we also know may be transmitted via genetics and so the support for brain structures being involved in schizophrenia is strengthened. Differences have been observed in healthy neurons compared those neurons of an individual with schizophrenia. As discussed in chapter 2, nerve cells or neurons are integral to the functioning of the brain as they transmit information to and from other areas and provide the 'glue' to strengthen this transfer of information. Some researchers have observed smaller or fewer neurons whilst the earliest ideas were around disorganisation of those neurons. Most frequently this has been observed in the hippocampus.

There are currently many authors who believe that schizophrenia arises in part as a response to damage to the frontal areas of the brain, hippocampus and temporal lobes (see chapter 2 for a further explanation of these areas). These ideas are based on studies of neurobiological functioning and in more recent times accurate scans of the brain (Kircher & Thienel, 2005). Differences in brain activity have been highlighted in these frontal areas and linked to the cognitive deficits often associated with schizophrenia (Green, 2006). The frontal lobes are extremely important in allowing us to carry out higher order functioning tasks and when damaged can lead to all sorts of difficulties with executive functioning. Such tasks might include planning, manipulation of ideas, offering appropriate social responses or judgements

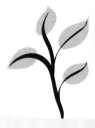

and being flexible in thinking to manipulate ideas. All such skills may be damaged in those with schizophrenia and indeed is commonly observed.

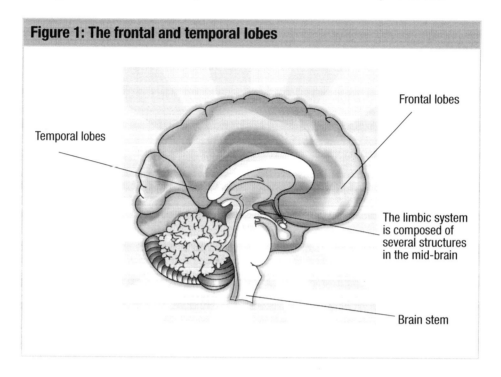

Figure 1: The frontal and temporal lobes

Frontal lobes

Temporal lobes

The limbic system is composed of several structures in the mid-brain

Brain stem

Those individuals who have experienced a frontal injury to the brain also often present with such difficulties. Areas of the frontal cortex and parts of the amygdala are important in controlling behaviour (Winstanley *et al*, 2004) and damage to this region has been associated with disinhibited or socially inappropriate behaviour and emotional changes (Berlin *et al*, 2004) (see also chapters 2, 3 and 4). As previously discussed, individuals with schizophrenia often exhibit socially inappropriate or disinhibited behaviour.

Thus the suggestion has been that where such difficulties occur there is likely to be some damage to the frontal parts of the brain, both in schizophrenia (Fujii *et al*, 2004) and in other disorders or injuries to the brain. Whilst this similarity between head injured and patients with schizophrenia looks similar in some respects the evidence is still circumstantial, although brain imaging is helping to further the understanding of this relationship. Indeed criticism has been made of the assumption that executive functioning is damaged in greater amounts in those with schizophrenia as compared to healthy adults and some go so far

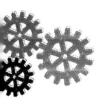

as to say that the literature has overestimated the importance of damage to the frontal systems (Zakzanis & Heinrichs, 1999).

Brain structure and size

There have been findings relating to differences in brain structure and size of certain areas in the brain. A study by Steen *et al* (2006) looked at magnetic resonance imaging (MRI) studies which found a reduced volume of the whole brain as well as specifically within the hippocampus (see chapter 2).

In trying to consider the cause and path of schizophrenia in relation to brain examination, children with schizophrenia have been examined. In a recent MRI study (Zahn *et al* 1997; Rapoport *et al*, 1997) teenagers with the illness were compared to those without it in terms of their brain structure. What the authors found was reduced cerebral volume and enlarged ventricles (see chapter 2) not dissimilar to that found in the adult brain. These ventricles continue to enlarge as the disease progresses when compared to healthy controls which show no ventricle enlargement.

Possible reduction in grey matter

As well as the size of ventricles discussed in the previous section, a loss of grey matter in the brain is also postulated as a potential hypothesis for understanding schizophrenia. Grey matter is an important part of the brain (see chapter 2). It is actually a gray-brown color which comes from the blood vessels and neuron cell bodies within it. It is thought that some of the networks in the brain within the grey matter have a potential for disconnection (Ellison-Wright & Bullmore, 2009) as well as a general reduction in the amount of grey matter seen in people with schizophrenia. It is thought that those with the greatest tissue loss demonstrate the greatest number of and perhaps more severe symptoms.

Neurotransmitters

Neurotransmitters are important chemicals deep within our brain, which can cause changes in behaviour. A neurotransmitter is a chemical which sends a signal to a particular cell from a neuron across a synapse (see chapter 2). In the case of schizophrenia, it is thought that the pathway of a specific neurotransmitter, namely dopamine, is altered in some way, perhaps producing more than is necessary. Drugs which block this pathway in the brain are found to reduce psychotic symptoms.

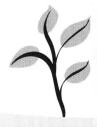

Having said that, there are now newer atypical antipsychotic medications that reduce the symptomology. However, by working on serotonin function as well as the dopamine function, this perhaps suggests that other neurotransmitters may also be involved, thus complicating the situation further. Another neurotransmitter, glutamate, has in more recent times also been hypothesised to be involved in schizophrenia. In this instance, however, it is not an excess but a lack of glutamate receptors that is thought to be the problem. Further, glutamate is thought to affect dopamine functioning; glutamate function is found to be reduced in those who have difficulties with cognitive tasks involving frontal activation (Tuominen *et al*, 2005).

Although we can safely say that people with schizophrenia have some differences in their brain structures when compared to healthy controls, we are still unclear if this is a 'chicken or egg' situation. Did the brain structures alter and produce schizophrenia or did the disorder itself cause changes in the structure of the brain?

It seems that current ideas support the notion that brain differences develop in childhood leading to schizophrenia, but there needs to be more developmental research in the areas if we are to be clearer about this. Some authors today suggest that schizophrenia may not be a disorder, but more of a response to brain injury at an earlier time (Pincus & Tucker, 2003).

Links between mental illness and cognitive or neuropsychological functioning

As already seen in chapter 5, disease or damage to areas of the brain that control emotion can also cause disabilities of a social and emotional nature and we have discussed above how parts of the brain are related to functioning in schizophrenia. Often social functioning is impaired in those with schizophrenia and emotions are often blunted or can be extreme. Unusual beliefs may be held by the individual and they may find it difficult to relate to other people. It is a perplexing disease for which we currently do not have all the answers, but certainly neuropsychology and cognitive function have something to offer. From a neuro-behavioural perspective, there does seem to be broad agreement that there is neuropsychological impairment frequently seen in those with schizophrenia. Indeed some authors (Green & Nuechterlein, 1999) suggest that the absence or disturbance of certain neuropsychological or cognitive functioning could allow consideration of a different set of neuropsychological symptoms to be considered in the case of schizophrenia.

There are psychological ideas or theories that can help increase our understanding of schizophrenia. There are some psychological theories that focus more on unconscious communications and relationships. There are others, however, which offer cognitive ideas that sit nicely with apparent structural changes in the brain. 'Cognitive bias' is one such mechanism that has been highlighted in those with schizophrenia (Lewis, 2004). Such biases result in a tendency to consistently view the outside world in a particular or 'skewed' manner which could include impaired reasoning, excessive attention to possible threat, making attributions or jumping to conclusions (Kurtz, 2005). Further, some evidence considers that the content of delusional experiences can reflect emotional causes and that how a person interprets their experiences can influence their symptomology (Kuipers *et al*, 2006).

Further, it is believed that a person can learn to cope with and challenge their delusional or hallucination experiences by the use of cognitive behavioural therapy (CBT). This is recommended within the National Institute of Clinical Excellence (NICE) guidelines for treating people with schizophrenia. Such is the weight of evidence at present that this is recommended treatment for people to receive within the NHS. Given then that a psychological treatment that is partly cognitive in nature is recommended for people with schizophrenia, one perhaps must consider the importance of this cognitive aspect of functioning.

Cognitive deficits in schizophrenia

Assessing neuropsychological functioning in individuals with a psychiatric disorder is not an easy task. Most psychiatric disorders include disturbance of emotions which may impact upon cognitive abilities. However, there are a number of common difficulties seen in those with schizophrenia which are discussed in the case study below. Here you will also meet Mark and James, two young men with schizophrenia whose cognitive deficits are evident in their day-to-day behaviour and functioning.

Case study 2

Mark was a student at high school and was a high achiever who had obtained good GCSEs and was expected to gain four A-levels and go on to attend university. He first reported that he started feeling 'funny' just before his 17th birthday. He described feeling like he was removed from other people and that he no longer saw the world in the same way that others did. He described often feeling confused and as not always

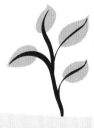

being able to follow the conversation, finding himself getting lost or 'stuck' on a particular piece of information. He also described finding it difficult to remain attentive during school lessons and found he was able to recall little from his classes. On occasion he found it difficult to generate the word he was looking for, leaving him feeling embarrassed. Mark found all this extremely distressing and consequently his school grades fell and he withdrew from his friends and rejected the support of his teachers. He found it difficult to relate to his family and friends and became very socially isolated.

As the illness progressed, Mark began to 'hear voices' and experience delusions (or false beliefs) which finally prompted him to self-harm and cut his arms in an attempt to make the 'voice' go away. He was eventually diagnosed with schizophrenia.

Difficulty with clear thinking is an integral part of the symptomology of schizophrenia. As well as those symptoms described as hallucinations, an individual with schizophrenia may experience a range of other difficulties. Generally, such difficulties are seen in cognitive functioning across a broad range of areas. Neuropsychological assessment (and observation) reveal difficulties (or poorer performance) with attention and concentration, ability to consider abstract thought, problem-solving, cognitive flexibility (for example, being able to shift from one idea to another idea, learning something new or different, or changing a response in a given situation etc.), verbal skills and manipulation and memory (Heinrichs & Zakzanis, 1998).

Some authors argue that difficulty in cognitive functioning is the essence of schizophrenia as it determines day-to-day functional performance. Indeed this is supported by studies which have found evidence that children and adolescents with poor cognitive abilities might be at increased risk of schizophrenia (Macabe, 2008). If this is the case, then we can argue that poor cognitive function is associated in some way with causing the disorder.

These deficits in cognitive functioning were so consistent and often observed in people with schizophrenia that much therapeutic endeavour has been focused on developing therapies such as cognitive remediation therapy (see Wykes *et al*, 1999) that specifically target this area. The target is the cognitive domain and functioning and such therapy is now thought to produce consistent improvements (Mcgurk *et al*, 2008). In the last decade this development of non-pharmacological treatments has been growing. What now seems to be agreed is that cognitive deficit is a relatively stable feature of schizophrenia. Often, even when the psychotic symptoms are well controlled, deficit in cognitive functioning remains (Sharma & Antonova, 2003).

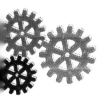

Medication

Medications used to reduce symptoms of schizophrenia are called antipsychotics and they are most commonly used for helping those with symptoms of psychosis. They are known within two groups called typical and atypical antipsychotics. The atypical antipsychotics are those that have been more recently developed and the typical antipsychotics are those developed in the 1950s (such as clozapine). Both groups of medication tend to block receptors in the brain's neural pathways, most commonly dopamine but antipsychotic drugs include a wide range of receptor targets. Those antipsychotic medications developed for the treatment of schizophrenia have been thought to exert some influence on cognitive functioning in those who take them. Initially the findings were fairly negative in that they made some cognitive functioning worse. However, some of the newer medications available (atypical) have been found to exert a more positive influence in improving concentration and other functions.

Development of neuropsychological tools

These observations of difficulties in cognitive functioning in individuals with schizophrenia led to the use of neuropsychological 'tools' to help us understand these deficits and how they may impact on someone's overall functioning. By understanding the specific problems and what is previously therapy/rehabilitation/remediation can then be targeted. Tools or tests have been developed to help assess cognitive functioning so as to support an individual to cope with problems in their daily life.

See the case of Mark on p327 and discussion of the more common cognitive difficulties found in those with schizophrenia below. Note though, that although four of these areas are discussed separately, as highlighted in chapter 1, these are not distinct from one another and often a deficit in one area may be linked to difficulties in another. For example, as can be seen below, if someone has difficulties with attention, then this will likely impact on their ability to remember things; if they have difficulties with cognitive flexibility, it is likely that their executive functioning will be impaired.

Overall cognitive functioning

Overall it is thought that people with schizophrenia perform well below the average person across a range of domains including attention, memory, motor speed and executive functioning. These difficulties will then likely impact

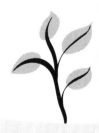

on ability to communicate and build relationships with others. Memory, for example, plays an important part in day-to-day functioning and consequently wider cognitive abilities. Memory and attention are used in learning, understanding and communication. Although a range of neuropsychological tests will be considered to help to understand specific aspects of functioning, some batteries of tests have been proposed to be suitable for focusing on the deficits seen in schizophrenia. Two such tests are the Repeatable Battery for the Assessment of Neuropsychological Status (RBANS) and the Brief Assessment of Cognition in Schizophrenia (BACS). The BACS is a recent instrument that assesses the aspects of cognition found to be most impaired and most strongly correlated with outcome in people with schizophrenia whilst the RBANS, although initially developed for assessing older people, is capable of providing reliable and valid assessments of people with schizophrenia (Gold *et al*,1999; Wilk *et al*, 2002) (see also chapter 7).

Some specific cognitive areas

Memory

Case study 3

Jane is an ordinary 31-year-old woman with three children who works four days a week. She continually has to use her cognitive abilities to plan, organise and execute her day in the most efficient way possible. This may mean that she will plan to make only one journey to the shop and collect all that she needs for food for the rest of the week, while remembering that one child is on a school trip on Friday and needing a packed lunch. She may also find herself going away overnight with work and so will need to arrange child care for Wednesday and all this has to be considered before she gets to work on Monday. Once there she may have to look up a telephone number, remember it for a minute or so before she dials; or she may have to use her previous experience to enable her to deal with a presenting problem.

The description above is not dissimilar from many people's lives – many of the tasks are familiar to all. Even in this short description of a couple of hours of Jane's morning, we can see the amount of cognitive manipulation, memory and effort that is used even for the very small, daily tasks. It is only when people find they have difficulty doing or remembering something that deficits show.

There are a number of different types of memory. Essentially there is conscious or explicit memory and unconscious or implicit memory. Within each of these there is short-term, immediate or working memory, and long-term memory. Generally, difficulties with memory function seem to be common in those with schizophrenia. Memory for events that have happened, so called 'episodic' or 'declarative' memory which is conscious and explicit has been the area where most dysfunction has occurred and can perhaps be considered a robust and consistent marker of schizophrenia (Bilder, 2009). This is the area of memory that allows us to learn and recall information from previous experiences and to build on that. In a review of studies (Cirillo & Seidman, 2004), verbal declarative memory was found to be significantly impaired in schizophrenia and as largely accounted for by deficits in the encoding stage. Subtle impairments in increased rates of forgetting were found to be also present, but were mild compared to amnesic disorders. Thus this deficit has led some authors to argue that in fact it is so specific to schizophrenia that it perhaps should be a marker for the disorder.

Implicit memory is a type of memory which we are not conscious of. It is things we learn without consciously recalling them to know how to behave in light of them. This type of memory does not appear to be highlighted in the literature as an area specific or distinct within schizophrenia.

Memory difficulties within schizophrenia are not thought to be mainly due to forgetting the information. It is more likely that it is to do with difficulties in retrieving the information from the memory banks. Alternatively, it may be due to not laying down and storing the memory properly in the first place. People with schizophrenia find it difficult to remember things even when prompted with a clue or the start of the word thus suggesting that it is with the encoding and retrieval of information that may be problematic. Further, with healthy individuals if one is prompted by saying 'it's an animal' then often we will be able to get the correct word, however, people with schizophrenia do not find this helpful and they remain still unable to retrieve the information or word. It was this finding that led to the belief that encoding and retrieval problems were the cause of the problem (Stone *et al*, 1998).

In relation to short-term memory, it is possible that this may be compounded by the symptomology that the individual experiences and the impact of this on their ability to attend to something to be able to recall it at a later state. You will remember the case of Mark who describes himself as being unable to recall information from his school classes (to a far greater degree than previously and in comparison to other teenage boys).

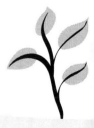

Generally reviews of the literature support the notion that there is significant memory impairment in schizophrenia. An analysis of the literature in 1999 suggested that the impairment was stable, wide ranging, and not substantially affected by potential moderating factors such as severity of psychopathology and duration of illness (Aleman *et al*, 1999).

Assessing memory functions

Observation of behaviours

As discussed earlier, neuropsychologists assess memory functions in two ways. One way is to observe the person struggling to recall things such as a conversation or remember information previously learnt (as with James the dentist previously). They may be observed finding it hard to plan or make decisions; they may report a wide range of functional difficulties which are dependent upon memory functioning such as forgetting appointments, telephone calls or conversations.

Declarative memory, as discussed above, is that form of memory that allows for recall of previous experiences and to learn from them. If someone is unable to remember they would not learn what was dangerous in life and what is not and thus be unable to adjust their behaviour accordingly. Such memory is hugely important in social and occupational functioning as well as in independent living. Working memory is also important in those circumstances. Remember Jane's simple couple of hours in a morning and the working memory tasks that she needed to perform for her family, occupation and daily living? An individual with schizophrenia would very likely struggle with all of those tasks described.

Tests and testing

There are many ways to assess memory function, from using the very simple tools to using much more complicated ones. There are many well used and researched individual tests which measure a range of different memory functions used by occupational therapists and psychologists. These include the Rivermead Behavioural Memory Test; the California Verbal Learning Test and the Wechler Memory Scales. Such tools can be very useful but in some instances can be too long for the person with schizophrenia. Consequently, neuropsychologists may choose only parts of these tests which allow assessment of the specific domains highlighted.

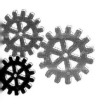

Part of the brain thought to be responsible for function:

Working memory processes appear to be associated with part of the frontal cortex (Buchsbaum & Hazlett, 1998) and imaging studies show that this part of the brain is active when performing working memory tasks. It is thought that impairments of working and semantic memory are primarily due to dysfunction of the frontal and temporal lobes and hippocampus. The temporal lobe is also thought to be a brain region crucial for long-term memory function (Cirillo & Seidman, 2004). Refer to **figure 1** as a reminder of where in the brain this memory is taking place.

Executive functioning/higher order problem-solving (including cognitive flexibility)

Overview

Executive functioning covers a wide range of skills and activity. It is this area of the brain that is responsible for those tasks which may be considered abstract or those which are required to generate a solution to a problem. The other important areas considered to be part of executive functioning are the ability to monitor your own and others actions; to plan and execute a response to novel situations and to have cognitive flexibility. Cognitive flexibility is an important function which allows us to problem solve, learn and make sense of information presented to us.

So let us reconsider the case of Mark. You will remember, one of the things he describes is *getting lost or 'stuck' on a particular piece of information*. By this he means he finds it difficult to move from one train of thought or idea to another. Often he may not even realise he is stuck but finds it difficult to shift to any other ideas. This made studying for academic qualifications really challenging for Mark, as he would become pre-occupied with some aspect of what he was learning rather than learning a range of ideas he needed for an examination.

Observations of behaviours

Executive dysfunction, like memory dysfunction can be debilitating and disabling, while disrupting both occupational functioning and independent living skills. In terms of what can be observed, a range of problems in learning, planning, multi-tasking and coping with novel situations may

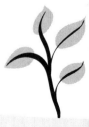

be evident. People may have problems at work managing their time or workload, prioritising tasks and executing them. They may have difficulties with independent living such as managing their financial affairs, organising themselves, or failing to get minor tasks or errands carried out. Initiation and motivation are both difficulties considered to be part of executive functioning and it is often these difficulties that impact on occupational and daily functioning.

Testing for problems with executive functioning

Like all areas of behaviour some executive functioning problems can be observed. However, in schizophrenia some very subtle difficulties can be present, which the observer may not notice at a first glance. There are a number of tools which can help us get a clearer picture of executive functioning and what exactly the specific difficulties might be. All these tasks have some sort of planning, organising or abstract thought aspects to help narrow down the focus.

The most common tools a psychologist will administer to assess executive functioning include the Stroop Colour Word Test, which looks at ability to inhibit wrong answers; the Trail Making Test for flexibility of thinking; the Tower of London task, which looks at ability to plan and monitor behaviour and the Wisconsin Card Sort Test involves shifting strategies and cognitive flexibility. In addition, they all require some sort of monitoring function to complete.

Patients with schizophrenia vary in the amount of dysfunction they experience in relation to executive functioning, however, most do show deficits on the tools described above. If one is unable to monitor one's own behaviour and performance then it must be difficult to recognise when one is unwell (Sharma & Antonova, 2003).

Part of the brain thought to be responsible for this executive function

It has been known for many years that the part of the brain responsible for these higher order functions are the frontal lobes. Indeed, following head injury and damage to the frontal lobes, changes in patients are observed that include difficulties with planning and organisation, prioritising and self-awareness.

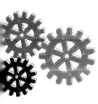

If the centre in the brain which allows us to monitor ourselves is damaged in those with schizophrenia, then it is not at all surprising that one of the symptoms often seen is a lack of self-awareness. This shows itself in all sorts of ways including the common problem of not taking medication. This could, in part, be due to the memory difficulties described above, but could also be due to a lack of awareness that one needs to take the medication to stay well.

Summary of this section

It is clear that neuropsychological methods can help us understand this debilitating and little understood disorder. Neuropsychological dysfunction or deficit has been reported in many studies and some have found widespread cognitive difficulties whilst others have found evidence for the selectivity of problems. Those domains that have received a particular focus include attention, memory and executive functions. They appear to be served by those neural networks that link together frontal and temporal regions of the brain.

Attention

Overview
Clearly, common sense would tell us that if we did not attend to something properly, we may be in danger of misunderstanding it, or not learning or taking it in properly; it is thus closely linked with memory. Attention is that group of skills which allow us to focus on a particular thing when there may be other things going on around us thus being selective; and it allows us to focus on something for a period of time until we have completed the task or processed the information. Some people find it more difficult than others to divide their attention between more than one task and indeed people with mental health problems may find all such tasks more difficult than others.

Consider the case of James (page 320) who described hearing 'whispering'. Imagine that you were trying to read a book with a constant commentary right in your ear talking about what you were doing, or criticising the way you were reading or telling you that you were stupid. Do you think you would be able to get to the end of the chapter and remember what it said? How do you think you may feel emotionally – upset perhaps? As with other areas of cognitive functioning, emotion will impact upon attention as for other skills.

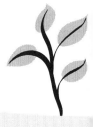

Some have suggested that the focus and meaning that people with schizophrenia often give to what appear to be very small amounts of irrelevant information may be linked to the experience of and in an attempt to make sense of delusions (Garety & Hemsley, 1997).

Alternatively, there may be an attentional bias that then makes processing other information difficult. Lastly, there is the higher order attention that can be considered the attentional supervisory control system. It is this function that allows us to keep track of and monitor our own performance in context and respond accordingly. This is a control strategy which can determine, for example, when attention needs to be shifted from one stimuli to another. Without this monitoring system our behaviours may be more erratic, less efficient and far less adaptable to the world around us. We can see difficulties with control in those with schizophrenia.

So, attention can include those skills of being able to focus on something specifically; to divide concentration between tasks or select between stimuli. It is required over short bursts as well as more sustained periods of time. Individuals with schizophrenia have difficulty in sustaining attention over long periods of time as well as dividing it between tasks.

Observation

Attention, as for memory is crucial for daily living and for occupation. One is often required to sustain attention for long periods of time to be able to hold down a job. An individual with attentional difficulties may focus on or get stuck on one particular piece of information; they may be easily distractible either by their own train of thought or by external information (such as noise) and may not pay attention long enough or with enough quality to help learn new information. A person who is unable to monitor their own behaviour may struggle in social situations finding it difficult to follow the rules of interaction.

Testing for attention is always going to be a difficult task as it can only be considered indirectly. The speed at which information is processed will also affect the ability to maintain attention. Further, this is linked (as discussed earlier) with working memory as well as executive functioning in the idea of a supervisory attentional system to monitor one's behaviours.

Attention is closely related to perception and alertness and appears to be something that is considered in terms of degree. Imagine sitting in a very boring and long lecture; you may find it difficult to maintain your focus on what the speaker is saying over a period of an hour, however, you may be able to attend to an engrossing film which is far longer. Fatigue also has an impact on the ability to maintain concentration and attention is further complicated by the dimension of effort considered within it. This may be the ability to maintain specific and focused attention on a particular task for a short period of time to achieve a goal. Thus, given the different components of attention, it is difficult to give it one clear definition, which in turn makes measuring it very difficult.

However, rather than consider the categories or type of attention that actually do not help us understand more clearly, it is perhaps more helpful to gain an understanding specifically of what the issues and difficulties are. An example would be an inability to follow instructions in a noisy environment; an individual losing their 'train of thought' over a sustained period of time, or falling asleep in a lecture. Observation can also be useful in gathering information about attention.

Testing

We can, however, more formally carry out tests for different aspects of attentional functioning if needed for clarification. One may argue that there are no tests of pure attention as it is not a discrete and singular skill. Timed visual search tasks can be used; tests of sustained attention perhaps using a sound or repeated task over time; divided attention can be assessed by consideration of the ability to attend to two different rules at once or engage in two different tasks within a given space of time. Tools that assess focused attention or distraction can be used to specific particular difficulties. Most often this will be to confirm what we suspect already.

Many of the tests discussed in relation to executive functioning can be said to aid understanding of attention as it is often considered to be part of that group of high order functions. Processing speed may be slowed if someone is having difficulties with maintaining attention, which in turn will cause problems in memory and thus learning. There are specific tests available, which include the Test of Everyday Attention (considering a range of attentional aspects), the Stroop-Colour Word Task (measuring distraction and speed of processing) and the Paced Auditory Serial Addition Task (PASAT), which is a combination of two tasks in one test measuring divided attention. Many attentional tasks, however, can be assessed with limited formal tools.

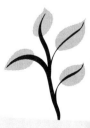

Part of the brain thought to be responsible for this function

The areas of the brain that control attention are those involved in the executive system and these are discussed in more detail below. Essentially, they are the frontal areas of the brain and have wide connectivity across the brain to other regions. It is clear that attention does not belong to one area or cerebral structure alone because of the range of functions and processes considered within it. As well as the executive system, the brain stem must also be involved given the idea that alertness is important. The brain stem (see **figure 2**) is responsible for the basic functions such as wakefulness and mental state; consequently it has a large role in attentional aspects of behaviour. Given that attention is not located in one area of the brain, diffuse rather than specific damage may be more problematic to attentional systems, as much of their work is about connectivity between systems.

It has been discussed above that attentional bias, where attention and focus is given to a specific bit of information, can be evident in those with schizophrenia. It has also been considered how attention is important for feedback from our environment and to allow us to regulate certain behaviours. In given situations we must also maintain attention to give a certain goal or understanding and thus we can see how easily this can be disrupted.

Anxiety disorders including obsessive compulsive disorder and post-traumatic stress disorder

Overview

Anxiety disorders range in terms of their extremes as well as in their behavioral output, and they are extremely common in the adult population. Essentially, anxiety disorders refer to the abnormal and sometimes pathological fear and anxiety, which only came to the attention of psychiatry toward the end of the 19th century.

Anxiety itself is actually a very normal response to stress or danger. At times it is can be helpful because it can help prepare the body for action, and it can improve performance in a range of situations say just before an exam or public speaking. This anxiety is short-lived and reduces usually quite quickly. Anxiety also gives a person extra energy to deal with a dangerous situation or to flee from one, and only becomes a problem when it is experienced intensely, when it interferes with a person's daily life and functional ability.

Unlike the relatively mild, brief anxiety caused by a stressful event (such as public speaking or sitting an exam), anxiety disorders last at least six months and can get worse if not treated. People often find their own way of coping with their anxiety which may mean staying at home, organising things in their own specific way, avoiding certain situations or using drugs and alcohol to cope.

The term 'anxiety disorder' is considered to include disorders of emotion, but it has been argued that certain types of anxiety disorder such as generalised anxiety disorder (GAD) are in fact a cognitive dysfunction (McNaughton, 1997). The cognitive system is essentially there to mediate emotional perception and emotional states, which can have a profound effect on cognitive functioning.

We will look at the cognitive aspect of some of them in more detail below. Broadly, anxiety disorders include panic disorder, obsessive compulsive disorder, post-traumatic stress disorder, social phobia and generalised anxiety disorder.

Post-traumatic stress disorder

Overview

Post-traumatic stress disorder (PTSD) is an anxiety disorder that can develop after experiencing a traumatic event. It develops after a terrifying ordeal that may have involved physical harm or the threat of physical harm. The person who develops PTSD may have been the one who was harmed, or the harm may have happened to a loved one, or the person may have witnessed a harmful event that happened to loved ones or strangers. Basically, this fear or threat overwhelms the individual's ability to cope and PTSD can develop. This development can lead to changes in behaviour, affect and cognition and the behavioural aspect of this disorder includes re-experiencing the traumatic event (such as a car crash, sexual assault) by way of flash backs, which can be sounds, smells, images etc. or nightmares. They may also experience distressing thoughts.

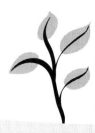

Case study 4

Sarah is a 57-year-old healthy woman who has retired and spends two days a week caring for her two-year-old granddaughter Katie. She has cared for Katie since her daughter went back to work when Katie was six months old. One day, not long after Sarah had started looking after Katie, they were in the car on the way to the local shops a few miles away from their home, and as they went about their day, a small white van speedily came over the hill towards their car and it was on the wrong side of the road. Sarah had to serve off the road in order to miss it. Luckily there was very little else on the road and other than being shocked and enduring a few scratches and bruises, everyone was alright. Katie suffered no injuries at all and Sarah had some bruising and a cracked rib from her seatbelt.

Eighteen months later, Sarah will not drive a car with a baby in it; she will only go out on the roads when they are not busy and she suffers from extreme anxiety whenever she sees a small white van on the road. She tends to avoid doing the shopping at all, her sleep is disrupted and she is generally more 'on edge' than she was previously. She also finds concentrating difficult other than when it is for short periods of time.

Diagnosis

The diagnosis of PTSD includes such symptoms as re-experiencing the original traumas via flashbacks or nightmares as well as avoidance of experiences linked with the trauma. Increased arousal, such as difficulty falling or staying asleep, anger, and feeling overly alert, is also a symptom considered. Diagnostic and Statistical Manual (DSM-IV) criteria require that the symptoms last more than one month and cause significant impairment in social, occupational or other important areas of functioning.

As you can see from the case of Sarah above, such behaviours can be evident. It is not the issue of the actual outcome of the experience (she and Katie are both fine) but more the possibility or perception that it could have been fatal and at the time believed to be life threatening. Indeed it is believed that in the more serious cases where an accident has resulted in brain trauma and thus loss of memory in the event, people are less affected with PTSD than those with a memory of the experience (Warden *et al*, 1997). The resulting outcome for Sarah is that her daily life has altered significantly, impairing her ability to socialise and carry out her usual daily errands.

Cognitive aspects of PTSD

As for the other mental health problems, there are often a range of cognitive problems associated with the disorder. Cognitively, there appear to be difficulties in learning new material and memory in many cases of those with PTSD. Anxiety is often associated with distractibility and poor attention (see previous discussion on attention) and generally mental efficiency such as processing speed may be slowed. Given what we have already considered in relation to memory and attention in schizophrenia, we know that they are linked and that if disrupted they can impact upon a number of different functions. The issues are thus largely similar here.

Observation

The person suffering from PTSD may show a range of behaviours including avoidance of anything that may remind them of the ordeal. People with PTSD may startle easily, become emotionally numb (especially in relation to people with whom they used to be close), lose interest in things they used to enjoy, have trouble feeling affectionate, become irritable, more aggressive, or in extreme cases violent. The affective and behavioural nature of the difficulty can make occupational functioning and daily living extremely difficult.

Testing

As described previously, a neuropsychologist may assess the relevant functions of a disorder in order to understand and help rehabilitate specific cognitive deficits. In the case of PTSD, those symptoms described as attentional difficulties, memory and learning difficulties can all be considered with the tests highlighted in the previous section.

Part of the brain thought to be involved in anxiety PTSD

There is not as much literature and research into possible brain dysfunction in anxiety disorders as there is in schizophrenia. However, the part of the brain responsible for fear and anxiety more generally are thought to be the orbito-frontal cortex on the inferior frontal lobes of the brain along with the amygdala which receives input from all the sensory systems.

There are three main areas thought to have altered function in PTSD. These are the prefrontal cortex (as highlighted above); the amygdala and the hippocampus. Several MRI studies have now demonstrated that PTSD is

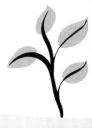

associated with a reduction in volume of the hippocampus, an area crucially involved in new learning and memory (Bremner, 1999). It is possible that such difficulties could also stem from the continued release of the stress hormone on the hippocampus. As considered at the beginning of this chapter, most brain functions are linked due to their need to pass information to other areas. As discussed above, the amygdala receives input from all sensory systems. It is thought that the amygdala is strongly involved in the formation of emotional memories, especially fear-related memories. Possible over arousal of the amygdala due to poor control by the prefrontal cortex and the hippocampus is proposed as an explanation (Milad *et al*, 2009).

Figure 2: A Picture of the brain stem, highlighting the limbic system including hippocampus and amygdala

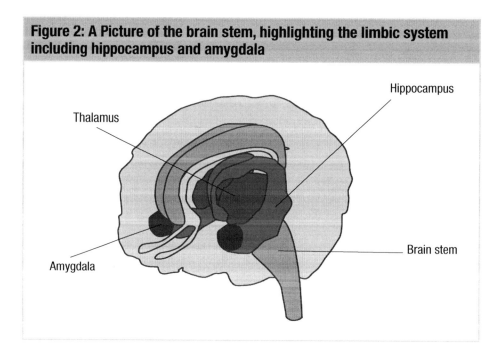

It is also more recently proposed that memory systems are also involved in the processing of trauma and thus resulting disorders, which is known as the dual representation theory.

Neurotransmitters

As with the other mental disorders, PTSD displays biochemical changes in the brain. It is possible that low cortisol levels may predispose individuals to PTSD because cortisol is normally important in restoring balance after a stress response, and it is thought that trauma survivors of trauma with

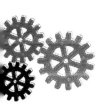

low cortisol experience may have the predisposition to develop PTSD. It is the impact of cortisol which has been highlighted as one of the possible contributors to deficits in cognitive functioning (Vasterlin & Brewin, 2005). However, there is considerable controversy within the medical community regarding the neurobiology of PTSD. A review of existing studies on this subject showed no clear relationship between cortisol levels and PTSD. Only a slight majority have found a decrease in cortisol levels while others have found no effect or even an increase (Lindley *et al*, 2004).

Serotonin is another important neurotransmitter to be considered in PTSD. Serotonin receptors can be found in many brain regions including the amygdala, hippocampus and the pre-frontal cortex. Serotonin is thought to play a role in the functioning (inhibition and excitation) and regulation of these areas. It is possible that changes in the regulation of these areas contribute to the symptoms of PTSD by for example contributing to the misinterpretation of emotionally laden information. Alterations in serotonin levels are also thought to be involved in fear-related behaviours (Vasterlin & Brewin, 2005).

Obsessive compulsive disorder

Overview

Obsessive compulsive disorder (OCD) is a disorder about controlling anxiety, no mater what that anxiety may be about. It is considered amongst the top most debilitating illnesses by the World Health Organization in terms of loss of income and decreased quality of life and is thought to affect roughly 2–3% of the UK population. People with OCD experience persistent, upsetting thoughts or obsessions that may be around a range of things, but most commonly dirt or germs. They develop and use rituals or compulsions to control the anxiety that these thoughts produce. When a particular ritual is carried out the level of anxiety the individual experiences in most cases falls. For how long the effect lasts, depends on the severity of the individual's anxiety and ritual controlling behaviour but it is always temporary. There are many examples of OCD, ranging from very minor to those which severely disrupt life and occupational functioning.

For example, if a person is obsessed with tidiness, they may not be able to leave the house until every single thing is symmetrical on a shelf; or cushions are facing exactly the right angle; and all their clothes have exactly the same space between them on the hangers and so on. Those

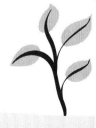

obsessed with germs may develop a compulsion to wash their hands over and over again or use antibacterial hand gel repeatedly. There are also other common rituals such as a need to repeatedly check or touch things. Some common obsessions include having frequent thoughts of violence and harming loved ones, persistently thinking about performing sexual acts the person dislikes, or having thoughts that are prohibited by religious beliefs.

Aggressive and sexual obsessions are also seen in OCD and can be particularly horrifying to those who experience them. For some people, obsessive fears of committing a terrible act in the future compete with fears that they may already have done something awful in the past. Therefore, they feel compelled to constantly check. These obsessions can involve violent or graphic imagery that is upsetting and disgusting to the person, such as rape, physical assault or even murder.

Of course all of us have our daily routines we carry out, or we may be someone who likes to 'double check' the door is locked or that the windows are shut. OCD is somewhat different with the impact that it has on everyday life.

Diagnosis

To be diagnosed with OCD, a person must have obsessions, compulsions, or both, according to the DSM IV. It is suggested that several features characterise obsessions and compulsions and these are recurrent and persistent thoughts, impulses or images that are experienced as intrusive and that cause increased anxiety or distress. These thoughts, impulses or images are of a degree or type, which are different to the usual range of worries about everyday problems.

Cognitive aspects of OCD

Some studies indicate that OCD is associated with higher IQ when compared to the general population whilst others argue that there are few neuropsychological differences between OCD and healthy participants. Generally, the specific cognitive deficits seen in OCD include executive and non verbal difficulties.

Neuropsychological investigations of adults with OCD also show impairment on complex measures of executive functioning and strategic memory. These problems may not be apparent in childhood because normal children do

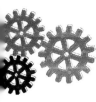

not have fully matured prefrontal networks and consequently show less developed executive functioning (Savage & Rauch, 2000). Other patient studies confirm that patients with OCD show specific cognitive deficits on tasks of executive and visual memory function (Purcell *et al*, 1998). In a more recent study looking at executive and spatial functioning, OCD patients showed controlled fluency, visual-spatial construction, learning and memory deficits (Boldrini *et al*, 2005). In a review of the literature in 1997, Tallis found that there is modest evidence for the presence of non-verbal and praxic memory deficits in patients with OCD. These deficits are consistent with contemporary theories of frontal functioning and may represent the cognitive substrate of doubt-related phenomena such as checking; the demonstration of specific memory impairments in OCD were also found (Tallis, 1997). A more recent systematic review of the literature (Kuelz *et al*, 2004) confirms general deficits in cognitive functioning as well as specifically in memory and impaired organisation of information, which is the executive functioning.

Observation

Individuals with OCD can be seen performing certain behaviours in a repetitive manner and they may choose not to leave the house as they spend too much time performing their rituals. Alternatively they may take many hours to perform a simple task or errand due to the interfering rituals.

Compulsions may also be repetitive mental acts that the individual feels driven to perform. The aim of such thoughts is to reduce the likelihood of a bad event happening, but often the thought or mental act has no bearing on the probability of the event occurring. For example, the mental act of an individual repeating the word 'no' 100 times to prevent a loved one being involved in a car crash may be compulsive but has no bearing on the likelihood of a car crash taking place. Thus much mental energy is required to control or ignore the experience.

Inattention to space external to the person most often following head injury or damage is termed neglect, as this is not commonly seen in those with schizophrenia it will therefore not be considered in this chapter.

Testing

The pattern of cognitive deficit in OCD seems less distinct than that highlighted in schizophrenia. As for attention, specific testing with a focus on discrete tasks is necessary, but it is clear that experiencing the compulsions

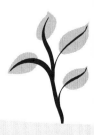

and obsessions as described above would of course impact on the ability to attend to and learn new information. If one's focus is on carrying out a specific ritual then one's cognitive functioning and effort may be tied up in this task leaving little capacity for anything else. Testing can aid the specific cognitive aspects and help rehabilitate those areas which would include in this case executive functioning tests, memory tests and specific tests of attention.

Areas of the brain

Studies of images of brains have revealed that abnormalities in the orbito-frontal cortex (see previous section) may be common in OCD. Deeper structures such as the basal ganglia and thalmus are also involved, thus it is suggested that the communication between these parts of the brain is not functioning correctly. When anxiety rises in the OCD sufferer, a circuit of inappropriate response happens between these parts of the brain. The pattern of impaired performance found in these patients has been found to be qualitatively similar to the performance of patients with frontal lobe problems and subcortical pathology suggesting that the underlying pathophysiology of OCD could be conceptualised as reflecting dysfunction of these frontal systems (Purcell *et al*, 1998).

Neurotransmitters

As for the other disorders discussed, neurotransmitters are also thought to be involved in the production of OCD. Serotonin is often the neurotransmitter highlighted in relation to OCD. It is a chemical that allows nerve cells to communicate with each other by working in the space between nerve cells in the synaptic cleft. Serotonin also helps connect nerve cells right across the brain in a number of different ways, thus a change in serotonin levels may alter the connectivity influencing behaviours such as OCD.

Glutamate, which was discussed in the case of schizophrenia earlier in the chapter, has also recently been implicated in the functioning of OCD, as recent studies have found evidence suggesting there is an excess of glutamate in the physiology of OCD (Chakrabarty *et al*, 2005).

Summary of chapter

This chapter has considered mental health difficulties and the cognitive aspects involved in their presentation and functioning. It has looked at the disorder of schizophrenia in some detail and of anxiety disorders to a lesser degree, and what should be made evident while reading this chapter is that all the areas of cognitive functioning are related and not clearly distinct from each other. This is because the brain, where cognition takes place, is made up of many areas with different roles which are both functionally and physically linked. Consider also the similar neurotransmitters discussed in relation to these disorders.

Mental health problems, as you have seen, show similarities in areas of deficit and common themes emerge. Aspects of executive functioning and memory seem to be a common area of deficit in all of the disorders discussed. Further, all mental health difficulties, to a greater or lesser degree involve difficulties with emotion and emotional processing. This is because in turn this is related to and mediated by cognition resulting in a given behaviour. Thus the endeavour of treatment for these difficulties includes medication and some form of cognitive therapy alongside specific remediation or rehabilitation techniques. But the challenge for assessment is to help pinpoint the specifics of the damage. It is undoubtedly a complex process, but by understanding the patterns related to each type of illness, we can help aid diagnosis and rehabilitation. It is clear that the brain is involved in the production of behaviour and therefore makes sense that it has a role when aspects of our behaviour are altered or lost. Within the brain, it is also clear that the structures involved in cognition are disparate and may involve areas of the cortex, midbrain and limbic system all interacting with each other.

In relation to testing, there is a range of tests available to assess cognitive functioning and these can be applied to those with mental health problems noting the common issues with lack of motivation and initiation common to many. Tests available vary widely and are constantly under review, and those discussed here are by no means exhaustive and there are many others that may be suitable or helpful. Cognitive models can help conceptualise the difficulty in an alternative way to the medical model alone providing greater analysis and understanding of the presenting issue and area of dysfunction specific to that individual.

The importance of observing function via daily tasks cannot be underestimated and referral to a neuropsychologist of such deficits are observed. Scientists and researchers do not all agree fully on aspects of functioning in the relevant areas, but deficits are broadly agreed. The frontal lobes and the connectivity between major areas of the brain such as the amygdala and hippocampus appear to be most sensitive to the development

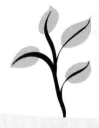

of such disorders. What we also know is that many of these deficits in function makes occupational and daily life very difficult and many mental health sufferers have to have extra support to allow them to get by.

Figure 3: Areas of the brain connected in production of behaviour: from nerve cells to the limbic system to the frontal lobes

Information is passed through the mass of neurons in the brain to other areas of connectivity

Information passes to and from the limbic system (dealing with emotion)

From the limbic system to other areas of the brain such as the frontal lobes (and back again)

Quiz

1. What is schizophrenia?

2. How does it develop?

3. Why does neuropsychology help us understand the disorder?

4. What cognitive deficits are typically associated with schizophrenia?

5. How would you test for cognitive deficits without the use of formal tests?

6. What behaviours might someone with schizophrenia exhibit?

7. How is the brain different in someone with schizophrenia than that in a healthy person?

8. What cognitive deficits might you expect to see in someone with an anxiety disorder?

9. Where in the brain is memory located?

10. Why is it important to consider motivation when assessing someone cognitively who has a mental health problem?

11. How easy is it to define specific areas of the brain in relation to a specific mental health difficulty?

12. Why is emotion considered to have an important impact on cognitive functioning?

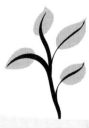

References

Aleman A, Hijman R, de Haan EHF & Kahn RS (1999) Memory impairment in schizophrenia: a meta-analysis. *American Journal of Psychiatry* **156** 1358–1366.

American Psychiatric Association (2000) *Schizophrenia. Diagnostic and Statistical Manual of Mental Disorders*. Washington: American Psychiatric Association.

Bender L (1942) Schizophrenia in childhood. *The Nervous Child* **1** 138–140.

Bentall RP, Read JE & Mosher LR (2004) *Models of Madness: Psychological, social and biological approaches to schizophrenia*. Philadelphia: Brunner-Routledge.

Berlin HA, Rolls ET & Kischka U (2004) Impulsivity, time perception, emotion and reinforcement sensitivity in patients with orbitofrontal cortex lesions. *Brain* **127** (5) 1108–1126.

Bilder RM (2009) The Neuropsychology of schizophrenia circa 2009. *Neuropsychology Review* **19** (3) 277–279.

Boldrini M, Del Pace L, Placidi GP, Keilp J, Ellis S P, Signori S, Placidi GF & Cappa S F (2005) Selective cognitive deficits in obsessive-compulsive disorder compared to panic disorder with agoraphobia. *Psychiatrica Scandinavica* **111** (2) 150–8.

Boyle M (2002) *Schizophrenia, a scientific delusion?* New York: Routledge.

Bremner JD (1999) Alterations in brain structure and function associated with post-traumatic stress disorder. *Clinical Neuropsychiatry* **4** 249–245.

Buchsbaum MS & Hazlett EA (1998) Positron emission tomography studies of abnormal glucose metabolism in schizophrenia. *Schizophrenia Bulletin* **24** 343–364.

Chakrabarty K, Bhattachargya S, Christopher R & Khanna S (2005) Glutametergic dysfunction in OCD. *Neuropsychopharmalology* **30** 1735–1740.

Cirillo MA & Seidman LJ (2004) Verbal declarative memory dysfunction in schizophrenia: from clinical assessment to genetics and brain mechanisms. *Neuropsychology Review* **13** (2) 43–77.

Corcoran C, Walker E, Huot R, Mittal V, Tessner K, Kestler L & Malaspina D (2003) The stress cascade and schizophrenia: etiology and onset. *Schizophrenia Bulletin* **29** (4) 671–692.

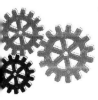

Ellison-Wright I & Bullmore E (2009) Meta-analysis of diffusion tensor imaging studies in schizophrenia. *Schizophrenia research* **108** (1–3) 3–10.

Fujii DE, Wylie AM & Nathan JH (2004) Neurocognition and long-term prediction of quality of life in outpatients with severe and persistent mental illness. *Schizophrenia Research* **69** 67–73.

Garety P & Hemsley DR (1997) *Delusions Investigations into the Psychology of Delusional Reasoning*. Hove: Psychology Press.

Gold S, Arndt S, Nopoulos P, O'Leary DS & Andreasen NC (1999) Longitudinal study of cognitive function in first-episode & recent-onset schizophrenia. *American Journal of Psychiatry* **156** 1342–1348.

Green MF (2006) Cognitive impairment and functional outcome in schizophrenia and bipolar disorder. *Journal of Clinical Psychiatry* **67** (9) 3–8.

Green MF & Nuechterlein KH (1999) Should schizophrenia be treated as a neurocognitive disorder? *Schizophrenia Bulletin* **25** (2) 309–319.

Harrison PJ & Owen MJ (2003) Genes for schizophrenia? Recent findings and their pathophysiological implications. *The Lancet* **361** 417–419.

Heinrichs RW & Zakzanis KK (1998) Neurocognitive deficit in schizophrenia: a quantitative review of the evidence. *Neuropsychology* **12** 426–445.

Kircher & Thienel (2005) Functional brain imaging of systems and cognitions in schizophrenia. The boundaries of consciousness. *Progress in Brain Research* **150** 299–308.

Kuelz A, Hohagen F & Voderholzer U (2004) Neuropsychological performance in obsessive-compulsive disorder: a critical review. *Biological Psychology* **65** 185–236.

Kuipers E, Garety P, Fowler D, Freeman D, Dunn G & Bebbington P (2006) Cognitive emotional and social processes in schizophrenia refining cognitive behaviour therapy for persistent positive symptoms. *Schizophrenia Bulletin* **32** (1) 24–31.

Kurtz MM (2005) Neurocognitive impairment across the lifespan in schizophrenia: an update. *Schizophrenia Research* **74** (1) 15–26.

Lindley SE, Carlson EB & Benoit M (2004) Basal and dexamethasone suppressed salivary cortisol concentrations in a community sample of patients with post traumatic stress disorder. *Biological Psychiatry* **55** (9) 940–5.

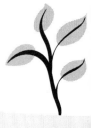

Lewis R (2004) Should cognitive deficit be a cognitive criterion for schizophrenia? *Journal of Psychiatry and Neuroscience* **29** (2) 102–113.

Macabe JH (2008) Population-based cohort studies on premorbid cognitive function in schizophrenia. *Epidemiologic Reviews* **30** 77–83.

Mcgurk SR, Twamley EW, Sitzer DI, Mc Hugo GJ & Musser KT (2008) A meta analysis of cognitive remediation in schizophrenia. *American Journal of Psychiatry* **164** 1791–1802.

McNaughton N (1997) Cognitive dysfunction resulting from hippocampal hyperactivity – A possible cause of anxiety disorder? *Pharmacology Biochemistry and Behaviour* **56** 603–611.

Milad MR, Pitman RK, Ellis CB, Gold AL, Shin LM, Lasko NB, Zeidan MA, Handwerger K, Orr SP & Rauch SL (2009) Neurobiological basis of failure to recall extinction memory in post traumatic stress disorder. *Biological Psychiatry* **66** (12) 1075–82.

Musser KT & McGurk SR (2004) Schizophrenia. *The Lancet* **363** (9426) 2063–2072.

O'Donovan MC, Craddock NJ & Owen MJ (2009) Genetics of psychosis; insights from views across the genome. *Human Genetics* **126** (1) 3–12.

O'Donovan MC, Williams NM & Owen MJ (2003) Recent advances in the genetics of schizophrenia. *Human Molecular Genetics* **12** (2) 125–133.

Owen MJ, O'Donovan MC & Harrison PJ (2005) Schizophrenia: A genetic disorder of the synapse. *British Medical Journal* **330** 158–159.

Pincus JH & Tucker GJ (2003) *Behavioural Neurology* (4th edition). Oxford: Oxford University Press.

Purcell R, Maruff P, Kyrios M & Pantelis C (1998) Cognitive deficits in obsessive compulsive disorder on tests of frontal striatal function. *Biological Psychiatry* **43** (5) 348–357.

Purcell SM, Wray NR, Stone JL, Visscher PM, O'Donovan MC, Sullivan PF & Sklar P (2009) Common polygenic variation contributes to risk of schizophrenia and bipolar disorder. *Nature* **460** (7256) 748–752.

Rapoport JL, Giedd J, Kumra S, Jacobsen L, Smith A, Lee P, Nelson J & Hamburger A (1997) Childhood-onset schizophrenia. Progressive venticular change during adolescence. *Archives General Psychiatry* **54** 897–903.

Savage CR & Rauch SL (2000) Cognitive deficits in obsessive compulsive disorder letter to the editor. *American Journal of Psychiatry* **157** 1182.

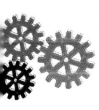

Schenkel LS, Spaulding WD, Dilillio D & Silverstein SM (2005) Histories of childhood maltreatment in schizophrenia: relationships with premorbid functioning symptomology and cognitive deficits. *Schizophrenia Research* **76** (2) 273–286.

Sharma A & Antonova L (2003) Cognitive function in schizophrenia deficits, functional consequences and future treatment. *Psychiatric Clinics of North America* **26** 25–40.

Steen RG, Mull C, McClure R, Hamer RM & Lieberman JA (2006) Brain volume in first episode schizophrenia: systematic review and meta-analysis of magnetic resonance imaging studies. *British Journal of Psychiatry* **188** 510–518.

Stone M, Gabrieli JDE, Stebbins T & Sullivan EV (1998) Working and strategic memory deficits in schizophrenia. *Neuropsychology* **12** 278–288.

Tallis F (1997) The neuropsychology of obsessive compulsive disorder: a review and consideration of clinical implications. *British Journal of Clinical Psychology* **36** (10) 3–20.

Tuominen HJ, Tiihonen J & Wahlbeck K (2005) Glutamatergic drugs for schizophrenia: a systematic review and meta-analysis. *Schizophrenia Research* **72** 225–34.

Vasterlin JJ & Brewin CR (2005) *The Neuropsychology of PTSD. Biological, cognitive and clinical perspectives*. New York: Guilford Press.

Warden DL, Labbate LA & Salazar AM (1997) Post traumatic stress disorder in patients with brain injury and amnesia for the event? *Journal of Neuropsychiatry and Clinical Neurosciences* **9** 18–22.

Wilk CM, Gold JM, Bartko JJ, Dickerson F, Fenton WS, Knable M, Randolph C & Buchanan RW (2002) Test–retest stability of the repeatable battery for the assessment of neuropsychological status in schizophrenia. *American Journal of Psychiatry* **59** (5) 838– 844.

Winstanley CA, Theobald DEH, Cardinal RN & Robbins TW (2004) Contrasting Roles of Basolateral Amygdala and Orbitofrontal Cortex in Impulsive Choice. *The Journal of Neuroscience* **24** 4718–4722.

Wykes T, Reeder C, Corner J, Williams C & Everitt B (1999) The effects of neurocognitive remediation on executive processing in patients with schizophrenia. *Schizophrenia Bulletin* **25** 291–307.

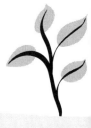

Zahn TP, Jacobsen LK, Gordon CT, McKenna K, Frazier JA & Rapoport JL (1997) Autonomic nervous system makers of psychopathology in childhood-onset schizophrenia. *Archives General Psychiatry* **54** 904–912.

Zakzanis KK & Heinrichs RW (1999) Schizophrenia and the frontal brain: a quantitative view. *Journal of the international Neuropsychological Society* **5** 556–566.

Further reading

Binder RM (2009) The neuropsychology of schizophrenia circa 2009. *Neuropsychological Research* **19** (3) 277–279.

Brune M, Abdel-Hamid M, Lehmkamper C & Sonntag C (2007) Mental state attribution, neurocognitive functioning and psychopathology: what predicts poor social competence in schizophrenia best? *Schizophrenia Research* **92** 151–159.

Cullen KR, Kumra S, Regan J, Westerman M & Schulz C (2008) Atypical antipsychotics for treatment of schizophrenia spectrum disorders. *Psychiatric Times* **25** (3).

Eddy KT, Dorer DJ, Franko DL, Tahilani K, Thompson-Brenner H & Herzog DB (2008) Diagnostic crossover in anorexia nervosa and bulimia nervosa: implications for DSM-V. *The American Journal of Psychiatry* **165** (2) 245–50.

Gold JM, Queern C, Iannone VN & Buchanan RW (1999) Repeatable battery for the assessment of neuropsychological status as a screening test in schizophrenia: I. Sensitivity, reliability and validity. *American Journal of Psychiatry* **156** (12) 1944–1950.

Goldner EM, Hsu L, Waraich P & Somers JM (2002) Prevalence and incidence studies of schizophrenic disorders: a systematic review of the literature. *Canadian Journal of Psychiatry* **47** (9) 833–843.

Green MF (2001) *Schizophrenia Revealed: From neurons to social interactions*. New York: Norton.

Jones HM & Pilowsky LS (2002) Dopamine and antipsychotic drug action revisited. *British Journal of Psychiatry* **181** 271–275.

Lezak MD, Howieson DB & Loring DW (2004) *Neuropsychological Assessment* (4th edition). Oxford: Oxford University Press.

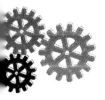

Marie-Josée B, Joyala CC, Godbouta L & Chantalb S (2009) Executive functions and the obsessive-compulsive disorder: on the importance of subclinical symptoms and other concomitant factors. *Archives of Clinical Neuropsychology* **24** (6) 585–598.

Peterson BS, Pine DS, Cohen P & Brook JS (2001) Prospective, longitudinal study of tic, obsessive-compulsive and attention-deficit/hyperactivity disorders in an epidemiological sample. *Journal American Academy Child Adolescent Psychiatry* **40** (6) 685–695.

Radua J & Mataix-Cols D (2009) Voxel-wise meta-analysis of grey matter changes in obsessive compulsive disorder. *British Journal of Psychiatry* **195** (5) 393–402.

Robinson DG, Woerner MG, McMeniman M, Mendelowitz A & Bilder RM (2004) Sympomatic and functional recovery from a first episode of schizophrenia or schizoaffective disorder. *American Journal of Psychiatry* **161** (3) 473–479.

Spreen O, Risser AH & Edgell D (1995) *Developmental Neuropsychology*. Oxford: Oxford University Press.

Zakzanis KK, Leach L & Kaplan E (1999) *Neuropsychological Differential Diagnosis*. Netherlands: Swets & Zeitlinger.

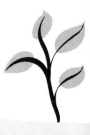

Chapter 13

Assessment of cognitive functioning for people who have learning disabilities

Suzie Beart and Rachel Mills

Aims of the chapter

This chapter aims to:

▶ help with understanding the importance of cognitive functioning in people with learning disabilities

▶ consider the barriers to cognitively assessing people with learning disabilities

▶ consider ways to overcome these barriers.

Introduction

This chapter is divided into four sections. The first gives a definition of 'learning disability' and the second gives a brief introduction to cognitive assessments with people with learning disabilities (see also chapter 7). The bulk of the chapter is taken up by sections three and four. Section three looks at the potential barriers to cognitively assessing someone with learning disabilities and how these barriers might be overcome and lastly, in section four, some examples of such assessments are given.

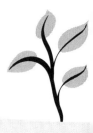

A definition of learning disabilities

This chapter will focus on the assessment of people with learning disabilities, a term that will be used throughout. The definition of a learning disability is:

'... *a significant impairment of intelligence and social functioning, acquired before adulthood.*' (Department of Health, 1998)

This definition incorporates the three criteria that are required to be fulfilled in order to be classified as having a learning disability:

▶ significant impairment of intelligence (IQ of 70 or below)

▶ significant impairment of adaptive/social functioning

▶ onset before the age of 18 years old (British Psychological Society, 2001)

A person's level of learning disability can range from mild disability to the more severe. The Valuing People white paper (2001) estimated that there were 1.2 million people with mild or moderate learning disabilities in England at that time, and 210,000 with severe learning disabilities. There is a wide variety of causes of such disabilities, which differ for each individual. These include the following factors.

Prenatal factors (before birth)

Biomedical issues, such as genetic disorders and chromosomal disorders, may be accountable for the development of a learning disability (Luckasson *et al*, 1992). The most well-known of such chromosomal disorders is Down syndrome, which will be explored further on in the chapter.

There is also a range of environmental factors that may be influential in the development of a learning disability before birth. These may include malnutrition of the expectant mother, the use of drugs by the mother during pregnancy, or illness suffered while pregnant.

Perinatal factors (during and immediately after birth)

Infections, such as rubella and bacterial meningitis, which may have a range of effects such as destroying brain tissue and affecting the central nervous system account for some learning disabilities (Berg, 1985).

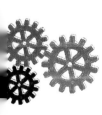

Complications during birth can also result in learning disabilities, the most common of which is asphyxiation (lack of oxygen). Other such problems can include premature birth and difficulties surrounding the umbilical cord (Stern, 1985).

Postnatal factors (after birth)

Illness and infection during childhood, such as meningitis, may also result in a learning disability (Emerson *et al*, 1999). Environmental causes can also play a big part in the development of a learning disability. Traumatic events during childhood, such as sustaining a head injury or long-term malnutrition, may also contribute to the development of a learning disability.

However, it is important to remember that no two people with learning disabilities are the same. As illustrated above, there are many different determining factors, thus each individual will have their own level of ability and skills. Some people may require minimal support in their everyday lives, whereas others may need a much higher level of care and support. It is not just the cause of the disability that can affect levels of support needed – a person's environment and the people around them can have a substantial effect on their abilities and skill levels.

As with everyone else, people with learning disabilities have their own individual personalities, regardless of the severity of their disability. This is often forgotten as the term 'learning disability' tends to put all people with learning disabilities into one homogenous group, and strips them of their identities. It is important to remember that people with learning disabilities have their own ideas, beliefs and hopes for the future – they may just need that extra support to achieve them.

Cognitive assessment for people with learning disabilities

Lezak *et al* (2004) state that the reasons for carrying out a cognitive assessment are as follows:

▶ to diagnose neurological conditions such as dementia

▶ to profile strengths and weaknesses (for care management)

▶ to plan treatment (what specialists are required, OT, speech and language therapy)

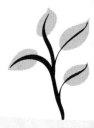

▶ to evaluate treatment (eg. neurosurgery/medication)

▶ research (eg. to relate brain to behaviour)

▶ forensic (eg. did brain dysfunction contribute to illegal behaviour?).

All of the above reasons apply as much to people with learning disabilities as to those without. People with learning disabilities suffer from the same neurological conditions as the general population. However, people with Down syndrome are more likely to have an Alzheimer's type dementia by the age of 60 than those without Down syndrome (Prasher, 2005). The British Psychological Society guidelines on people with learning disabilities with challenging behaviour recognise the importance of cognitive assessment stating: '*It's also good practice to have a clear picture of any specific neuropsychological difficulties the patient may have as a result of brain injury or impairment.*' (Ball *et al*, 2004).

In addition, understanding a person with learning disabilities using a cognitive/neuropsychological approach can provide a rich source of information to help understand the person and the challenges they face. It can also help to consider ways in which they might be supported, including to develop their areas of cognitive and functional strength and to compensate for areas of weakness. A cognitive/neuropsychological perspective can give a new and fresh perspective.

Unfortunately, there are real difficulties in offering people with learning disabilities the kind of cognitive assessment that is outlined in the other chapters. In order to understand an individual's strengths and weaknesses, most standard tests use comparisons with the general population, or 'norms', there are virtually no tests with norms for people with learning disabilities, therefore severely limiting what can be used to understand someone's cognitive strengths and difficulties. Issues around the consent of the person to be assessed need to be carefully thought through and often people with learning disabilities are simply not referred for cognitive assessment.

For many years people with learning disabilities have struggled to access services in the same way as those without learning disabilities. There is evidence that people with learning disabilities can struggle to have their physical health needs assessed and treated (Mencap, 2007) and to gain access to services such as talking therapies (Bender, 1993). We believe that offering people with learning disabilities a cognitive assessment for the reasons Lezak *et al* (2004) outline is part of their right to receive the

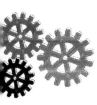

same services as people without learning disabilities. Outlined below are some of the potential barriers to offering people with learning disabilities a cognitive assessment, and ways to break these barriers down.

Potential barriers to cognitive assessment for people with learning disabilities

Limited literature

There is very limited literature on how to cognitively assess people with learning disabilities. A large number of studies do exist on specific aspects of cognitive functioning for people with learning disabilities, for example, verbal short-term memory in people with Down syndrome, (Vicari *et al*, 2004). These are often very interesting but are not especially clinically helpful as they do not immediately offer an insight about how to cognitively assess a person with a learning disability in a meaningful and helpful way. Finding research literature in this field that informs good clinical practice can be a difficult task.

However, the literature is expanding, especially around the assessment of dementia in people with learning disabilities and helpful, easily understandable guidelines have been produced. Papers have been written specifically focusing on which cognitive tests are useful to people with learning disabilities (eg. Martin *et al*, 2000; Rowe *et al*, 2006) and there are some thought-provoking papers about the use of the Wechsler Adult Intelligence Scale (WAIS-III and WAIS-IV) (Whitaker, 2005; Gordon *et al*, 2010). Lastly, people interested in this area can gain a great deal by reading a general text on neuropsychological models, such as Sohlberg and Mateer (2001), which considers models of different areas of cognitive functioning such as attention, memory and executive functioning. These models provide a basis for both test interpretation and for the observation of presenting behaviours.

Lack of referrals

One of the difficulties within learning disability services is that people are not always referred for cognitive assessment when this would be appropriate. This is for a number of reasons. The first is diagnostic overshadowing: a concept first described by Reiss *et al* (1982). They argue that the emotional problems of people with learning disabilities are often attributed to their cognitive difficulties rather than their psychosocial

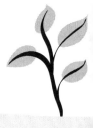

history, that is, to their brain differences rather than life experiences. The label of 'learning disability' is a very powerful one (Gillman *et al*, 2000) and research has shown that symptoms of schizophrenia in someone with a learning disability are much more likely to be underplayed than in an adult of average intelligence (Reiss & Szysko, 1983). Behaviours such as deterioration in memory or the appearance of challenging behaviour can be explained away as part of someone's overall disability.

Second, it can simply be harder for paid carers and family members to notice 'different' behaviour in a person that already behaves 'differently'. By definition people with learning disabilities need support in their day-to-day lives and this support may mask deterioration in skills (Oliver, 1999). For many people in the general population a change in cognitive abilities is noticed in subtle ways, such as them beginning to have mild word finding problems or getting slightly muddled making dinner. For many people with learning disabilities communication is difficult and extra word finding problems might be missed. Staff may not notice immediately that they are giving a person with learning disabilities extra prompts when they make a cup of tea.

Finally, many residential homes for people with learning disabilities have high staff turnover and, therefore, changes in someone's behaviour are simply missed.

Steps to overcome the above barriers need to focus on raising awareness in all those working with and caring for people with learning disabilities. Any change in behaviour should be taken seriously and it is important that those noticing this change do not dismiss it but ask themselves what the possible cause may be.

Case study 1

Henry was a 57-year-old man with Down syndrome living in supported living. A referral was made for a clinical psychology assessment after he had to be admitted to hospital because his legs were badly swollen. On discharge he did not appear to be 'his usual self' and an assessment with the help of care staff revealed a picture of memory problems and a decline in abilities over the previous two years. These included needing increasing help with self-care, for example, he suffered a deterioration in handwriting (evidenced by his weekly signing for his money) sleeping more; no longer coming down for breakfast; a loss of interest in his activities; becoming disorientated in the home he had lived in for four years. An assessment indicated that Henry was sadly in the late

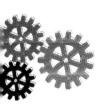

stages of a dementia of the Alzheimer's type. The supported living placement could no longer support him and he had to be moved as an emergency to a large residential placement with nursing care. It was here that he died six weeks later.

An earlier referral for Henry could not have stopped the dementia but it would have given more time for appropriate services to be put in place and to give him the best quality of life possible.

The main aim of this chapter is not to make the reader an expert on cognitively assessing people with learning disabilities, but instead to raise awareness that changes in the behaviour of people with learning disabilities should be taken seriously. Help from specialist services should be sought and cognitive assessments are one way of exploring observed changes in order to help the person being assessed to be supported appropriately.

Gaining informed consent for an assessment

Gaining consent for an assessment can sometimes be complicated as some people with learning disabilities may not have the capacity to make an informed decision. However, steps can be taken to ensure that the person with learning disabilities wishes to have a cognitive assessment or that such an assessment is in their best interest.

The first step is to ensure that the reason for referral is clear, along with what exactly the referrer is hoping to get out of any assessments or treatment. Any assessments or treatment should be to benefit the person with learning disabilities not to make things easier for those who support them (Emerson *et al*, 1999).

Referrals should always be discussed with the person with learning disabilities and, if this is not the case, the reasons for this should be clearly stated on the referral form, for example, limited communicative abilities.

The Mental Capacity Act (2005) is designed to protect people such as those with learning disabilities who may struggle to make their own decisions regarding issues such as consent. It is important that the guidance of the Mental Capacity Act (MCA) is followed whenever consent is being sought.

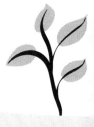

It is only if a person is judged as not having the capacity to make a decision that a decision can be made on their behalf, and the decision made should always be in the person's best interests.

If a person is found to have capacity to make a certain decision, then whatever they choose to do should be respected. A person with learning disabilities has just as much right as anyone else to make an unwise choice if they are capable of doing so, and they fully understand what this entails.

Implications of assessments should always be made clear, to both the referrer and the person being referred. Those carrying out such assessments should always be honest and very clear about why the test is being carried out, exactly what the test entails, and what the possible outcomes may be. All of this should be thoroughly explained to the person with learning disabilities in order for them to be able to give full and informed consent before completing the test. Before conducting cognitive assessments with people with learning disabilities, it should be made clear to them that they are entitled to stop doing the test whenever they wish. They should be reminded of this at regular intervals throughout the test.

Anxieties about cognitive assessments for people with learning disabilities

One of the barriers to offering cognitive assessments to people with learning disabilities is the anxiety held by paid carers, family members and even other professionals about the usefulness of such assessments. For the person with learning disability, a cognitive assessment can be incredibly anxiety provoking.

Lees-Haley and Fox (2001) have written a deliberately provocative paper about cognitive assessment for court work, arguing that some professionals – in the case of this book, two lawyers – often view such assessments with mistrust and suspicion. They write *expressions like "frontal lobe syndrome" and "executive functioning" are so diffusely and variably defined from one text to the next … that an expert could appear to explain anything with them'*.

The paper captures the negative feelings that can exist around cognitive assessment in general. For people with learning disabilities, it can be argued there has been a long history of misuse of such assessments.

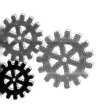

Noonan Walsh (2005) reflects on the history of trying to find meaningful activities for people with learning disabilities. She is critical of the high level of assessment that occurred 40 years ago for people with learning disabilities to establish what daytime 'work' activities they could engage in at day centres. She concludes: '*Many of the rigid boxes ferried through clinics, wards and dayrooms by psychologists in the 1960s, 1970s and 1980s helped seal the futures of unsuspecting men and women.*'

Noonan Walsh argues that in the recent past thousands of people with learning disabilities have been included or excluded from day services because of cognitive assessment results. She believes that such psychometrics have reinforced a medical model of care for people with learning disabilities so that the problem is seen to be within the person rather than in the way the environment supports or further disables them.

It can be argued that cognitive assessment within learning disability services has been tainted by the above history. This is particularly so in the still controversial area of IQ assessments.

Certainly it is all too easy to find examples of cognitive assessments acting as a 'gate-keeping' measure. The first criterion for accessing learning disability services is an IQ under 70. Noonan Walsh (REF) reports that since the mid-1990s, psychologists in Ireland have argued in court that children with severe learning disabilities cannot benefit from a school education. Lezak *et al* (2004) cite Folstein (1989) who describes how in the USA the Social Security Disability Insurance Agency set an IQ of 70 as the level above which someone could work. Folstein reports that many people with deteriorating conditions such as Huntington's disease would score above this threshold on IQ tests but functionally would no longer be able to hold down a job.

The authors' experience is that people with learning disabilities are often initially anxious about cognitive assessments as it can 'feel like school'. Most of our clients attended 'special school' and are often not confident about educational tasks.

It is important to recognise clients' anxieties and try and discuss these before and after the assessment, and to reflect in reports on how anxiety may have affected performance.

It is hoped that there is now the beginning of a culture change for cognitively assessing people with learning disabilities and that it will become something constructive, meaningful and person-centred.

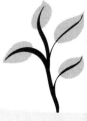

The difficulties with the concept of IQ

It is worth alerting the reader to the debates and difficulties around the concept of IQ, as an IQ below 70, as we have seen, is one of the criteria for accessing learning disability services.

The test most widely used to obtain an IQ score is the WAIS-III (the WAIS-IV is now published but is probably, at the time of writing, not as well used). Potentially the WAIS-III can be a useful tool in cognitive assessment within learning disability services. It is one of the few assessment instruments that has norms for people with learning disabilities and the profile of the scores from each of its 13 subtests can help to understand a person's strengths and difficulties. However, there are difficulties with the test itself and second, with the idea that intelligence, however defined, can be summed up in a composite score.

The test itself has been criticised for many reasons. Evans (1991) argues that like many cognitive tests it is culturally biased because it relies heavily on the skills and formal education knowledge taught in mainstream schools. For example, the WAIS-III has a section called 'Information' which has general knowledge questions of the type learned at school.

Whittaker (2005) criticises the WAIS-II for having instructions that are actually more complex than the item being tested and for its use of American English. The administration rules of WAIS-III state that some subtests are started on question 5, which is seen as being a 'comfortable' level of difficulty for the general population, allowing the lowering of anxiety. Only if a person fails an item in their first two attempts does the assessor then take that person back to earlier, easier questions. Leyin (2006) argues that this is not fair for people as they are less likely to succeed on these 'start' questions and therefore are less likely to benefit from early success and the confidence this brings. Compared to the general population, they are more likely to detail the 'start' questions and experience increased anxiety, which can affect performance.

Whittaker (2005) also argues that the WAIS-III had low numbers of people with learning disabilities included in the norm group. Whittaker argues that the lowest scores have been extrapolated and, therefore, the meaning of failing the easiest items is in doubt. Lastly, he points out that the WAIS-III assumes that low IQ scores follow a normal distribution, and this may not be the case.

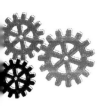

IQ is frequently misunderstood. The authors are often referred people with learning disabilities for IQ assessments on their 'ability to parent' and so the myth that IQ can tell you anything more about a person except for their likely performance in education still persists.

An IQ score alone is not helpful: it tells you nothing about a person's abilities, skills or strengths. It does not tell you if they will be a good parent or whether they will be able to hold down a particular job. IQ is a composite score that is several scores added together and the average taken and this average reveals nothing of use in a cognitive assessment. Lezak *et al* (2004) concluded that IQ as a score is inherently meaningless and not infrequently misleading as well. '*IQ, whether concept, score or catchword, has outlived whatever usefulness it may once have had and should be discarded.*'

It is important to remember that people with learning disabilities are a heterogeneous group who are diverse in their abilities, upbringings and personalities. Two people with an IQ of 100 (the average score) would not be expected to have the same strengths and needs in learning a new skill or in being a parent, but often two people with the IQ of 65 are treated as if they are the same.

Useful cognitive assessment allows us to see the person behind the IQ score. So, for example, a cognitive assessment for two people with learning disabilities who both want to be 'a good enough parent' might reveal that person A learns best through being shown what to do; relies on visual memory over verbal and has an organised, logical approach to new tasks. While on the other hand, person B may learn better when a task is broken down into steps and written down so they can read it several times to themselves; they may be good at staying on task but need prompting to move between tasks.

For all its potential problems, the WAIS-III can be a useful part of a cognitive assessment and contribute towards better understanding someone with a learning disability, and helping them toward a personally important goal.

In order to make a cognitive assessment useful and meaningful, it is important to remember to:

▶ always have a clear question in mind

▶ work in partnership with the person with learning disabilities, their family and/or support staff (Davis *et al*, 2002)

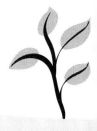

▶ be clear who will use the information from the assessment, and that it will be of benefit to the client (Emerson, 1999)

▶ guard against overanalysing psychometric test results; the results of psychometric assessments are helpful but they are a way to observe behaviour – they do not contain more truth than other observations

▶ challenge the myth that an IQ score tells you anything meaningful about a person.

Lack of suitable tests and normative data

There are very few tests that are based on norms of people who have learning disabilities. For example, Martin *et al* (2000) point out that no such memory tests exist. Therefore, for most people with learning disabilities the majority of tests are simply so difficult that they get a very low score. This is known as a 'floor effect'. This is not helpful for the assessor as it does not show the person's relative strengths and difficulties, instead the assessment just shows lots of very low scores. Also, it is extremely difficult to see changes over time, such as those associated with dementia, and so diagnosis in this area is very difficult. Ethically, it is clearly not useful to subject people with learning disabilities to cognitive assessment if only a minimum amount of information can be yielded from it.

There are three possible solutions to the above problem and these are considered briefly below.

1. Use tests that have included people with learning disabilities in their norm group (eg. WAIS-III) alongside tests that have been researched as being less likely to show floor effects for people with learning disabilities. For example, the Rivermead Behavioural Memory Test (RBMT) (Wilson *et al*, 1985) is a test which aims to assess day-to-day memory and to be ecologically valid, that is, reflecting everyday memory problems (eg. recognising faces). A paper by Martin *et al* (2000) explored how people with mild learning disabilities performed on this test. They concluded that the RMBT can be used to detect a change in memory functioning over time. Likewise, Rowe *et al* (2006) recommend that tests such as the Tower of London test (Shallice, 1982) may be useful in assessing executive functioning in people with Down syndrome. Such assessments used sensitively and qualitatively as well as for comparing scores can form the basis of a meaningful cognitive assessment for someone with a learning disability.

2. Lezak *et al* (2004) put forward what could be a controversial solution to the lack of normed tests for those people with 'severe cognitive impairment'. Lezak suggests that children's tests could be used and reported in terms of 'mental age'. Comparison between different tests would show where the person had particular cognitive strengths or difficulties, and comparison between tests over time could show evidence of any change in cognitive functioning.

   Theoretically this is a rather elegant solution to a real, clinical problem, however, learning disability services are dominated by the theory of Social Role Valorisation (SRV). SRV is the theory of Wolfensberger (1972) and is based on his own philosophy of 'normalisation'. Wolfensberger argues that people with learning disabilities are devalued in society and will only gain socially valued identities by adopting and being associated with the roles and behaviours of the dominant group in society. Here is not the place to engage in a critique of SRV, but it does mean that the use of children's tests would for many people with learning disabilities, their carers and many professionals be seen as at best unhelpful and at worst demeaning.

3. The third solution is for the assessor to use observation – their own and others' – within a clear neuropsychological framework (as set out in the other chapters). Even when carrying out cognitive assessments for people without learning disabilities, there are times when the use of psychometrics is inappropriate and often will not give the whole picture. In these cases the use of neuropsychological models may be a way forward in understanding a client's strengths and needs.

   Psychometric tests of executive functioning are a prime example of the point made above. Broadly speaking, such tests tap into the ability to keep information 'on line' and manipulate it (Manchester *et al*, 2004). However, executive problems also include personality changes and day-to-day problem-solving. For this reason Manchester *et al* caution against only using psychometric tests to detect the presence of executive changes.

As an example, Sohlberg and Mateer's (2001) model of executive functioning can be very helpful. Executive functioning has been described as: *'Those capabilities that enable a person to engage successfully in independent, purposive, self-serving behaviour'* (Lezak *et al*, 2004).

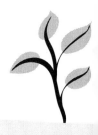

Sohlberg and Mateer break the concept into six areas. These are:

▶ initiating (starting behaviour)

▶ response inhibition (stopping behaviour)

▶ task persistence (maintaining behaviour)

▶ organisation of thoughts and behaviour

▶ generative thinking (being creative and flexible)

▶ awareness (monitoring and modifying one's own behaviour).

Sohlberg and Mateer (2001) argue that much can be learnt about executive functioning by observing the way a person carries out a multistep task such as cooking and, therefore, they advocate the importance of observation in assessment. There is no reason that this is less applicable to people with learning disabilities. The task should be chosen as not to demotivate or overly frustrate the person, but watching someone make toast or a cup of tea gives ample opportunity to assess planning, inhibition, initiation and self-monitoring abilities. Interviews with the client and those who know them well can also reveal the presence or absence of executive difficulties.

Therefore, having a clear model, in this case of executive functioning, is very useful when observing people with (or indeed without) learning disabilities do psychometric tests, everyday tasks, or when talking to care staff or family about the changes they have noticed in a person.

Case study 2

Eric was a 57-year-old man who had been to special school and had trouble with reading and writing all his life. He had done voluntary work in a charity organisation, for 20 years. He had always needed help with reading his letters and sometimes didn't seem to dress appropriately for the weather, but was a likable, hardworking man who did his work conscientiously. However, over the period of a year Eric became increasingly anxious about his letters and seemed to be forgetting how to do some of his tasks. A cognitive assessment and follow-up noted a decline in his memory, particularly his memory for what he had been told (verbal memory). However, through talking to those who worked with him, and through observing Eric in conversation, it also became apparent that he had very little self-awareness about the changes happening to him. Of course he may have always have been like this, but bearing the

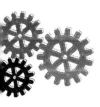

model of executive functioning in mind (particularly point six), the assessor asked more questions. It appeared that Eric's personality had changed: he seemed less inhibited and on a few occasions had said inappropriate things to charity shop customers, which was very unusual for this quiet, polite man. He also appeared to be less worried than a year ago by his memory problems, despite the fact they were becoming more noticeable. The information indicated a decline in his executive functioning as well as his memory.

The next section of the chapter looks at some examples of cognitive assessments for people with learning disabilities. Particular attention is paid to the process of assessing for dementia in people with learning disabilities as this is a particular issue for people with Down syndrome. Finally, there are two case studies of cognitive assessment; the first is for a young woman who wanted support to be a 'good enough parent' and the second, a woman who wanted to have the right support in her life.

Dementia assessment for people with learning disabilities

Dementia is an illness that affects the brain and is characterised by deterioration in a person's memory and daily living skills. It impairs a person's ability to function as they previously would; a decline which worsens over a period of months or years. For people with learning disabilities, the prevalence rate is higher than that of the general population. For people with Down syndrome, the figure doubles (Prasher, 2005).

Despite such high rates for people with a learning disability, there are a range of difficulties when it comes to assessment, especially for people with Down syndrome. Brain scans can prove difficult, especially as they can cause a great deal of stress and anxiety, and sedation would often be required. In addition, for people with Down syndrome, these scans do not reveal a great deal. This is because the plaques and tangles that form in the brain as a result of dementia may have already been present in a patient with Down syndrome. Therefore, they do not necessarily indicate the presence of dementia.

Tests that would be used to provide a baseline of cognitive function for someone without a learning disability are often unsuitable for use with a learning disability. The Mini Mental State Examination (MMSE) is often

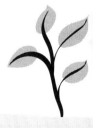

used to gain a baseline of skills and ability. However, for a person with a learning disability, this test shows very little as it assumes a certain level of ability, which someone with a learning disability may never have had. Their score without dementia may have been at the bottom of the scale, and thus using this exam to diagnose dementia in a person with learning disabilities is not helpful.

As we have already discussed, recognising the initial signs of dementia can also be a difficulty in people with learning disabilities. This is because changes in behaviour, or decline of skills and memory, may often be considered as being part of their learning disability. Symptoms of dementia can also be difficult to recognise in people with learning disabilities, whose behaviour may already be classed by those around them as being 'unusual' or against the norm.

Detection of the signs of dementia in people with learning disabilities requires those supporting or caring for them to know the person well and to be able to recognise changes in behaviour that may already be unpredictable.

Diagnosis of dementia in people with learning disabilities relies heavily on the information that can be provided by family members, carers and support staff.

It is important with dementia to recognise the early signs as soon as possible, and this is especially true of people with learning disabilities, as diagnosis can be that much more difficult and lengthy than with the general population.

Signs to look out for include:

▶ a decline in daily living skills (ie. personal care, dressing, eating)

▶ a decline in short-term memory

▶ becoming less sociable and interested in activities and hobbies previously enjoyed

▶ changes in sleeping patterns

▶ changes in mood

▶ a decline in communication skills (relative to previous communication abilities)

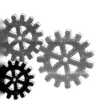

- ▶ restlessness and increased wandering

- ▶ increased confusion

- ▶ becoming less alert and aware of those around them.

Before undertaking an assessment of skills and abilities for a person with learning disabilities, it is important to consider other factors that might account for changes in a person's behaviour. There are a variety of health issues that can affect behaviour and need to be checked out. These include poor sight, reduced hearing capability, thyroid problems, heart defects, and seizures; all of which can have symptoms similar to that of early onset dementia, but are treatable.

In addition to such health issues, factors such as changes in environment, traumatic life events and changes in medication can also contribute to changes in behaviour that may look similar to the early signs of dementia, and so these also need to be considered. Any possible mental health difficulties also need to be investigated, as the presence of depression or anxiety may make the presentation of dementia-type symptoms even worse. All of the above need to be ruled out in order to aid a more accurate diagnosis.

Dementia and People with Learning Disabilities (British Psychological Society, 2009) recommends that clear pathways are drawn up to assist with investigations of dementia in people with learning disabilities. These focus on the most suitable and accurate assessments that can be used when investigating possible dementia in people with learning disabilities, and the timescales in which they should be completed. The following assessments are recommended.

Dementia Scale for Down Syndrome

The Dementia Scale for Down Syndrome (DSDS) is used to establish a baseline of skills and abilities, and explores the difficulties and changes that have been observed. It also explores other possible explanations for such changes as detailed above. The DSDS is usually carried out by at least two different people who know the person well. The pattern of change over time that may be highlighted by the DSDS can indicate whether dementia is present or not.

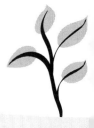

Severe Impairment Battery

The Severe Impairment Battery (SIB) examines performance by the client themselves on a number of low level tasks. It examines cognitive function in areas such as attention, language, and short-term memory. This test can establish a baseline of the person's skills, which can be repeated over time to assess decline in such skills.

Rivermead Behavioural Memory Test

The Rivermead Behavioural Memory Test (RBMT-II) focuses on common everyday memory difficulties that are associated with clients referred with a query of dementia. This test is also completed by the client and can be used to establish a baseline of the client's short-term memory, and can be repeated over time to measure any deterioration in this area.

(It is important to note that the SIB and the RBMT-II both rely on the client having a certain level of ability. For some clients, these tests may not always be suitable, and thus may not be completed. The reasons for this should be recorded).

Psychiatric Assessment Schedules for Adults with Developmental Disabilities

If there are indications of any underlying mental health problems, then the Psychiatric Assessment Schedules for Adults with Developmental Disabilities (PAS-ADD) can be used to assess this.

Results of the assessments should be fully discussed with the referrer and those who are involved in the client's life, and an action plan drawn up if appropriate. Any baseline assessments should be repeated after six months to establish if there is a dementia-type pattern.

It is important to try and recognise the early signs of dementia as quickly as possible in order to put in place a plan of action, which will help carers to support the person as best they can. Establishing structure and routine to a person's day can offer reassurance and comfort; a consistent approach to care will have a similar effect. The environment for a person with learning disabilities and dementia needs to be a calming familiar one and most of

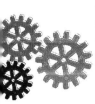

all, needs to feel safe for them. Establishing these things as soon as possible will help the person feel more comfortable and will hopefully give them a better quality of life.

A different way of thinking

Allowing for the difficulties and cautions mentioned previously about cognitive assessment with people who have learning disabilities, the neuropsychological and cognitive models set out in the previous chapters give us a different way of approaching, thinking about and understanding people with learning disabilities. Understanding a person from a point of view of the biopsychosocial model and neuropsychological domains, for example, attention, speed of processing, memory, language and executive functions, gives us an alternative way of highlighting a person's strengths and limitations, and in identifying ways in which they can be helped, supported and challenged.

The following two case studies are examples of cognitive assessment for people with learning disabilities.

Case study 3

Linda was a 25-year-old mother with two young children (aged two and four). She was in a long-term stable relationship with a supportive partner but she was having difficulty parenting and concerns had been raised to social services around whether, at times, Linda was neglecting her children. She clearly loved them but seemed to struggle to take on the health visitor's advice. Linda was given support but the support workers wished for guidance as how best to help her as she did not always seem to follow their advice.

Linda was initially very anxious about seeing a psychologist. As she became more comfortable with the situation, she became more talkative and relaxed. She explained that she had hated school where she was bullied; she had struggled to hear what the teacher was saying and even now found it hard to hear everything when there was background noise. Linda was still grieving after the loss of her grandmother who she had been very close to, and was beginning to have counselling for this. Linda agreed to a cognitive assessment but felt she would be nervous. This was discussed and breaks were built in between tests when Linda could have a cup of coffee and reflect on how she felt.

Linda's self-esteem was clearly very low. When she felt she was doing well on tests she looked very happy, even surprised and was chatty. When she began to struggle she would

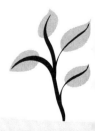

often begin talking to herself in a negative way, saying 'I'm stupid' and 'I bet other people can do this'.

Linda showed a huge discrepancy between her verbal memory and her visual memory. She was very good at recalling what she was shown, but could barely recall any of a short story from the Rivermead Behavioural Memory Test. Linda was very good at tests of non-verbal reasoning on the WAIS-III and carried these out in a focused, logical way. However, verbal reasoning tests were extremely difficult for her and made her anxious.

Initial language assessments showed that Linda did not understand negatives or words such as 'before' or 'after'. She understood two key words in a sentence but could not follow instructions with more than two steps at a time.

It was clear that Linda had a specific language difficulty and she was referred onto specialist colleagues in speech and language therapy, however a list of recommendations were given to those supporting Linda. For example, to allow her to learn by showing Linda how to do something and not just by telling her; to support Linda to have her hearing checked (it turned out that she did have reduced hearing in her left ear); to change sentence structure so to say: 'first give Ted (her son) his bath, then give him some milk' and not to say: 'after his bath, give Ted some milk', as this genuinely confused Linda; and to give one or two step instructions only.

With additional speech and language advice and an understanding support worker, Linda made good progress and her children's names were removed from the child protection register.

Case study 4

Denise was a 40-year-old woman with Down syndrome living with her very supportive sister. Denise had a range of interests and skills; she was very creative and enjoyed painting and singing. She worked in an organic garden and in a voluntary position in a café. Denise wanted to move out from living with her sister to living with housemates in supported living and her sister agreed with this but was naturally concerned that Denise's support needs were fully understood. We agreed with Denise and her sister that a cognitive assessment might help to understand what support Denise needed when she moved.

Denise liked the cognitive assessment. She concentrated hard but was exhausted after an hour and so the assessment was broken into shorter sections. She did extremely well on factual knowledge but had problems with social reasoning tasks. Her attention for staying on task was very good but she had problems in switching her

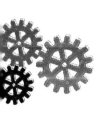

attention between tasks. Her memory was very good, especially her visual memory but she needed more time than most people to process verbal information. It was apparent that she had very real difficulties with day-to-day problem-solving and had problems monitoring her own feelings and her impact on others.

In conclusion, Denise had many strengths and was clearly a talented and skilful woman but she needed a great deal more support than was initially apparent.

Denise could not cope with day-to-day things like organising herself to go out, and her skills tended to exist in 'boxes' so, for example, without a great deal of prompting she could not transfer her gardening skills to her own garden at home. Denise also could not problem solve unplanned events such as a smoke alarm going off; and was frequently upset by people breaking social rules (eg. shouting on the bus). When her anxiety rose she withdrew and became more 'rigid' in her behaviour, and could appear as if she had autistic features although she did not meet the criteria for this diagnosis.

The assessment was able to recommend strategies that might help Denise such as establishing routines and 'down time' after busy or new activities. This was designed to stop her feeling overwhelmed by tasks that required a lot of executive involvement. Other recommendations included giving Denise time to process verbal information and backing this up with pictures or photographs (eg. a visual timetable of her day). Her new support staff were offered a workshop around Denise's strength with particular focus on understanding executive functioning difficulties. This allowed a person-centred support plan to be drawn up for Denise.

Take away message

There are often good reasons to assess cognitive abilities in people with learning disabilities and, if appropriate, they have the same rights to such assessments as anyone else in the general population. They can also provide a fresh perspective on a person's abilities and limitations. There are a number of potential barriers that may make having a meaningful and helpful cognitive assessment difficult, however, we believe that these barriers can be overcome. One of the key themes of this chapter is to be alert for cognitive changes in people with learning disabilities, and take these seriously. People with learning disabilities are often reliant on others to help them access the services, in this case cognitive assessment, that they need.

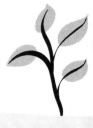

We would like to thank Ray St Ledger who has helped shape the ideas that this chapter is based on, and shared them in his usual generous way. Also, Jonny Powls for helping to make the link between people with learning disabilities and brain injury services.

Quiz

1. What are the three criteria for being diagnosed with a learning disability?

2. Name two possible causes of learning disability.

3. State two reasons for carrying out a cognitive assessment.

4. What is diagnostic overshadowing?

5. Name two reasons why people with learning disabilities may not be referred for a cognitive assessment.

6. What should you consider when accessing whether someone with learning disabilities has the capacity to consent to a cognitive assessment?

7. Name two criticisms of using the WAIS-III with people with learning disabilities.

8. How might you observe someone's level of executive functioning?

9. Name three possible signs of dementia in people with learning disabilities.

10. What other factors, excluding dementia, may be accountable for changes in a person's behaviour?

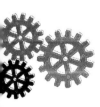

References

Ball T, Bush A & Emerson E (2004) *Psychological Interventions for Severely Challenging Behaviours Shown by People with Learning Disabilities:* Clinical practice guidelines. Leicester: The British Psychological Society.

Bender M (1993) The unoffered chair: the history of therapeutic disdain towards people with a learning difficulty. *Clinical Psychology Forum* **54** 7–12.

Berg JM (1985) Physical determinants of environmental origin. In: AM Clarke (1985) *Mental Deficiency: The changing outlook* (4th edition). Methuen: London.

British Psychological Society (2001) *Learning Disability: Definitions and contexts. Revised.* Leicester: BPS.

British Psychological Society and Royal Society of Psychiatrists (2009) *Dementia and People with Learning Disabilities. Guidance on the assessment, diagnosis, treatment and support of people with learning disabilities who develop dementia.* Leicester: British Psychological Society.

Davis H, Day C & Bidmead C (2002) *Working in Partnership with Parents: The parent adviser model.* London: Harcourt Assessment.

Department of Health (1998) *Signposts for Success in Commissioning and Providing Health Services for People with Learning Disabilities.* London: NHS Executive.

Emerson E, Hatton C, Bromley J & Caine A (1999) *Clinical Psychology and People with Learning Disabilities.* Chichester: John Wiley & Sons Ltd.

Evans IM (1991) Testing and diagnosis: a review and evaluation. In: LH Meyer, CA Peck & L Brown (2004) *Critical Issues in the Lives of People with Severe Disabilities.* Baltimore: Brooks Baltimore MD.

Folstein SE (1989) In: MD Lezak, DB Howieson & DW Loring (2004) Neuropsychological Assessment (4th edition). New York: Oxford University Press.

Gillman M, Heyman B & Swain J (2000) What's in a name? The implications of diagnosis for people with learning difficulties and their family carers. *Disability and Society* **15** (3) 389–409.

Gordon S, Duff S, Davidson T & Whitaker S (2010) Comparison of the WAIS-III and the WISC-IV in 16-year-old special education students. Accepted draft. *Journal of Applied Research in Intellectual Disability* **23** 197–200.

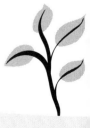

Lees-Hayley PR & Fox DD (2001) Isn't everything in forensic neuropsychology controversial? *Neurorehabilitation* **16** 267–273.

Leyin A (2006) Don't know if I'm going up or down… The WAIS-III and people with learning disabilities. *Clinical Psychology Forum* **163** 26–29.

Lezak MD, Howieson DB & Loring DW (2004) *Neuropsychological Assessment* (4th edition). New York: Oxford University Press.

Luckasson R, Coulter DL, Polloway EL, Reiss S, Schalock RL & Snell ME (1992) *Mental Retardation: Definition, classification, and systems of supports* (9th edition). Washington DC: American Association on Mental Retardation.

Manchester D, Priestley N & Jackson H (2004) The assessment of executive functions: coming out of the office. *Brain Injury* **18** 1067–81.

Martin C, West J, Cull C & Adams M (2000) A preliminary study investigating how people with mild intellectual disabilities perform on the Rivermead Behavioural Memory Test. *Journal of Applied Research in Intellectual Disabilities* **13** 186–193.

Mencap (2007) *Death by Indifference* [online]. Available at: www.mencap.org.uk/document.asp?id=284 (accessed December 2010).

Noonan Walsh P (2005) *Outside the Box: Assessments for life and work in the community Part One: Conceptual and textual issues. Assessing adults with intellectual disability. A service user's guide*. Oxford: Blackwell.

Oliver C (1999) Perspectives on assessment and evaluation. In: M Janicki & A Dalton (Eds) (1999) *Dementia, Aging and Intellectual Disabilities*. New York: Brunner/Mazel.

Prasher VP (2005) *Alzheimer's Disease and Dementia in Down's Syndrome and Intellectual Disability*. Oxford: Radcliffe.

Reiss S, Leviten GW & McNally RJ (1982) Emotionally disturbed, mentally retarded people: an under served population. *American Psychologist* **37** (4) 361–67.

Reiss S & Szysko J (1983) Diagnostic overshadowing and professional experience with mentally retarded people. *American Journal of Mental Deficiency* **87** 396–402.

Rowe J, Lavender A & Turk V (2006) Cognitive executive function in Down's syndrome. *British Journal of Clinical Psychology* **45** 5–17.

Shallice T (1982) Specific impairment of planning. *Philosophical Transactions of the Royal Society of London* **298** 199–209.

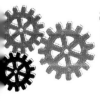

Sohlberg MM & Mateer CA (2001) *Cognitive Rehabilitation: An integrative neuropsychological approach*. New York: The Guilford Press.

Stern J (1985) Biochemical aspects. In: AM Clarke, ADB Clarke & JM Berg (Eds) (1985) *Mental Deficiency: The changing outlook* (4th edition). London: Methuen.

Vicari S, Marotta L & Carlesimo GA (2004) Verbal short-term memory in Down's syndrome: an articulatory loop deficit? *Journal of Intellectual Disability Research* **48** (2) 80–92.

Whitaker S (2005) The Uses of the WISC-III and the WAIS-III with people with learning disabilities: three concerns. *Clinical Psychology* **50** 37–40.

Valuing People (2001) *A New Strategy for Learning Disability for the 21st Century*. London: Department of Health.

Wilson BA, Cockburn J & Baddeley A (1985) *Rivermead Behavioural Memory Test*. Suffolk: Thames Valley Test Company.

Wolfensberger W (1972) *The Principles of Normalisation in Human Services*. Toronto: National Institute on Mental Retardation.

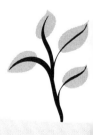

Glossary

Activities of daily living (ADL)
The day-to-day things people do to survive and to take care of themselves, such as dressing, personal hygiene, cooking and cleaning.

Amygdala
An almond-shaped body or a nucleus associated with aspects of memory and emotions especially fear.

Analgesics
Painkilling medications.

Anoxic/hypoxic
Describes a type of acquired brain injury that occurs when the blood pumped to the brain is either blocked or obstructed, or is otherwise insufficiently oxygenated (such as due to respiratory failure).

Anterior
Meaning towards the front.

Anticonvulsants
Anti-epileptic drugs, also sometimes prescribed for pain of neurological origin.

Antihistamines
Anti-allergy drugs, most commonly prescribed for hay fever.

Antihypertensives
Drugs prescribed to reduce high blood pressure.

Antispasticity drugs
Drugs prescribed to combat abnormalities of muscle tone commonly found in neurological conditions.

Aphasia
An acquired language disorder affecting one or more modes of language and this may include difficulties in speaking, understanding what is said, reading and writing.

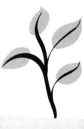

Asymmetries
A lack or absence of symmetry; a disproportion or dissimilarity in corresponding parts or organs on opposite sides of the body which are normally alike. For example, having one eye higher than the other, or having a mouth which droops at one side.

Axon
A part of a nerve cell or neuron that takes information from the cell body towards the next cell along. It is relatively quite long and covered in a white fatty substance known as myelin.

Basal ganglia
A collection of grey matter bodies or nuclei found in the white matter of the brain. It includes the caudate nucleus and putamen. The basal ganglia is closely associated with controlling motor tone and involuntary movements. Parkinson's disease is associated with changes in the basal ganglia as is Huntington's disease. The basal ganglia are also associated with learning skills and habits, for example, riding a bike or a handcraft.

Behavioural approaches
This aims to increase 'pleasant events' such as the amount of time people spend doing things they enjoy. The rationale is that if people are more often doing enjoyable activities then this will be rewarding and improve their mood. It is also called behaviour therapy.

Beta blockers
Drugs which have various effects and are used to treat a wide variety of conditions including angina, high blood pressure, some types of abnormal heart rhythm, heart failure, heart attack, anxiety, thyroid problems, glaucoma and migraine.

Biopsychosocial
A model or approach that encompasses the biological, psychological and social factors that influence the onset, course and outcome of an illness, disease or condition.

Brain stem
An important part of the brain through which the nerve connections of the motor and sensory systems from the cortex and limbic system pass to connect with the rest of the body. It includes nerve pathways, allowing the cortical areas to regulate body movement, and to receive information from the body

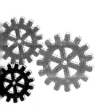

through touch and other bodily sensation (including pain and temperature). The brain stem also plays an important role in the regulation of heart and lung function. It also regulates the central nervous system, and is important in maintaining consciousness and regulating the sleep cycle.

Bronchodilators
Anti-asthma drugs.

Cerebral axonal dysfunction
Failure of axons in nerve cells in the brain to perform their normal function of passing information from one nerve cell to another.

Cerebellum
A part of the brain that lies below the main cerebral hemispheres and behind the brain stem. It is important for co-ordination of movements and also has been associated with some aspects of the new learning.

Chronic obstructive pulmonary disease
Breathing disorder most often due to chronic bronchitis or emphysema.

Circadian rhythms
The approximately 24-hour cycles in the biochemical, physiological and behavioural processes of all living things, including sleep–wake cycles.

Cognitive
Thought processes such as concentration, memory, information processing and problem-solving.

Cognitive rehabilitation
A therapeutic approach which is functionally oriented towards remediating or compensating for acquired cognitive deficits based on brain behaviour theories.

Compensation
A type of rehabilitation strategy that helps individuals to minimise their cognitive deficit by engaging in other learned behaviours.

Confabulation
A verbalisation or a story that is not based on external reality. This can often be seen in memory disorders where the person tries to 'fill in the gaps' to compensate for memory loss, for example, Korsakoff's disease.

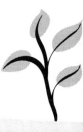

Corpus Callosum
A bundle of nerves that connects the two halves of the cerebral hemispheres.

Cortical
The outer layer of the brain primarily made up of grey matter forming the frontal, parietal, temporal and occipital lobes of the brain.

Corticosteroids
A type of drug most commonly used to reduce inflammation, suppress the immune system, or replace hormones in the body.

Cytokine
A number of different proteins, each of which are secreted by a specific type of cell (mostly in the immune system) that carry signals locally between cells, thereby having an effect on other cells.

Demographics
This term refers to the characteristics of a patient such as age, language spoken, cultural background, gender and handedness.

Dendrites
A part of a neuron that takes information from neighbouring cells.

Dorso-lateral frontal lobes
Dorso-lateral is a term meaning 'to the sides of' or 'the side of'. The dorso-lateral frontal lobes refer to the front and sides of the outer surface of the frontal cortex, which play a specific role in behaviour and motivation, such as planning and carrying out tasks, and flexibility in thinking.

Dysmorphic
A term used to describe a body characteristic that is abnormally formed.

Dyspraxia
The inability to carry out learned and purposeful movements for reasons other than to do with comprehension, sensation and muscle function. Almost any movement can be subject to a dyspraxia.

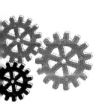

Ecologically valid
This term refers to how well a test can be reflected or related to everyday real life. Measures which are ecologically valid can be generalised beyond the setting they were carried out in and reflect the individual's behaviour, performance and abilities in real life.

Effort
This is the extent to which an individual exerts their full mental or physical energy in order to achieve a purpose or complete an activity.

Emotional lability
A term used to describe the often rapid and intense mood/emotional swings that may be associated with damage to the orbito-frontal lobes of the brain or psychiatric conditions.

Enablement
A process of helping someone achieve a previous or new goal.

Encephalitis
Inflammation of the brain due to infection, usually connected with a virus such as the herpes simplex virus.

Epidemiological
Studies into how often diseases or medical conditions occur in different groups of people, and why.

Epilepsy
Recurrent, unprovoked epileptic seizures.

Erythrocyte sedimentation rate (ESR)
A blood test used to help diagnose conditions associated with acute and chronic (that is, short or long duration) inflammation, including infections, cancers and autoimmune diseases.

Flynn effect
The Flynn effect describes an increase in the average IQ test scores over generations – an effect seen in most parts of the world. Attempted explanations have included better nutrition, a trend towards smaller families, better education and greater environmental complexity.

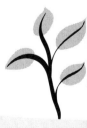

Full blood count (FBC)
A broad screening blood test used to check for such disorders as anaemia, infection, and many other diseases. It is actually a panel of 10 tests that examine different parts of the blood.

Gastro-oesophageal reflux
Leakage of acid from the stomach up into the gullet (oesophagus) causing heartburn and other symptoms.

Glasgow Coma Scale (GCS)
A way of measuring the extent to which someone is conscious, for example, after a significant brain injury. It is a 15-point scale, which assesses the response of someone's eye, what they are able to say and what they are able to do. The lowest possible Glasgow Coma Scale score is three, which indicates a deep coma and the highest 15, which indicates that the person is conscious.

Glial cells
These are cells that surround and support nerve cells or neurons.

Goal planning
The planning required to work towards achieving an agreed end point or outcome of the rehabilitation process.

Group rehabilitation
Rehabilitation that is delivered in a group format which may include one or more facilitators to address a common cognitive deficit.

Haemorrhage
The term that describes a burst blood vessel and resulting bleed, which is a common cause of acquired brain injury, and can occur spontaneously (such as from a weak or malformed blood vessel, or extremely high blood pressure), or traumatically (such as from a high speed accident). A haemorrhage can cause additional trouble if a haematoma forms, which is a formed blood clot that occupies additional space inside the enclosed skull cavity, sometimes crushing other brain structures.

Half-life
A measure of the duration of action of a drug, and the period of time required for the concentration or amount of drug in the body to be reduced by one half after a single dose has reached its highest level in the bloodstream.

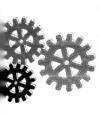

Hindbrain
This is the description used for the pons, cerebellum and medulla collectively.

Hypnagogic
The transition between sleep and wakefulness.

Hippocampus
This is part of the limbic system and is found on the inside of the temporal lobes. It is very important in memory function and is vulnerable to a number of brain disorders including Encephalitis and Alzheimer's disease.

Hypnotic medications
Drugs prescribed typically to treat insomnia.

Hypothalamus
Is involved in the regulation of body functions such as temperature, sleep, appetite and exerts a lot of control over the pituitary gland.

Infarct
Is an area of the brain that has died because the supply of blood has not been sufficient. This can happen due to a lack of nutrients or a build of waste products that are not carried away properly.

Immune modulators
Drugs influencing the immune system.

Interleukins
A group of cytokines particularly involved in the activity of white blood cells.

International Classification of Functioning, Disability and Health (ICF)
A model proposed by the World Health Organization that classifies health in relation to functioning and disability. Components include bodily functions and structures, activities, limitations and participation restrictions, and environmental factors in relation to health.

Intervention
A set of actions or processes aimed at improving a person's difficulties or circumstances.

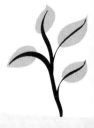

In utero development
An individual's pre-birth medical history and development.

Korsakoff's disease
A disease that arises from vitamin B1 (Thiamine) deficiency and is often associated with chronic abuse of alcohol because of the lack of proper diet in people who are addicted to alcohol. It is associated with a number of difficulties in cognition especially disruption of recent memory but also can involve difficulties with orientation, hallucinations and confabulation.

Limbic system
Refers to parts of the brain lying between the cortex (the outer layer of the brain primarily made up of grey matter) and sub-cortical areas (primarily made up of white matter), which contains both cortical and sub-cortical areas. As well as being a part of the brain through which information passes between cortical areas, and between the cortex and sub-cortical parts of the brain, rather like a telephone switchboard. It also contains a number of important structures directly and indirectly involved in various aspects of cognition, perception, memory, mood and behavioural regulation, hormone release and regulation of bodily functions such as blood pressure, heart rate, hunger, thirst, sexual arousal and the sleep–wake cycle.

Medico-legal
Relating to or concerned with both medicine and law, frequently related to people seeking compensation following a road traffic accident, or an accident at work.

Medial/mesial
Both terms mean 'middle' and are often used to describe locations in the brain such as the medial frontal lobes or the medial temporal lobes.

Medial frontal lobes
When the medial frontal lobes are damaged bilaterally (ie. on both sides) the person can have difficulty generating spontaneous activity and quite often be placid and immobile. They may become apathetic and seem disinterested in life. Sometimes this is mistaken for either depression or someone being 'lazy'.

Medial temporal lobes
The bilateral inner middle areas of the temporal lobes that mainly house the amygdala and the hippocampus.

Medulla
Part of the brain stem lying between the spinal cord and the pons.

Meningitis
An infection of one of the layers of tissue surrounding the brain (the meninges).

Midbrain
A sub-cortical part of the brain stem below the limbic system that provides important connections between the cerebral cortex and the rest of the brain stem. It passes messages into the spinal cord to control sensory processes such as vision and movement.

Milieu therapy
A holistic neuropsychological rehabilitation programme that examines the individual in their environment and involves intensive participation from the therapist and patient. It involves the prescription of specified activities and social interactions for patients.

Mood
A pervading state of mind or feeling.

Myelin
A fatty substance surrounding most axons that allows for the faster conduction of electrical charge through the axon. It is the myelin covering or sheath that is damaged in multiple sclerosis.

Neuro-behavioural
An aspect of problematic behaviour or activity caused solely or substantially by injury to the brain.

Neuro-behavioural disability
Disability caused by problematic behaviour or activity caused solely or substantially by injury to the brain.

Neuroimaging
These are sophisticated x-rays of the brain, which include techniques such as angiograms and computerised tomography (CT), magnetic resonance imaging (MRI) and positron emission tomography (PET) scanning that are done in a radiology department.

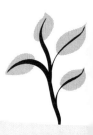

Neurological conditions
Conditions affecting the neurological system including the brain.

Neurological system
The body's electrical system, which includes the central nervous system (the brain and spinal cord).

Neuron
Another name for a nerve cell.

Neuropsychological
Psychological functions (emotions, cognition, or behaviour) directly associated with the brain.

Nocturia
The need to get up in the night to urinate.

Norm
Norm-referenced tests compare an individual's performance on a test to their peers (people of the same age, ethnicity, background etc.). Such a test will tell you how your performance compares to similar people on a given set of skills and knowledge.

Normed
A normed test is one which (during development) has been tried out on a wide range of people from the general population or from a specific patient group. This process results in tables of normal scores for each age group. These tables are then used to compute the level of an individual's performance on a test in comparison to other people from the same population.

Obstructive sleep apnoea
The most common type of sleep-disordered breathing, the symptoms of which most usually include snoring, repeated momentary cessation of breathing during sleep and daytime tiredness.

Orbito-frontal lobes
The area beneath (or the under surface of) the frontal lobes (about level with the eyes) which shares thousands of connections with the limbic system and plays a large role in moderating or controlling emotions and emotional behaviours. Damage to the orbito-frontal lobes often results

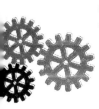

in impulsive behaviours, emotional lability, caring less about negative consequences of one's own behaviours, irritability and aggressiveness.

Pituitary gland
The most important gland in the endocrine system, which is the system of sending chemical messages from the brain around the body; it is controlled by the hypothalamus.

Pons
Part of the brain stem lying between the medulla and mid-brain which acts as a bridging point between two halves of the cerebellum.

Posterior
Meaning towards the back or rear.

Post-traumatic amnesia (PTA)
The inability to remember continuous events after sustaining a head injury, which causes an alteration of consciousness – even when the person is apparently awake. It is normally a temporary state of altered cognition and behaviour associated with a concussive-type injury, generally following a period of unconsciousness.

Progressive neurological condition
A neurological condition that is expected to worsen over time.

Prosody
A component of speech that includes tone, pitch and volume, and plays a role in the expression and interpretation of emotional content or meaning.

Psychological adjustment
A process of developing new outlooks or behaviour in the context of changed circumstances.

Psycho-social disability
Disability caused by the interaction of a psychological condition and an adverse social circumstance.

Quality of life
An assessment of how satisfactory life is based on internal and external measures such as independence, autonomy, self-esteem, recreation, employment, social functioning and relationships.

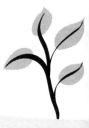

Reliability

This refers to how consistent a measuring device is. A measurement is said to be reliable or consistent if the measurement can produce similar results if used again in similar circumstances.

Reporter bias

An interpretation of an event or condition which relies on a reporter's perception of the important aspects. This interpretation may be different from how other people view it.

Restitution

A type of rehabilitation strategy that typically involves breaking down a cognitive function into its constituent parts and retraining each of these with drill and practice (ie. repetitive) training.

Reticular activating system (RAS)

Is a network of nerves most closely associated with the brain stem, and the function of which is to regulate attention and levels of arousal.

Ruminative thinking

Brooding over something without being able to reach conclusions or solutions, with a sense that you cannot switch these thoughts off, or distract yourself from them in any way.

Selective serotonin reuptake inhibitors

The newer type of antidepressants which are less sedating and more energising than the older tricyclic and tetracyclic forms.

Striatal-thalamic-frontal cortical system

An interlinked part of the brain involving parts of the striatum and thalamus in the limbic system, and parts of the frontal cortical areas involved in serial decision-making and mood regulation, among other functions.

Sub-cortical

Parts of the brain lying beneath the cortex (primarily made up of white matter) linking the cortical areas (frontal, parietal, temporal and occipital lobes) to each other and the nerve supply to organs and limbs. This includes much of the limbic system, the midbrain, brain stem and the cerebellum.

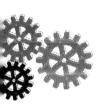

Supported communication
Strategies used to support and facilitate expression and understanding in people with aphasia.

Self-regulation
The ability to be aware of one's own emotions and behaviour, and to influence them positively.

Sensitivity
An index of the performance of a test. A test is sensitive to the impairment if it is able to accurately identify those individuals with a genuine impairment.

Specificity
An index of the performance of a test. A test is specific if it identifies impairment in only a small percentage of those people who do not actually have an impairment.

Symptom validity tests
Frequently referred to as 'effort tests', these are methods to determine the accuracy or truthfulness of the individual's behavioural presentation, their performance on neuropsychological measures, or self-reported symptoms.

Synapse
The gap between two nerve cells in which chemicals known as 'neuro-transmitters' pass information from one nerve cell to the next.

Thalamus
A very important 'relay centre' for information moving up from the spinal cord and cerebellum and between different parts of the brain. Damage here can affect many functions including language, and the ability to plan, executive and monitor behaviours.

Theories and models
Ideas about how things work based on an empirical or systematic study of them.

Tinnitus
A perception of sound in the ears (often a buzzing or ringing-type noise) in the absence of any outside source of noise.

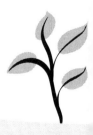

Tumour necrosis factor
A cytokine involved in the regulation of cells in the immune system to kill other cells to reduce inflammation, stop viral replication or inhibit the growth of tumours.

Validity
The extent to which an assessment instrument is measuring what was intended ie. a memory test should be measuring memory and not attention.

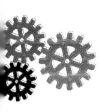

For further information please contact the editors:

Dr Declan Mc Nicholl
Department of Clinical Neuropsychology
Lodge Two
Leicester General Hospital
Gwendolen Road
Leicester
LE5 4PW

Robert Poppleton
Dept of Neuro-psychology
Royal Leamington Spa Rehabilitation Hospital
Heathcote Lane
Warwick
CV34 6SR

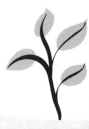